Charles-Edouard Brown-Séquard

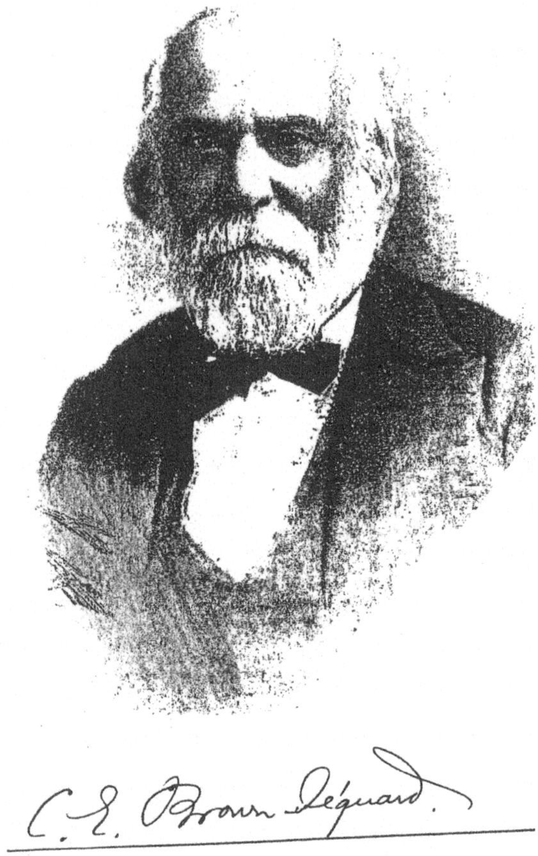


Photo taken in Brighton, England in the early 1890s © Celestin

Louis-Cyril Celestin

# Charles-Edouard Brown-Séquard

## The Biography of a Tormented Genius

Springer

Louis-Cyril Celestin
London
UK

ISBN 978-3-319-03019-7 ISBN 978-3-319-03020-3 (eBook)
DOI 10.1007/978-3-319-03020-3
Springer Cham Heidelberg New York Dordrecht London

Library of Congress Control Number: 2013953211



Printed on acid-free paper

Springer is part of Springer Science+Business Media (www.springer.com)

*Si la science n'a pas de patrie,
l'homme de science doit en avoir
une et c'est à elle qu'il doit
reporter l'influence que ses
travaux peuvent avoir dans le
monde.*

Louis Pasteur
Discours prononcé à l'inauguration
de l'Institut Pasteur
Paris, 14 novembre 1888

*If Science has no Motherland,
the man of science must have one
and it is to her that he must
credit the influence that his
work may have in the world.*

Louis Pasteur
Speech delivered on the inauguration of
the Pasteur Institute in Paris on 14th
November 1888

*This book is dedicated to*
*the memory of my father*
*Louis Abel Célestin*
*C.B.E., M.C., M.D.*

# Acknowledgments

Credit for this book goes to Brown-Séquard himself. His diaries, letters, notes, and scientific writings and likewise the letters and reminiscences of his relatives, friends, countrymen, colleagues, patients and acquaintances have been scrupulously consulted in preparing this book. Indeed, it is his personal and private papers composing the impressive Goody-McCausland Collection in the Archives of the Library of the Royal College of Physicians of London (abbreviated GMcCC in the footnotes) as well as his published books, lectures, and innumerable articles which have been extensively used in presenting his life and scholarly achievements. However, this is not to say that thanks are not due to all those who have been engaged in the realization of this book, which has been written and constantly revised over a period of 20 years.

First and foremost of these is Kenneth E. Curtis who has painstakingly read through the typescript and made a number of valuable suggestions that have all been implemented. His gracious help is gratefully acknowledged here. However, he is not, in any way, responsible for any fault that remains.

Since 2005, I have enjoyed the friendship and support of Bianca Bellissima and Samuele Lodato and truly, this book would not have seen the light of day without their encouragements. My special thanks to both of them.

Mr. Jeffries Davenport, the Librarian; Ms. Julia Allum, the Assistant-Librarian; and Ms. Teresa Sutton, the Librarian's Secretary at the Library of the Royal College of Physicians of London, have been of inestimable help in providing all the archive material relating to Brown-Séquard which was consulted, in the course of daily visits to the Library, from September 1993 to July 1995.

The Library staff of the Wellcome Institute for the History of Medicine gave me much help in tracing and providing medical books and periodicals of the nineteenth century. Their courtesy and helpfulness were greatly appreciated in the course of weekly visits to the Institute from September 1994 to June 1995.

Finally, the works of many Authors, past and present, listed in the 'Secondary Sources' or referred to in the 'footnotes' have been of great assistance, and every effort has been made to give proper credit to them.

London, September 2013 Louis-Cyril Celestin

# Contents

# Chapter 1
# Physiology in the Nineteenth Century

This book tells the story of the eventful life of Charles-Edouard Brown-Séquard and outlines his lifetime achievements. He was at the forefront of physiological research in the nineteenth century. It is impossible, however, to look at his life and work in isolation, as he must be seen in the context of the burgeoning discipline he entered. We introduce his life then with a brief account of the considerable advances that physiology made in that century, when France and Germany led the world—a history in which Brown-Séquard plays a significant role.

Experimental physiology, based on laboratory findings, was pioneered by François Magendie. On his appointment as Professor of Medicine at the **Collège de France** in 1830, he founded there the first Laboratory of experimental physiology. Of his many contributions to this field, his major achievement was the classification of the motor and sensory functions of the ventral and dorsal spinal nerve roots.[1] His German contemporary, Johannes Peter Müller, published his **Handbuch der Physiologie des Menschen**, which was a landmark in physiological research. He was a great teacher whose pupils were to make substantial contributions to the progress of physiology.

The use of instruments in physiological research featured, significantly, in the works of the three Weber brothers. Ernst Heinrich studied the behaviour of fluids flowing through cylinders to work out the characteristics of the flow of blood through blood vessels. Wilhelm Eduard studied locomotion, while the youngest, Eduard Friedrich, together with his eldest brother, demonstrated that stimulation of the vagus nerve slows and even stops the heart. In France, Jules Marey, who held the Chair of Natural History at the Collège de France, invented the **sphymograph**, an instrument for recording the strength and variations in the rate of the arterial pulse. He also pioneered cinematography by photographically recording and analysing animal movements.[2]

---

[1] Magendie F (1822) Expérience sur les fonctions des racines des nerfs rachidiens. J Physiol Exp Pathol (Paris) 2: 276–279.

[2] Marey EJ (1882) Emploi de la photographie instantanée pour l'analyse des mouvements chez les animaux. C R Acad Sci (Paris) 94: 1013–1020.

L.-C. Celestin, *Charles-Edouard Brown-Séquard*,
DOI: 10.1007/978-3-319-03020-3_1, 

During the 1840s, a group of German physiologists, who had been pupils of Johannes Peter Müller, were very active. These were: Emil Du Bois Reymond, the founder of electro-physiology; Ernst Wilhelm von Brücke, who did a considerable amount of research into phonetics; Herman Ludwig Ferdinand von Helmholtz, who invented the ophthalmoscope, an instrument for examining the interior of the eye through the pupil and Karl Friedrich Wilhelm Ludwig, a remarkable researcher and an influential teacher, whose profound mark on physiology was made by the many international students who attended his laboratory in Leipzig. To name but a few, these were Angelo Mosso, an Italian, who devised an ergograph for recording the amplitude of muscular contractions; Ivan Petrovitch Pavlov from Russia, the first winner of the Nobel Prize for Physiology in 1904, well-known for his work on conditioned reflex: an automatic response to a stimulus that does not really cause it, and Henry Pickering Bowditch, who opened the first physiological laboratory for students in America at the Harvard Medical School.

Advances that were made in Chemistry contributed to the progress of physiological chemistry, especially in the field of metabolic processes. Justus von Liebig classified foodstuffs according to their chemical composition into carbohydrates, proteins and fats. With Friedrich Wohler, he made a study of protein metabolism by determining the amount of nitrogen in the urine. Along the same lines, Louis Joseph Proust analyzed the composition of carbohydrates and found that they contained carbon, hydrogen and oxygen, while Michel Eugène Chevreul showed that lipids were composed of fatty acids and glycerol and Charles Adolphe Wurtz isolated by-products of protein metabolism such as uric and hippuric acids.

Overshadowing all the physiologists of the nineteenth century, however, was Claude Bernard. In 1841, two years before graduating as a doctor in medicine, he became François Magendie's assistant at the **Collège de France**. In 1852, a chair of Physiology was created especially for him at the Sorbonne, the seat of the University of Paris. Three years later, he succeeded Magendie as Professor of Medicine at the Collège de France and, in 1868, he was given a well-equipped laboratory at the **Muséum national d'histoire naturelle** with a newly created chair in this establishment. The most honoured French scientist of the nineteenth century, he was elected to the **Académie des sciences** in 1854 and nominated a member of the prestigious **Académie Française** in 1869.

He did pioneering work in many areas of physiology, but was most eminent in the field of digestion. His finest discoveries were: the role played by the pancreatic juice in the digestion of fats[3]; the glycogenic function of the liver[4]; the importance of erythrocytes in the transportation of oxygen and carbon dioxide by the blood, and he was one of the first to describe some of the properties of the vasomotor nerves.[5]

---

3 Bernard C (1856) Mémoire sur le pancréas et sur le rôle du suc pancréatique dans les phénomènes digestifs, particulièrement dans la digestion des matières grasses neutres. Paris.

4 Bernard C (1853) Recherches sur une nouvelle fonction du foie considéré comme organe producteur de matière sucrée chez l'homme et les animaux, Paris.

5 Bernard C (1879) Influence du grand sympathique sur la sensibilité et la calorification. C R Soc Biol (Paris) 3: 163–164.

Bernard had a large following. Scientists from all over the world attended his lectures and frequented his laboratories. He was the mentor for many who achieved eminence in their own rights. These were men like: John Burdon-Sanderson and Walter Holbrook Gaskell from England; Silas Weir Mitchell, the Father of American Neurology; Ivan Mikhailovitch Sechenov, the founder of the Russian School of Physiology and the German, Isidore Rosenthal, who occupied the chair of neuropathology in Vienna. Amongst Bernard's French pupils were Jacques Arsène d'Arsonval, Louis Pasteur, Louis Ranvier and Paul Bert.

Bert was the most illustrious of Bernard's pupil-physiologists, succeeding his mentor to the Chair of Physiology at the Sorbonne in 1868. His research was mainly concerned with the physiological effects that variations of atmospheric pressure have on living organisms. In 1878, he published his book, **La Pression barométrique: Recherches de physiologie expérimentale**,[6] a classic, unsurpassed to this day. His findings were ignored for 65 years until, during the Second World War in 1943, when his book was translated into English[7] because of the immense bearing it had on aviation physiology. For example, he had shown that anoxaemia, which is the absence of oxygen in arterial blood, causes syncope at high altitude, and that the effects of oxygen and other gases in the blood are not dependent on their proportions, but on their partial pressures.

Of course, there were many other eminent physiologists of the nineteenth century, too many for each to be mentioned here. However, an understanding of physiology, in that century, would be incomplete without touching upon the research that was done in two fields: the study of the functions of the endocrine glands and of the nervous system.

Concerning the endocrine glands, the German Moritz Schiff showed that the thyroid gland was essential to life. His compatriot, Arnold Adolf Berthold, drew attention to the possibility of the existence of an internal secretion by showing that the effects of castration were negated by transplanting the testes to another part of the body. In France, Alfred Vulpian found that venous blood issuing from the adrenal glands contains an active substance, which was later identified as adrenaline. This was the first indication of an hormonal secretion.[8]

In neurophysiology, Charles Bell, in England, differentiated between the motor and sensory action of nerves, while his countrymen, Marshall Hall, discovered the phenomenon of spinal reflexes and Charles Sherrington carried out pioneering research into the function of the neuron. Marie Jean Pierre Flourens, Professor of Natural History at the **Muséum national d'histoire naturelle**, identified the cerebellum as the point where the coordination of body movements originates and

6 Published by G. Masson, Paris, 1878.

7 Translated into English by Hitcock MB & Hitcock FA (1943) Barometric Pressure. Researches in Experimental physiology. Columbus, Ohio.

8 Vulpian A (1856) Note sur quelques réactions propres à la substance des capsules surrénales. C R Acad Sci (Paris) 43: 663–665.

that the function of the semicircular canals of the inner ear is the sensing and maintenance of balance; moreover, he located the noeud vital (the respiratory centre) in the medulla oblongata.

The localization of cerebral functions was the subject of much research. Jean-Baptiste Bouillaud and later, Pierre Paul Broca, located a speech centre.[9] From his clinical observations of focal epilepsy, John Hughlings Jackson deduced that functions were located to areas of the cerebral cortex.[10] Jean-Martin Charcot localized areas of the brain affected by diseases, and argued that the encephalon is made up a "federation of organs."[11]

These two additions to the science of physiology: the functions of the endocrine glands and those of the nervous system, lead us to Charles-Edward Brown-Séquard, a most unpredictable scientist. He carried out pioneering work on the physiology of motor and sensory pathways in the spinal cord[12]; he rivalled Claude Bernard in the discovery of the functions of the vasomotor nerves[13]; he elaborated his own theory of localization of cerebral functions. A theory which was recently revived. He proved the vital importance of the adrenal glands[14] and heralded the era of **Organotherapy** and **Hormonal therapy**.

He has been described as an inventor, and

> some of his fundamental ideas, considered to be strange and almost insane at the time he expressed them, in the confused state in which he so often left them, have yet shown an originality as marked, perhaps, as those of Pasteur or of Claude Bernard. He left a profound mark on the biological field, because he had conceived a very high ideal of science, which he pursued in spite of all obstacles with a passionate devotion, sacrificing to it the idols ordinarily worshipped by men: money, positions and honours. In his material life there was the same instability, the same lack of measure as in his intellectual pursuit, and he spent an existence as wandering and agitated as that of a scholar of the sixteenth century. His life was passed between two races, French and Anglo-Saxon, to both of which he belonged by family ties, incessantly journeying along the routes of the world, from the Indian Ocean, which had witnessed his birth, to the seas of Europe and America. Sometimes an experimenter, sometimes a consulting physician, sometimes a scientific journalist, and sometimes a professor at Paris, at London, at Dublin, at New York and at Boston.[15]

---

9 Broca PP (1861) Perte de la parole, ramollissement chronique et destruction partielle du lobe antérieur gauche. Bull Soc Anthro (Paris) 2: 235–238.

10 Jackson HJ (1881) Epileptiform convulsions from cerebral disease. Trans Int Med Con 2: 6–15.

11 Charcot J-M (1893) Oeuvres complètes, vol 4. Progrès médical et Alcan, pp. 3–4.

12 Brown-Séquard CE (1849) De la transmission des impressions sensitives par la moelle épinière. C R Soc Biol (Paris) 1: 191–194.

13 Brown-Séquard CE (1852) Researches on the influence of the nervous system upon the functions of organic life. Med Exam Phila 8: 481–504.

14 Brown-Séquard CE (1856) Recherches expérimentales sur la physiologie des capsules surrénales. C R Acad Sci (Paris) 43: 422–425 & 542–546.

15 Berthelot MPE (1898) Notice sur la vie et les travaux de M. Brown-Séquard. Typographie de Firmin-Didot et Cie, Paris.

# Chapter 2
# The Birthplace

Brown-Séquard was born in Mauritius. As this island is far from being a household name, a geographical and historical outline is called for. Few are those who can locate it on a map of the world. It is often confused with Mauritania, a republic of the African mainland, or thought to be somewhere in the Caribbean Sea. Queen Alexandra, the consort of Edward VII, once addressed a letter to "Mauritius, West Indies."

This island of volcanic origin is not more than a pin-prick, in the middle of the Indian Ocean, on a world map. About the same size as the County of Surrey, it is pear-shaped and occupies an area of 1,865 $km^2$. Its greatest length and breadth are 60 and 48 km respectively. It comprises a central plateau, the floor of a large extinct volcano, which gently slopes down to a coastal plain. The island is surrounded by a coral reef which, though broken in many places, provides lagoons and long sandy beaches.

Mauritius lies 20° south of the Equator, slightly north of the Tropic of Capricorn. It is 800 km east of the Democratic Republic of Malagasy, 3,600 km from the Cape of Good Hope at the southern tip of the African mainland, and 4,600 km from Bombay in India. Its nearest land neighbour is La Réunion, its sister island, which lies 220 km to the southeast (Fig. 2.1).

At the turn of the eighteenth century, France was in possession of three islands, forming the Mascarene Archipelago, in the southwest Indian Ocean. These islands were then named the Isle de France (present day Mauritius), the Isle Bourbon (present day La Réunion) and the island of Rodrigues, some 550 km east of Mauritius.

The Isle de France had been known to Arab seafarers as early as the tenth century and had been charted by them as Dina Arobi. It was visited in the early part of the sixteenth century by Portuguese mariners and named Ilha de Cirné (Island of the Swan) in 1511, by one of their navigators, Domingo Fernandez Pereira. In 1598, Mauritius received its current name after being claimed for Holland by Admiral Wybrandt Van Warwyck and named after its ruler, Maurits Van Nassau. The island was settled by the Dutch in 1638 and abandoned by them in 1710. Five years later, on September 20, 1715, it was annexed by Captain

L.-C. Celestin, *Charles-Edouard Brown-Séquard*,
DOI: 10.1007/978-3-319-03020-3_2, © Springer International Publishing Switzerland 2014

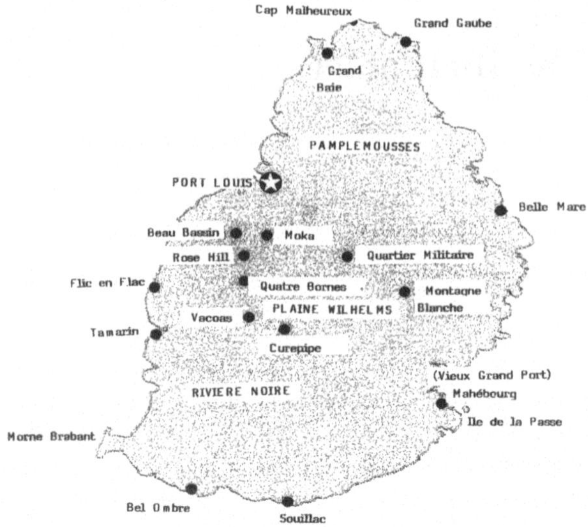


**Fig. 2.1** Map of Mauritius © Celestin

Guillaume Dufresne d'Arsel, in the name of France and her king, Louis XV, and renamed Isle de France.

Louis XV ceded his rights over the Mascarenes to the Compagnie des Indes orientales. In 1642, France had taken possession of the Isle Bourbon and the first settlers arrived there in 1665. The colonization of the Isle de France began on December 24, 1721 "by 12–15 inhabitants of the Isle Bourbon, a lay priest and a surgeon under the command of Major Duronguët Le Toullec."[1] In January 1722, arrived the recently appointed Administrator of the Mascarenes, the Chevalier de Nyon. He had left France the previous June with "a Swiss platoon of 210 men with 20 women and 30 children, several officers, engineers, clerks and workmen."[2] However, during the journey, many of the Swiss soldiers died and "the number landed on the Isle de France, possibly, did not exceed 100."[3]

By 1735, when Bertrand François Mahé de La Bourdonnais, a Breton sea captain, appointed general administrator of the Mascarenes arrived, there were 850 inhabitants on the Isle de France, of whom 650 slaves, living in a state of anarchy. It was a situation that would not last long. Within five years of his arrival, La Bourdonnais had founded Port Louis on the northwest coast of the island. In the natural harbour there, he built docks equipped with shipyards, warehouses, arsenals and fortifications. Roads were built from Port Louis to the island's interior. Land was cleared for the growing of cotton, indigo plants and sugar cane.

---

[1] Kucznski RR (1977) Demographic Survey of the British Colonial Empire, vol 2. The Harvester Press, England, p. 748.

[2] *Ibid.*

[3] *Ibid,* p. 749.

La Bourdonnais left the Mascarenes in 1746 and was succeeded, in turn, by four other administrators of the Compagnie des Indes orientales. Over a period of 20 years, they encouraged immigration from the French trading posts along India's coast and from France, while greatly increasing the forced labour population by bringing slaves from India and Madagascar.

The Seven Years War, 1756–1763, had disastrous consequences on the economy of the Mascarenes which, in turn, affected the **Compagnie's** finances by hampering its trade with the East. To add to their difficulties, the Archipelago became a haven for privateers operating—with the consent of the French government—against British shipping as well as that of other nations. In the end, the **Compagnie des Indes orientales** went bankrupt and had to sell the islands to the French Crown, whose control became effective on July 14, 1767.

Under Crown rule, from 1767 to 1788, the Mascarene Archipelago was administered by governors-general who appointed intendants to be responsible for local affairs. Two of the latter, Pierre Poivre and François de Souillac, deserve special mention for their improvements of the harbour facilities of Port Louis. The Archipelago prospered; Port Louis became a major free port attracting traders from Europe and the United States, as it stock-piled an infinite range of goods. Furthermore, it offered repair facilities, rigging and supplies to the French naval forces operating in the Indian Ocean. In addition to all this, during the American War of Independence, 1778–1783, Port Louis was a base for 30 American warships which harassed both the British navy and its commercial fleet. During this 20-years period, the population of the Isle de France doubled. Eighty percent of this number was made up of slaves who were being imported from the east coast of Africa.

In 1789, on the eve of the French Revolution, the Isle de France was the most westernized place, and Port Louis the most fashionable city, east of Africa. By 1794, however, the slave-owners had rebelled against and rejected the authority of the French government, refusing to enforce the Law of February 4, 1794, voted by the National Convention in Paris, declaring the abolition of slavery in all the French colonies. From then on, until 1803, the Mascarenes enjoyed a period of autonomy. However, slavery was re-established by Napoléon on May 19, 1802 and, to restore order in the Archipelago, he appointed one of his generals, Charles Mathieu Isidore Decaen, as governor of the Mascarenes.

It was during the Wars of the French Revolution, 1793–1802, and the Napoleonic Wars, that the Isle de France reached its apogee as a trading centre. Indeed, between 1786 and 1810, nearly 600 American ships, amongst several thousands of those of other nations, called at Port Louis. Privateering, however, was experiencing a similar boom. It was being financed by the local community, since the bounty it brought back attracted American trading ships and many others from neutral powers.

England's subsequent action against the Mascarenes was not solely prompted by the privateers' continual harassment of her commercial fleet; she felt threatened by the growing relationship between the Indian princes and General Decaen who, previously, had served in India. To safeguard her interests in that country, and to be in absolute command of the sea, she had to put an end to the island empire that France had built in the Indian Ocean.

England started a naval blockade of the Mascarenes, immediately after wrestling the Cape of Good Hope from the Dutch, in 1806. The blockade lasted 4 years and eventually proved effective. In 1809, British troops from India gained control of Rodrigues and used it as a stepping stone to launch attacks against the other two islands. On July 7, 1810, a British force captured the Isle Bourbon.

Once in possession of the Isle Bourbon, the British tightened their stranglehold on the Isle de France. In August 1810, sailors from a British naval force occupied the Isle de la Passe, an islet guarding the entrance to the harbour of Grant Port, on the south-east coast of the main island. They managed to entice four French warships inside the harbour by flying the French tricolour over the islet. The two sides battled non-stop for three days and nights. In the end, the British struck their colours. This naval battle was the only French sea victory of the Napoleonic era. Known locally as **La Bataille du Vieux Grand Port**, it is inscribed on the Arc de Triomphe in Paris as **Bataille de l'ile de la Passe**.

Four months after this glorious episode, on November 22, 1810, General John Abercrombie, the commander-in-chief of Bombay, left Rodrigues for the conquest of the Isle de France. He landed at Cap Malheureux, the northernmost tip of the island, with a force of 12,000 men and marched on Port Louis. The French were short of equipment and ammunition and, more fatally, they were grossly outnumbered. They fought a rearguard action, while the main portion of their forces protected Port Louis. However, when a second British force landed south of Port Louis, Decaen realised the futility of the situation and capitulated on December 3, 1810.

The terms of surrender were most benevolent. No prisoners of war were taken. The British undertook to safeguard all the rights enjoyed by the islanders; namely their laws, their customs, their language, their religion and their children's education. The Treaty of Paris, signed in 1814, reaffirmed all the conditions of surrender. The Isle Bourbon was returned to France. The treaty, however, extended British jurisdiction not only to the Isle de France, but to all her dependencies: Rodrigues, Seychelles, the Saint Brandon Islands and the Chagos Archipelago. France was thus deprived of naval bases in islands scattered over thousands of kilometres of the Indian Ocean. The name of the Isle de France reverted to Mauritius. "Although the Union Jack waved over Mauritius for 160 years, the island never effectively became British… Mauritius never ceased to be the Isle de France."[4] French culture prevailed during the whole period of British rule, which ended in 1968.

[4] Tinker H (1977) Between Africa, Asia and Europe: Mauritius: Cultural marginalism and political control. African Affairs 76: 304–323.

# Chapter 3
# The Forebears

Less than three years after the capitulation of the Isle de France, on July 28, 1813, an American, Charles **Edward Brown** and a local girl, Henriette Perrine **Charlotte Séquard**, were joined in marriage, in Port Louis. It was a non-religious ceremony. The couple exchanged their vows in the presence of the Chief Superintendent of Police, who was also the Head of the Registrar General's Office. The bridegroom presented an affidavit affirming his date and place of birth and declaring that he had not, previously, contracted marriage.[1] The bride submitted a baptismal certificate[2] originating from the Roman Catholic Parish Church of St. Louis of Port Louis, dated April 24, 1790, testifying to her birth 21 months previously.[3]

Edward Brown was born on October 29, 1784 in Philadelphia, U.S.A., the son of George Brown and his wife, née Gale Ryan.[4] His family originally came from County Galway, Ireland, settling in New York and Philadelphia in the eighteenth century.[5] He was a captain in the merchant navy, but had "served several years, when young, as a midshipman in the United States Navy."[6] Though both his parents were dead, his maternal grandparents were still alive in America. They were a wealthy elderly couple who had investments in company stocks and real estate in Dublin.[7] Captain Brown was in regular correspondence with Canon Henry Feltus, the husband of his maternal aunt, and the curate of St. Anne's Church in Brooklyn. Little is known of Captain Brown's years of service in the United States Navy, apart from conflicting reports that "he entered the American naval services in 1812, was engaged in different actions and sent to Mauritius on an expedition which France was to have

[1] Marriage certificates of Edward Brown and Charlotte Séquard. The Registrar General's Office, Port Louis, Mauritius.

[2] Joint baptismal certificate of Charlotte Séquard amd her sister Gillone. St Louis Cathedral, Port Louis, Mauritius.

[3] Registrar General's Office, *op. cit.*, note 1, above.

[4] GMcCC, Ms 999/7, p. 30 & Ms 951/128.

[5] Brown-Séquard CE (1856) Letter to the Boston Medical & Surgical Journal 55: 254.

[6] *Ibid.*

[7] Feltus HJ (1816) Letter to Charles-Edward Brown. GMcCC, Ms 981/145. 1st May.

L.-C. Celestin, *Charles-Edouard Brown-Séquard*,
DOI: 10.1007/978-3-319-03020-3_3, © Springer International Publishing Switzerland 2014

helped, but did not."[8] Or that "he was in action against the British between 1812 and 1814, and was sent before the peace was signed to intercept East Indiamen plying between the ports of India and Great Britain."[9]

Charlotte Séquard was born in Port Louis on August 23, 1788. She was the daughter of Pierre Paul Séquard and his wife, née Marie Jeanne Elizabeth Geneviève Nativel. Her parents had married on June 12, 1787, in Port Louis, in the Roman Catholic Parish Church of St. Louis.[10]

Pierre Paul Séquard, Charlotte's father, was born in 1753 in Marseille, France. He bore the same forenames as his father and his mother's maiden name was Marie Anne Grosse.[11] He was a merchant who emigrated to the Isle de France in 1783.[12] In 1791, the Governor-General of the Mascarenes, David Charpentier de Cossigny de Palma appointed him as secretary to a three-member executive committee responsible for the internal affairs of the Isle de France.[13] He served in this post until 1799, during which time, he was responsible for the issue and distribution of paper money.[14] On leaving this post, he resumed his former occupation as a merchant.

Geneviève Nativel, Charlotte's mother, was born at Saint Pierre, Isle Bourbon, between 1765 and 1767. She was the daughter of André Nativel and his wife, née Marie Leichnig. André Nativel was from France and was an officer in the National Guards regiment garrisoned in the Isle Bourbon. Marie Leichnig was the daughter of Wilhelm Leichnig or Lechenig, a German sailor, marooned on the Isle de France, soon after the departure of the Dutch in 1710. He was found living a Robinson Crusoe lifestyle by the first settlers who came from the Isle Bourbon in 1721.[15] It is said that the district of Plaine Wilhelms, the "only district of Mauritius to bear the name of a man"[16] was named after him. Geneviève died in 1792, having given birth to three daughters. The eldest, Marie Joseph Petronille—born out of wedlock in May 1786[17]—and the youngest, Marie Louise Gillone died before their mother passed away.[18] The second daughter, Henriette Perrine Charlotte was brought up by her father and his black female slaves.

---

[8] The Daily News (1894) Obituary of Brown-Séquard. London, 3rd April.

[9] The New York Daily Tribune (1894) Brown-Séquard. The story of his life. New York, 22nd Apr.

[10] Marriage certificate of Pierre Paul Séquard and Geneviève Nativel. In: Rouget FA (1930) Brown-Séquard et son oeuvre. Esquisse biographique. General Printing & Stationary Office, Port Louis, Mauritius, p. 97.

[11] *Ibid.*

[12] The date of his arrival in the Isle de France is recorded in the population census of 1796.

[13] Rouget, *op. cit*, note 10, above, p. 48.

[14] *Ibid*, p. 87.

[15] Barnwell PJ, Toussaint A (1949) A Short History of Mauritius, Longman Green & Co., p. 44.

[16] *Ibid.*

[17] Role A (1977) La Vie étrange d'un grand savant: le professeur Brown-Séquard. Plon, Paris, p. 21.

[18] Rouget, *op. cit,* note 10, above p. 49.

The marriage of Edward Brown and Charlotte Séquard was not the result of a chance encounter. It was a much more mundane affair: an arrangement that suited both father-in-law and bridegroom. The latter, who owned a ship, carried goods bought in Asia for Pierre Paul Séquard, who was a wealthy,[19] sixty-four old widower with an only daughter. He was well connected with the local business community and also mixed with the upper echelons of the Civil Service. He was engaged in the bulk import of cloth, grain, legumes and rice from the Asian sub-continent. In Port Louis, he had storage warehouses, a chain of retail shops and a large and beautiful house cared for by more than half a dozen slaves.

However, on a September night in 1816, disaster struck Pierre Paul Séquard. By the morning, he was, just about, completely ruined. Indeed, a great fire broke out in the commercial and residential quarters of Port Louis, destroying his warehouses, his shops and his town house.[20] Urgent measures were taken to lessen the impact of this disaster and to provide help to all the victims. All the dry food stocks had been destroyed. A great number of inhabitants were without shelter, 700 houses having burnt down.

A huge operation was mounted to avoid famine and in early October, Captain Charles Brown duly set sail for Madras, where he was to fetch a cargo of rice. A sailing ship leaving Mauritius for Madras should arrive at its destination within three weeks at the most, as the Indian Ocean is the most navigable of all oceans. For the first six months of the year, the northeast monsoon blows away from Asia towards the Tropic of Cancer. Conversely, for the second half of the year, the southwest monsoon, blowing from the equatorial region, traverses the entire ocean to reach Asia. In the first week of November, Captain Brown's ship set sail from Madras bound for Port Louis with its cargo of rice. The ship was expected back by the end of the month. It never arrived.[21] As time passed, it became clear that the ship was lost with all souls on board and that the circumstances of their plight would never be known.

Needless to say, tragedies such as these are always deeply felt by their seafaring communities. But disappearances at sea always give rise to fantastic tales of survival. Stories went round that Captain Brown had taken his ship to America; that he had been captured by pirates in the Bay of Bengal,[22] despite the fact that this bay was relatively free of marauders.

The wildest tale of all the disappearance stories was told, many years after the event, by foreign journalists, with a manifestly scanty knowledge of the history and geography of Mauritius. They wrote that Captain Brown's ship had been "attacked by pirates within sight of his father-in-law's villa, which stood on a mountain over Port Louis,"[23] and that the Captain "had to walk the plank."[24] It is true that Signal Mountain overlooks Port Louis, but its slopes were bare of

---

19 Brown-Séquard CE (1852) Letter to Lady Blanche. GMcCC, Ms 977/1, 17th December.

20 Barnwell, Toussaint, *op. cit,* note 15, above.

21 Brown-Séquard, *op. cit,* note 19, above.

22 The Daily News, *op. cit,* note 8, above.

23 The New York Daily Tribune and The Daily News, *op.cit,* notes 8 and 9 above.

24 *Ibid.*

habitations and its summit was occupied by a signalling post for the harbour's sea traffic. What is more, no pirate had operated in the Mascarenes' waters since Olivier Le Vasseur,[25] alias "La Buse" (The Buzzard), was brought to the scaffold in the Isle Bourbon in 1730. In fact, the sea around Mauritius was, from 1813 to 1835, guarded by British warships, deployed to stop the illegal landings of slaves under the Slave Trade Abolition Law, which came into force in Mauritius in 1813. Finally, the journalists' stories are rendered apocryphal by the fact that the Captain's father-in-law was homeless at the time. His town house, which was not far from the harbour, had been destroyed by the Great Fire of 1816.

The only reasonable conclusion that one can reach, regarding the fate of Captain Brown and his crew, is that they came to grief in a hurricane. The Mascarene Archipelago lies within a cyclone belt. These tropical storms are caused by depressions which travel westward from the Brandon Islands; they appear every year from December to April, but not all of them hit the islands. Many blow themselves out at sea where they prove a great menace to shipping.

So, as 1817 progressed, prospects looked very bleak for Charlotte Brown. She was barely thirty and her husband was missing, presumed dead. Eighteen months previously, she had lost her firstborn child, a baby daughter, Marie.[26] Her father was, in terms of local life expectancy, an old man at sixty four years of age, with little hope of recouping the losses he had suffered as a result of the fire. The only ray of hope in Charlotte's life was the birth of another child, expected in early April (Fig. 3.1).

These were the circumstances which surrounded the birth of Edouard Charles Brown—the future Brown-Séquard—at eleven o'clock on the morning of April 8, 1817. The Health Officer, Ferdinand Desjardins, acted as accoucheur and, in the absence of the boy's father and, in compliance with the law, put his signature to the birth certificate before that of the boy's grandfather, Pierre Paul Séquard. The certificate was drafted in French, but Edouard Brown was a British subject by birth.[27] Six years previously, in 1811, his mother and grandfather had become British subjects through conquest, and had taken an oath of allegiance to King George III of England.[28]

Edouard was baptised in the Roman Catholic Parish Church of St. Louis of Port Louis. His godparents were Emile Gausseran and Mme. Patée, who was either the sister or the first cousin of the godfather.[29]

Despite the fact that Edouard was the descendant of Irish-Americans on the paternal side, and that both his maternal grandfather and great grandfather were French from metropolitan France, he was not purely of European stock.

[25] Le Vasseur and Taylor, alias "The Terror of India" were responsible for the capture of 'La Vierge du Cap', the biggest loot in the history of piracy. Le Vasseur was arrested in 1730 and hanged in the Isle Bourbon.

[26] Brown-Séquard, *op. cit*, not 19, above.

[27] Birth certificates of Edouard Charles Brown. Registrar General's Office, Port Louis, Mauritius.

[28] The registers bearing the signatures of the inhabitants who swore allegiance to George III were available as early as 1811.

[29] The Standard (1894), London, 3rd Apr. Also: Brown-Séquard (1838) Letter to Emile Gausseran, 17th July and Letter to Mme Patée 25th Jan 1839 GMcCC, Ms 994/16.

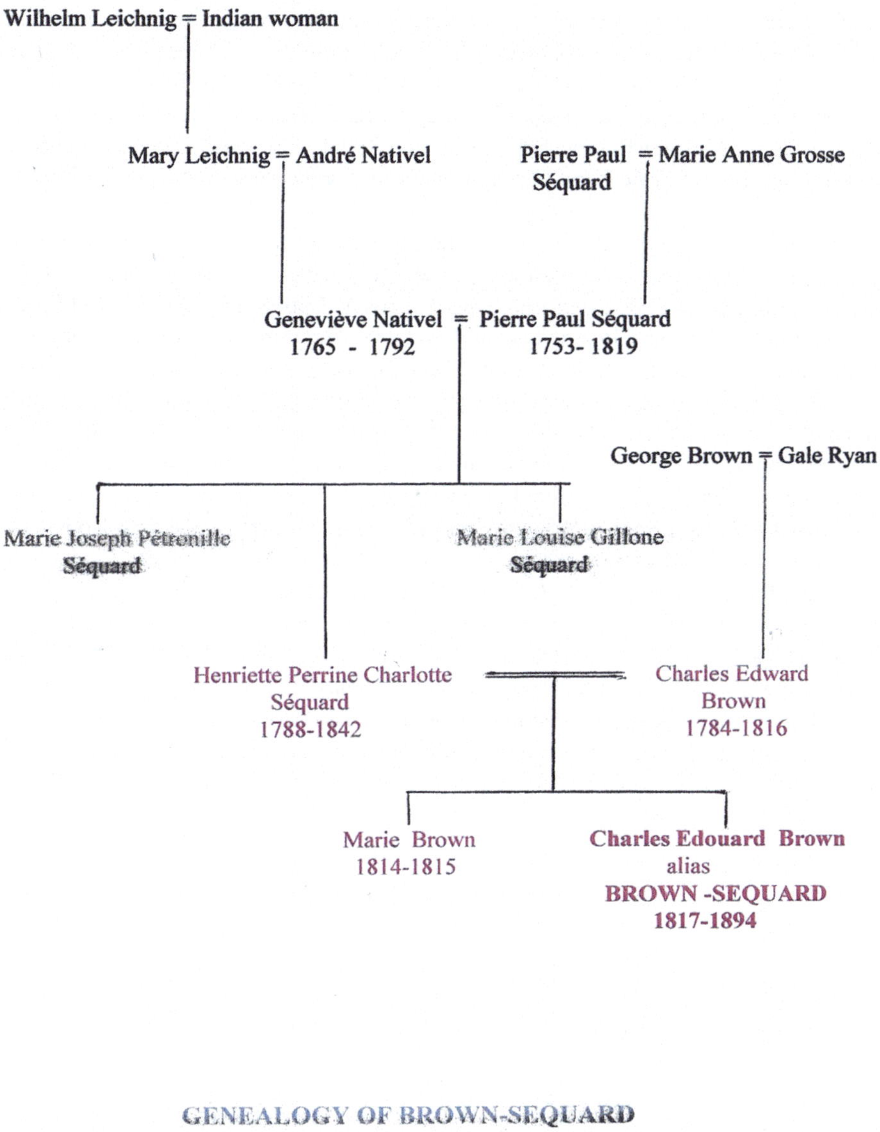


**Fig. 3.1** Genealogy of **Brown-Séquard** © Celestin

His maternal great grandmother, Marie Leichnig, the wife of André Nativel, was the daughter of an Indian woman, a native of the Malabar Coast,[30] the southwest coast of India which stretches from Goa in the north to Cape Comorin in the south. Unfortunately her name has not been recorded. Edouard was born in a community

[30] The New York Daily Tribune, *op. cit.*, note 9, above.

which is referred to by historians of Mauritius as the Free Coloured Population. This is a largely middle and upper-middle class community, predominantly Roman Catholic, which identifies with French culture and whose origin includes a mix of European and Indian or Malagasy blood. The Malagasies are not of black African origin, but of Malayo-Polynesian stock, and speak the Austronesian language. They emigrated to uninhabited Madagascar, some two centuries before the birth of Christ.

The Free Coloured Population of the Mascarenes dates back to the very beginning of the French colonization of the Archipelago. In the Isle Bourbon, the earliest settlement, in 1665, was made up of various European men, mostly French, but also Dutch, German, Portuguese and Spanish. The women were predominantly Indian and Madagascan. Indeed, only 2 out of every 9 women at that time were French from metropolitan France.[31] Twenty years later, the ratio had slightly changed to 7 out of 12. The percentage of women married to Frenchmen were then: 35 Madagascans, 33 Indians from Goa, the French trading posts of India and the Malabar Coast and 28 French from France.[32] The Isle de France was first settled in 1721, by third and fourth generation descendants of the Isle Bourbon's inhabitants of mixed ethnic origin.[33]

Edouard had some of the physical characteristics of his Indian ancestry: the black wavy hair, "the flashing black eyes" and a dark complexion. He himself acknowledged the fact that one of his forebears, on the maternal side, "was a Malabar woman."[34] His Indian traits were quite marked as Pierre Eugène Marcelin Berthelot, the distinguished chemist, who met him when he was 30 years old, described him as having "the physical characteristic of the Indian creole."[35]

---

[31] Scherer A (1990) La Réunion. Presses Universitaries de France, p. 11.

[32] Kuczynski RR (1977) Demographic Survey of the British Colonial Empire, vol 2. The Harvester Press, England, p. 747.

[33] *Ibid.*

[34] The New York Daily Tribune, *op. cit.*, note 9, above.

[35] Berthelot MPE (1896) Notice sur la vie et les travaux de M. Brown-Séquard. Typographie Firmin-Didot, Paris, p. 6.

# Chapter 4
# The Formative Years: 1817–1837

In the wake of the Great Fire of Port Louis, a Communal Board was set up to speed up the reconstruction of the commercial and residential quarter that had been destroyed and to re-house the great number of homeless inhabitants. So, shortly after Edouard's birth, his mother and grandfather moved into a house in the reconstructed area, in the centre of the town. Their new home was on the corner of rue Royale and rue de La Rampe.[1] They lived next door to a family called Chauvin and, within a short walk of the house of Augustine Maisonneuve, a very close friend of Charlotte Brown, Edouard's mother.

Pierre Paul Sequard died shortly after his grandson's birth,[2] some time in 1819. The exact circumstances of his death are not known, but he could have been a victim of the 1819–1820 cholera epidemic which ravaged the island from November to January and killed at least 6,000 inhabitants.

Charlotte was left to fend for herself and for her son. Having been tutored at home, she had learnt, among other things, embroidery and crochet. So, when Edouard was still an infant, she was able to supplement her income, made up of returns on investments her father had left her, with paid embroidery work which, when completed, was delivered by her maid. This black woman may well have been her nanny and was now Edouard's, as she had a lot of affection for this slave.[3] Besides this nanny, there were several other slaves, their spouses and children in Charlotte's home; likely to be the cook, the chambermaid, the errand boy, the gardener and the coachman: the normal complement of servants in a well-to do Mauritian home. These slaves, Charlotte had inherited from her father.

Charlotte's neighbours, the Chauvins, had young children, including Jules who was about the same age as Edouard, and with whom he used to play. Life was certainly not the one of wealth that Charlotte had known when her husband and

---

[1] Rouget FA (1930) Brown-Séquard et son oeuvre. Esquisse biographique. General Printing and Stationary Office, Port Louis, Mauritius. p. 23.

[2] Brown-Séquard CE (1852) Letter to Lady Blanche. GMcCC, Ms 977/1, 17th Dec.

[3] Brown C (1839) Letter to a friend in Mauritius. GMcCC, Ms 972/2, 16th July.

L.-C. Celestin, *Charles-Edouard Brown-Séquard*,

DOI: 10.1007/978-3-319-03020-3_4, 

father were alive, nor was it a life of poverty. She devoted herself entirely and selflessly to the well-being of her son.[4] As Edouard grew older, she reduced her workload of embroidery and opened her home as a boarding house for the British officers, who came to Port Louis, on leave from posts in the remoter parts of the island. The Mauritians, who had taken the occupation very well, had welcomed to their homes the officers who were stationed in military posts around the coast.[5]

As the garrison reduced in size, Charlotte found new lodgers in naval officers and the passengers of ships which stayed in the harbour.[6] In later life, Edouard was to comment that "the French language was the only one that was spoken in my Family and amongst the families who were friends of ours."[7] However, with so many English-speaking guests accommodated at his mother's home, he became as fluent in English as he was in French.[8]

Edouard attended the privately-owned Faraguet primary school, and from his earliest schooldays, studied alongside his two best friends: Jules Chauvin and Joseph Désiré Tholozan. When he was 8 years old, he began his secondary education. He attended the Singery School, a private, fee-paying school which taught the Classics, Ancient History, Philosophy, Mythology, French, French History and Literature, Geography and Mathematics. The principal and owner of the school was M. Singery, a well-known and reputable man. He was a dedicated teacher, whose schooling produced two generations of Mauritians who distinguished themselves in literature, the arts and sciences in France and other French-speaking parts of Europe.[9]

All the teaching at the Singery School was in French. The curriculum brought the pupils to the level of the **Baccalauréat-ès-Lettres**: an examination which, in the nineteenth century, was the equivalent of a university bachelor's degree and not, as nowadays, a secondary school examination qualifying successful candidates for higher education. It was not possible to sit for this examination in Mauritius; so, any young man, who wanted to continue his education had to go to France to sit for this examination. Furthermore, should he wish to study a scientific subject, he would have to take the **Baccalauréat-ès-Sciences**.

From the start of his schooling, M. Singery was impressed by Edouard's exceptional intelligence, so much so, that "he developed a passion for his pupil, for he discovered in him extraordinary gifts for a child of his age and urged him on in his studies."[10]

---

[4] Laurent F (1898) Biographie de Brown-Séquard. In: Le Blanc Brown-Séquard. Imprimerie Roussel et Cie. Port Louise, Mauritius, p. 1.

[5] Barnwell PJ, Toussaint A (1949) A short history of Mauritius. Longmans Green & Co, London, p. 128.

[6] The New York Daily Tribune (1894) Brown-Séquard. The Story of his life. New York, 22nd April.

[7] Brown-Séquard (n.d.) Autobiographical letter. GMcCC, Ms 999/7, p. 42.

[8] The New York Daily Tribute, *op. cit,* note 6, above.

[9] Laurent, *op. cit,* note 4, above, p. 2.

[10] *Ibid.*

Apart from the exposure to the English language that he had at home, it is likely that Edouard also received some form of English tuition at the Singery School. Many privately-owned teaching establishments had introduced English in their later-years' curricula, as it was in great demand on the island. With the presence of British rule, English traders were regularly visiting Port Louis. Furthermore, English shopkeepers had set up businesses in various towns and English was the only language permitted in higher law courts.[11] Mauritius's first English primer appeared in 1812.[12] It was so popular that, within 20 years, it had been through seven editions.

By the age of 15, Edouard had completely exhausted his school subjects and could be taught no more. Not only was he an academically precocious child, but he was very popular with his schoolmates. At the Singery School, he forged friendships which were to last a lifetime and even extend to the sons of his schoolmates.

It had always been his childhood ambition to study medicine. We know this both from himself and from Mme. Lantour, a widow, who was an intimate friend of his mother. In a letter to him, when he was a qualified physician, she recalled his early aspirations:

> I have always hoped that God would reward you for the perseverance that you have never stopped displaying, in a very tedious work, in order to attain the goal that you had set yourself since an early age.[13]

It was an ambition that he shared with his mother and both strove, through their difficulties, to achieve it. Leaving school at such an early age, Edouard was still too young to start thinking seriously about going to France, to continue his studies. Moreover, he needed a lot of money for such a long stay abroad. He, therefore, took a job and began to help his mother with the upkeep of the home and to add to the money that she was saving for his education in France. He worked, as a shop assistant, in one of the stores in Port Louis. This general store, situated on the Place d'Armes, fronting the harbour, sold

> foodstuffs from India and China, rhetorical treatises, fine clothes, trinkets, the work of Voltaire, court shoes to Paris's latest fashion, vintage wines and other goods prized by local people with refined tastes.[14]

This store was also the meeting place for a circle of writers. Many of these men of letters were relatives of Edouard's schoolmates—families such as that of the Lolliots' who, at that time, boasted of a novelist, a poet, a musician and an editor of an historical and artistic review. Edouard became acquainted with a wide range of contemporary local authors and their works: the comedies of Victor Jubien, the

---

[11] French was used for the first time in the Law courts in the 1850.

[12] Léchelle A (1827) Cours d'exercices anglais, avec des notes grammaticales et une table des verbes irréguliers. Imprimerie Vallet et Cie, Port Louis, Mauritius.

[13] Lantour, Mme (1852) Letter to Brown-Séquard. GMcCC, Ms 980/4 & Ms 999/6, pp. 15–16.

[14] Dupuy E (1894) Notice sur M. Le professeur Brown-Séquard, ancient Président de la Société de biologie. Revue Scient (Paris) 2: 737–743.

epic poems of Hubert Louis Lorquet, the essays and parodies of François Chrestien to name but a few. The most accomplished of a plethora of writers then, was Léoville L'Homme who was also the editor of a daily newspaper, Le Journal de Maurice. Writing is a pastime which Mauritians indulge in. Since the beginning of the nineteenth century to the present day, 250 authors based in Mauritius have published over 750 works between them. In recent years, several Mauritian writers, who moved to Paris, have made a name for themselves. Among the best known of these are Loys Masson and his brother André, Marcelle Lagesse, Jean Fanchette, Marie Thérèse Humbert and a large group of poets like Raymond Chasle, Emmanuel Juste, Edouard Maunick, Kenneth Nathaniel and Jean-Georges Prosper.

Not only was Edouard greatly influenced by this literary clique, but he soon began to write himself. The verses, plays, novels and philosophical dissertations he wrote, won him praise. So much so that he started entertaining aspirations of a literary career for quite a while. One of his writing is extant, dating from 1837: a poem inspired by a verse from one of Alfred de Musset's poems and, whatever its literary merit, it reveals the author as a very knowledgeable 20 years old youth.[15]

Literature, however, did not occupy all of his spare time. He was greatly and emotionally involved in the burning issue of the day: the anticipated law on the abolition of slavery. This was a major political theme in Mauritius in the period from 1813 to 1835 and, naturally, of great interest to this liberal-minded young man. The subject was debated endlessly between him and his friends. He also read the works of the French authors who were opposed to slavery. These were writers like Pierre Marivaux, Guillaume Raynal and Voltaire; not forgetting the, then locally popular novelist, Bernardin de Saint Pierre, author of the romance Paul et Virginie who, in his Voyage à l'île-de-France expresses in strong terms, his abhorrence of slavery.

Apart from the intellectual pursuit, which he shared with his friends Jules Chauvin, Eugène Cloarec, Auguste Laporte, Emile Dubois and Joseph Désiré Tholozan, he used to maintain a healthy physical life. On the advice of his mother, he would swim in the sea twice a day, everyday of the year. She believed that this would give him a strong constitution and "increase his below average height."[16] At weekends, he went to the southwest coast of the island, to Petite Rivière Noire which, with its lush green gorges and the Piton de la Rivière Noire, Mauritius's highest mountain, is undoubtedly one of the most scenic places in the island. There, he would go with his friend Emile Dubois and stay with M. Faciolle, a distant cousin of his mother, or with M. and Mme. Dubois, who were Faciolle's in-laws.[17]

---

[15] Brown-Séquard CE (1837) Pages of poetry. GMcCC, Ms 999/82.

[16] Brown-Séquard CE (n.d.) Letter to Emma Doherty. GMcCC, Ms 976/162.

[17] Brown, *op. cit.*, note 3, above.

By the end of 1837, Charlotte had saved enough money to send her son to university in France. Although, she had sufficient funds to see him through 3 years in Paris,[18] she decided to go with him, so as to give him some practical assistance during his time there. Finally, their departure was planned as an emigration. Mother and son had no intention of returning to Mauritius. Edouard confirmed this decision when, from Paris he wrote to a Mauritian friend: "I shall never more return to Mauritius."[19] Charlotte sold her house.[20]

Apart from the proceeds from the sale of her house and the money that she had painstakingly put aside, Charlotte received, in 1836, a sum of around 250 sovereigns—the equivalent today of £30,000—by way of compensation, from the British government, for freeing her slaves.[21]

On January 8, 1838, mother and son set sail from Port Louis, bound for Nantes.

[18] Brown-Séquard, *op. cit.*, note 2, above.

[19] Brown-Séquard CE (n.d. probably 1838) Letter to Jules Chauvin. GMcCC, Ms 994/16.

[20] Brown-Séquard CE (1838) Letter to Emile Gausseran, GMcCC, Ms 994/16, 17th July.

[21] When slavery was abolished in 1835, the British government paid £2,100,000 to the Mauritian slave-owners for some 80,000 slaves. The 1821 Census returns record the composition of Charlotte Brown's household: herself, her son, her slaves, their spouses and their children.

# Chapter 5
# The Medical Student: 1838–1846

Charlotte and Edouard Brown reached Nantes in April 1838, where they stayed for a few days, at the home of Bertrand Hercule Blevec,[1] a relative of Edouard's godfather, Emile Gausseran. From Nantes, they travelled to Tours, staying at the home of another Mauritian, M. Rousseau.[2] Then, they made their way to Paris, where they took temporary accommodation in the rue Jacob,[3] near the ruins of the Abbey of St. Germain des Près. Whilst living there, Charlotte began to look for a town house in the Latin Quarter, as she planned to open a boarding house for provincial students who were following courses in Paris. She had to get a place ready for the new academic year in the autumn, so she eventually leased a house at number 28, rue Férou, which runs south from Place St. Sulpice into the rue de Vaugirard.

The house which they moved into, in early August,[4] was chosen because "it had an advantage, very rare in Paris, of possessing a courtyard and a garden for our sole use."[5] It had enough rooms to accommodate five or six students, including Edouard.[6] Charlotte made do with one downstairs room as her bedroom, which also served as a daytime lounge for her guests.[7]

Meanwhile, Edouard's first preoccupation was with the literary world. The praises that he had won from the group of authors who met in the Port Louis store, not only had given him confidence in his literary ability, but had awakened in him a strong aspiration to become a writer. As he himself wrote:

> I loved literature with passion and I had written I do not know how many dramas, tragedies, poems, light verses and philosophical pieces. I had left my native land with the intention of, not only studying medicine in Paris but also, with the desire and the hope of

1 Brown-Séquard CE (1838) Letter to Blévec. GMcCC, Ms 994/16, 18th Nov.
2 Brown-Séquard CE (1838) Letter to Rousseau. GMcCC, Ms 994/16, 13rd Aug.
3 Brown-Séquard CE (1838) Letter to Eugène Cloarec. GMcCC, Ms 994/16. 13th Aug.
4 Brown-Séquard, *op. cit.*, note 2, above.
5 *Ibid.*
6 Brown-Séquard (1838) Letter to Jules Bouchet. GMcCC, Ms 994/16.
7 Brown C (1839) Letter to a friend in Mauritius. GMcCC, Ms 975/2, 16th July.

L.-C. Celestin, *Charles-Edouard Brown-Séquard*,
DOI: 10.1007/978-3-319-03020-3_5, 

indulging after sometime, in literary activities. I had hoped that I would have been able to live and help my mother with the proceeds of my publications.[8]

So, even before he began his studies for the **Baccalauréat-ès-Lettres**, he approached "a fellow countryman already well known amongst the men of letters of the then flourishing romantic school''[9] for an introduction to Charles Nodier, who was the focal point of a group of disciples of the Romantic School known as the **Cénacle**. An excellent critic, he was himself a distinguished author of fictional works.

Edouard had brought most of his writings with him from Mauritius and gave his best pieces to Nodier to read. The latter made it clear to him that he had no professional future in literature. His first visit to this man of letters was

> a disappointment. Nodier told him, in a paternal way, but bluntly that he should acquire a profession in order to live and not to believe that there was, in what he had read, anything yet that foreshadowed a writer, let alone a dramatist, and he had read his very best excerpts.[10]

Nodier's verdict was, no doubt, a very painful blow for Edouard. He sought the opinion of several other critics and received no further encouragement. As he wrote himself:

> I went to see several eminent men of letters,… all told me that, even should I be the greatest poet of the century, I would not be able to earn money for several years.[11]

In the end, he decided to get rid of all his writings he had brought from Mauritius:

> I then took a courageous decision which caused me to shed many tears. I burnt all that I had written, except for some dramas left in my country and some verses forgotten in a drawer.[12]

A great disappointment maybe, but his experience was not unique. Some years earlier, Claude Bernard who, as a physiologist, he would eventually emulate and succeed, had taken some work to Saint-Marc Girardin, professor of poetry at the Sorbonne. It was a five-act play called Arthur de Bretagne, and was told to abandon all hope of literary fame. However, in both their cases, as intimated by the biologist, Maurice Arthus. "nobody knows what literature lost, but everyone knows what science gained."[13]

---

[8] Brown-Séquard CE (1852) Letter to Lady Blanche. GMcCC, Ms 977/1, 17th Dec.

[9] Dupuy E (1894) Notice sur M. Le professeur Brown-Séquard, ancient Président de la Société de biologie. Revue Scient (Paris) 8: 737–743, p. 737.

[10] *Ibid.*

[11] Brown-Séquard, *op.cit.*, note 8, above.

[12] *Ibid.*

[13] Arthus M (1898) Brown-Séquard et son oeuvre. In: Le Blanc M Brown-Séquard. Imprimerie Roussel et Cie. Port Louis, Mauritius, pp. 10–11.

In order to pursue his medical studies, Edouard had to sit both Baccalauréats. On November 13, 1838, he passed the Baccalauréat-ès-Lettres and was able to enrol in the Faculty of Medicine.[14] A letter from his mother, addressed to Augustine Maisonneuve in Mauritius, dated December 9, 1838, gives a good impression of his daily routine and shows his determination to achieve his ambition. It reads:

> I am happy to see the conduct of my son, so young and yet able to endure so many sacrifices. He has been to a Show only once and it was M. Dubois who took him. He knows none of the pleasures of Paris, goes only to where his work calls him and, furthermore, for the past month he has gone everyday to take a lesson in chemistry and from there to the hospital to learn how to dissect.... He is determined to learn this profession.
>
> And always, with pleasure and passion, he would like to know everything immediately.[15]

Charlotte's first lodgers were not French students, but young Mauritians. As we know, this had not been her original intention, but she apparently "had no other option than to take Creoles for board and lodging."[16] Word had gone round the Mauritian community of Paris that Mme. Brown had rooms to let, through the good offices of Gabriel Désiré Laverdant, a writer and a business man. The son of a wealthy Mauritian sugar-cane planter, who was well established in Paris and had access to a great many people. Shortly, after the Browns's arrival in Paris, he left for a long visit to Mauritius but, prior to his departure, he had introduced Charlotte and Edouard to many of his closest friends. These included: M. Amiel, an artist painter; M. Laviron, a business man; Victor Considérant, a social reformer[17] who, in turn, introduced Edouard to the architect César Denis Daly .

So, in September 1838, Charlotte received her first group of Mauritian students. Among them, was Julien Faure, who had just submitted his thesis for the Doctorate of Medicine and was on the point of leaving Paris to practise in Mauritius; Emile Dubois, the school friend of Edouard, who was studying to be a notary; Alexandre Bonnefin, a medical student, the eldest of three brothers, who all studied medicine; Cloarec, the brother of Edouard's schoolmate, Eugène; Cantin, a medical student who befriended the Browns in Paris and a "mulatto son of Mr. Staub of Mauritius."[18] The rooms were let unfurnished,[19] except in the case of Emile Dubois, who had come straight from Mauritius, and had not yet acquired any furniture.[20]

Charlotte employed a cook and a chamber-maid.[21] Her dining table, which could sit 12 guests, was regularly attended by other Mauritian students who were

---

[14] Brown-Séquard CE (1838) Letter to Jules Chauvin. GMcCC 994/16. 14th Nov.

[15] Brown C (1838) Letter to Augustine Maisonneuve. GMcCC, Ms 975/1, 9th Dec.

[16] Brown, *op. cit.*, note 7, above.

[17] Brown-Séquard CE Letter to Laverdant, 30th Sept, 22nd Dec, 1838; Apr & July, 1839. GMcCC, Ms 994/16.

[18] Brown-Séquard, *op. cit.*, note 8, above.

[19] Brown, *op. cit.*, note 15, above.

[20] Brown, *op. cit.*, note 7, above.

[21] Brown, *op. cit.*, note 15, above.

living in Paris.[22] One of the regular diners was d'Arifat, who partnered Edouard in the dissecting room.[23] There were other Mauritian students in Paris, whom Edouard made contact with in the late 1830s. There were 12 studying Medicine, 5 Pharmacology and 10 Law.

For these young Mauritians at Charlotte's house, these evening reunions were a good opportunity to talk about and share the news from home.[24] After dinner, the company would disperse, the diners would leave and the lodgers went to study in their rooms.[25] Sometimes Edouard would study in his mother's room, where she would sit reading a newspaper or a book, darning socks, repairing clothes or sewing a dress for herself.[26] These private moments between mother and son were not prolonged until late at night as, after his success in the Baccalauréat-ès-Lettres, Edouard had developed a routine which he would follow for most of his life. He would wake up at three o'clock in the morning and read in bed until daybreak, then he got up, got dressed and studied until breakfast time. He then revised his science subjects until one o'clock before going for private tuition to prepare for his Baccalauréat-ès-Sciences and then to the hospital to dissect. He returned home for dinner, which was served at six and would be free until nine.[27]

Most days, Charlotte was visited by two very good Mauritian lady friends. These were Mme. Lantour, who called either with her granddaughter, Délice Baudiac[28] or with another elderly woman, Mme. Chandelier[29] Edouard, on the other hand, was a loner, who felt more at ease in the company of older men. Loneliness is a recurrent theme in his letters to his friends in Mauritius, as seen in this one to Désiré Laverdant who was thinking of staying for good in Mauritius:

> Have you no hope of returning to France, Laverdant?... If you have may it soon be fulfilled! How happy I should be then... Both for mamma and for myself. I have not a single friend here, not one. That is the truth. There are, in the world, three persons whom I love at least as myself and two are far away, you and Jules Chauvin. Only one is here, my mother, who is very old through worries, affliction and age.[30]

He particularly missed the company of women so much, that his lack of sexual outlet became a problem for him. This too, was an incessant subject in his letters and, though they are veiled in figurative language, his references are easily recognizable:

---

[22] Brown-Séquard CE (1838) Letter to Laverdant. GMcCC, Ms 994/16, 30th Sept.

[23] Brown-Séquard, *op. cit.*, note 14, above.

[24] Brown, *op. cit.*, note 15, above.

[25] *Ibid.*

[26] *Ibid.*

[27] Brown-Séquard CE (1839) Letter to Jules Chauvin. GMcCC 994/16. 10th Feb.

[28] Brown-Séquard CE (1839) Letter to Mme Patée. GMcCC 994/16. 25th Jan.

[29] Brown, *op. cit.*, note 15, above.

[30] Brown-Séquard CE (1838) Letter to Laverdant. GMcCC, Ms 994/16, April.

> I would be very well, were it not that I am constantly troubled by the blood. I need to be less continent than I am, but I am lacking time and money. I fear I may be a long time suffering.[31]

In another letter, he wrote: "I do not have a mistress nor a friend, I, who am stirred by strong passions."[32] His comments about a stereotyped Parisian woman are tinged with sexual overtones, for example:

> It is a woman… whose eyes intensely bright and fiery reveal a passionate nature. If you have, sometimes, formed a mental picture of Semiramis, the Queen of Babylon, then you have that of a Parisian woman—a woman who enjoys life three times more than other women of the world and thus, her organs promptly wear out and old age sets in accompanied by numerous and swift infirmities.[33]

In an effort to subdue his carnal desires, he used to exercise in the gymnasium once a week, accompanied by his mother's boarder, Cloarec or by M. Laviron, the business man. They went to a gymnasium on the Champ Elyssés, where he was particularly attracted by a very brilliant and numerous society "men of letters and scientists who seek to regain back the energies that they have spent through arduous work staying up at night".[34]

He, sometimes, went out to meet various acquaintances: M. Amiel, the artist-painter; M. Laviron and particularly, Victor Considérant.[35] It was with the latter and also with Désiré Laverdant that he was introduced into Fourierist circles and, consequently, into a very much wider group of acquaintances which included representatives to the **Chambre des Députés**, higher civil servants, freethinkers, artists and scientists. Several Parisian newspapers drew attention to his association with Fourierists. In 1894, one wrote that "he kept company with phalansterians, although younger, by several years, than most of them,… to remain their friends until their deaths."[36] He was invited to Fourierist lectures and debates and also to their balls, banquets and meetings. Less than six months after his arrival in Paris, on October 1st, 1838, he was invited to attend a commemoration of the first anniversary of the death of Marie Charles Fourier. This is what he wrote to Désiré Laverdant, in Mauritius:

> M. Considérant wrote me a charming letter asking me to join with his friends and other persons who are giving a banquet tomorrow on the occasion of the anniversary of the death of the modern Jesus: Fourier. He tells me that, apart from standing in for you, I will also be there for my own sake.[37]

---

[31] *Ibid.*

[32] Brown-Séquard CE (1838) Letter to Laverdant. GMcCC, Ms 994/16, 16th July April.

[33] Brown-Séquard CE (1838) Letter to Eugène Cloarec. GMcCC, Ms 994/16, 31st July.

[34] *Ibid.*

[35] Brown-Séquard, *op. cit.*, note 22, above.

[36] Paris (1894) Brown-Séquard. Une grande figure scientifique. Paris, 4th Apr. Also L'Eclair (1894) Brown-Séquard. Quelques notes intimes sur le célèbre physiologiste. Pairs, 4th Apr.

[37] Brown-Séquard, *op. cit.*, note 22, above.

The terms **Fourierist** and **phalansterian** need some explaining. The former derives, of course, from the name of the founder of the movement, Marie Charles Fourier, a utopian philosopher who dreamt of a universal socialist system, which came to be known as Fourierism. The second term refers to the formation of phalanxes or communities, which was central to the Fourierist movement. A phalanx was a group of people, known as phalansterians, living together, like one big family in phalansteries: vast buildings or communes and holding property, in common. These phalansteries were the forerunners of the kibbutzim and the hippies' communes. The phalansterians were led and taught by apostles and sages, whom they had elected.

Among the members of the Fourierist society in Paris, whom Edouard frequented, Victor Considérant, Désiré Laverdant and César Daly were apostles[38] and he was referred to as a phalansterian.[39] The Fourierists held a materialistic outlook on life. They were mostly atheists or freethinkers who could, politically, be described as liberal-minded, left-wing republicans. They vehemently opposed slavery and advocated universal suffrage. Moreover, they were, at that time, strongly opposed to the monarchical government of Louis-Philippe.

There were, in the 1830s and 1840s, a great many believers in Fourier's Utopian new world. In 1831, Alexandre François Baudet-Dulary, a physician of E-tampes, who was the deputy of Seine-et-Oise, tried to set up a commune at Condé-sur-Vesgre, in the forest of Rambouillet. However, the project had to be abandoned. Monthly journals, such as Le Nouveau Monde and La Réforme Industrielle were founded in 1832. The readership was so large, that these publications were expanded into a review La Phalange, which had an enormous success. The Fourierists collected large sums of money and propagated their doctrine through lectures, concerts, banquets and balls. On Fourier's death in 1837, Considérant was chosen as the head of the movement.

Prosper Victor Considérant's chequered career began in a military academy and he served as a captain in the army until 1832. He, then, gave up his army post to spread the word of his teacher, Fourier. He founded the review **La Phalange** and rallied the Republican Party during the Revolution of February 1848, proclaiming in his manifesto that "All socialists are republicans, all republicans are socialists." Prior to that Revolution, the tenets of French socialism had been "the right to work", which Considérant advocated himself. He was elected the deputy of the Seine in May 1849 and had opposed, the previous December, the election of Louis Napoléon as President of France. Together with Alexandre Ledru-Rollin and others, he had drafted the Call to Arms, which resulted in the riots of June 13, 1849. As a result, he was accused of insurrection and fled abroad.

Leaving for the moment Edouard's involvement with Fourierism, there is no doubt that he could not have chosen any better place than Paris to study, as it was the centre of the medical world in the 1830s and 1840s. The Paris medical teaching scene was dominated by three men: Andral, Chomel and Louis. Gabriel Andral

---

[38] Dupuy E (n.d.) Letter to Charlotte McCausland. GMcCC, Ms 986/8.

[39] Friedlin J (1853) Letter to Alex Harrison. GMcCC, Ms 986/8, 11th Apr.

devoted much of his time establishing the origin and mechanism of diseases; Auguste François Chomel was a brilliant expositor both in his teaching and writing and Pierre Charles Alexandre Louis was a keen observer, who had a great and lasting influence on American medicine. The Parisian hospitals boasted a galaxy of eminent physicians and surgeons and the Paris Medical School, many dedicated teachers. These were scholars like François Magendie, who laid the foundations of experimental pharmacology; Jean Cruveilhier, renowned for his treatise of pathological anatomy: **Anatomie pathologique du corps humain**; Jean-Baptiste Bouillaud who discovered the association between stenosis of the mitral valve of the heart and acute rheumatic fever (nowadays associated with infection by a haemolytic group A Streptococcus) and between aphasia and the frontal lobes of the brain; Armand Trousseau, the top clinician of his day and many others, such as Pierrre François Olive Rayer, an expert on renal diseases. Experts as they were, these savants were not limited to their medical science. They also had strong cultural backgrounds and were steeped in the Classics. They were not out of place in the flourishing literary salons of which there were so many in Paris, in those days. Finally, they were greatly admired and respected for their humane and humanistic attitudes.

The doctorate of the Medical Faculty was then opened to holders of both Baccalauréats. The studies lasted 4 years, assessed by five annual examinations and a thesis in Latin or French on a medical or medically-related subject. Students started their hospital training from the day they entered the Faculty. Every morning, they attended a hospital and were coached by a physician or surgeon. In the afternoon they attended lectures and practical demonstrations at the Medical School. The whole course was free of charge, apart from a modest annual registration fee and the purchase of books. So the main expenses, for the students, were those incurred in the day to day cost of living.

At that time, the Paris Social Service: **L'Assistance publique** held two competitive examinations each year, in December. They were called the **Concours de l'externat des hôpitaux** and the **Concours de l'internat des hôpitaux**. Run independently of the Medical Faculty's examinations, their purpose was to select candidates for the posts of Externes and Internes, to work in the Paris hospitals' wards. The Externes undertook minor medical and surgical tasks, under the supervision of qualified medical staff. Normally, medical students sat the Externat after completion of their second year in the Faculty and worked in that capacity for 3 years. The Internat was attempted, after the Faculty's third year examination, by the Externes only. This meant that a candidate, successful at both these Concours. would present his doctoral thesis after 6–8 years of medical and clinical studies. The Externes were not residents in the hospitals, whereas the Internes were, earning a modest salary, but the importance of reaching such a level was that it was the sesame to a future career as a hospital physician or surgeon.

In November 1839, Edouard successfully sat the Baccalauréat-ès-Sciences,[40] despite being hindered in his studies by contracting measles shortly before.[41]

---

[40] Brown-Séquard, *op. cit.*, note 14, above.

[41] Brown, *op. cit.*, note 7, above.

At the end of 1840, after completing his second year in the Medical School, he was taken as a pupil-assistant by Dr. Martin-Magron, who ran his own private research laboratory. It was customary, in those days, for research-minded scientists to set up their own laboratories and minimise their expenses by taking on student-assistants. Although, he did not make any lasting contribution to medical science, Martin-Magron was, nevertheless, highly esteemed by his colleagues and was, moreover, an able physician, keenly interested in experimental physiology.

Though Edouard had largely grown out of his teenage dream of becoming a writer, he was still nostalgic about having failed to make the grade as evidenced by the following passage of a letter to his childhood friend, Jules Chauvin of Mauritius:

> At times, my heart bleeds, but my spirit at least is subdued. I have no more dreams of literary glory, or unrestricted longings to make a name for myself in literature, dreams and longings which followed me for quite a while. I have rid myself completely of all that, and now aspire to nothing, but my diploma in medicine.[42]

In fact, it was in Martin-Magron's laboratory that he had a revelation of his genuine calling. It seems that the point to where his passion for physiology can be traced is his second year of work in that laboratory, when he began to think about carrying out research of his own. His passion was married to a keen desire for knowledge, an ambition he mentions in a letter to Zulma Laporte, the daughter of his godfather, Emile Gausseran:

> I have so much work to do that it is absolutely necessary for me to live like a savage, like a bear. I want to know something more than all the Physicians of Mauritius who have just enough knowledge to bleed you when you have a plethora and to purge you when you have too much bile.[43]

His work in Martin-Magron's laboratory had to be combined with teaching commitments. In 1840, he started work in a school, teaching Physics, Chemistry and Natural History, preparing pupils for the Baccalauréat-ès-Sciences. He was also, working in 1841, as a laboratory assistant to a professor who taught Physics and Chemistry, acting as substitute teacher when the professor was absent.[44] By 1842, he had extended the subjects he taught to include Anatomy and Physiology.[45] They were all fruitful activities for him and, an added bonus was the substantial sum of money he was earning. As he said,

> he had felt the necessity to create in Paris a position such that by the sole products of my work, I might be able to live in comfort with my mother.[46]

---

[42] Brown-Séquard CE (1839) Letter to Jules Chauvin. GMcCC, Ms 994/16, 6th Apr.

[43] Brown-Séquard CE (1839) Letter to Zulma Laporte. GMcCC, Ms 994/16, 24th July.

[44] Brown-Séquard, *op. cit.*, note 8, above.

[45] *Ibid.*

[46] Brown-Séquard CE (1840) Letter to Auguste Laporte. GMcCC, Ms 994/16, 1st Sept.

> Such necessity, however, has matured me early, and while metamorphosing me from a child into a man, has unfortunately, made me slightly sad, slightly gloomy.[47]

Gone for ever the days when he had hoped to live from his pen, with which, he would have inscribed his name on the "Temple of Glory and Immortality."[48]

Meanwhile, by then, Charlotte's boarding house was well established. She was never short of Mauritian lodgers, whom she looked after as if they were her own sons. At this time, she was anticipating the arrival of her Mauritian friend's son, Jules Maisonneuve, who was coming to Paris, to study Arts. His impending arrival brought out her maternal instincts. She wrote to Jules's mother, Augustine, describing the room that he would occupy, promising to make sure he was properly clothed in winter, discussing the sum of money he would need to live as a student, and undertaking to approach M. Amiel, the artist-painter, whom she would ask about the best Art School for Jules to attend. Her final words reveal the true warmth of her nature:

> My good old friends be reassured on your child's lot. Here, he will find a mother who loves him and a brother who cherishes him. Is he not my child? It was in my arms that he was placed when he came into the world. I wait for him everyday this dear child.[49]

In due course, Jules came to Paris and stayed at Charlotte's house, while he attended an Art school. His studies over, he returned to Mauritius, where he was in demand as an artist and lithographer. In 1870, he emigrated to The United States. There, in 1873, he was re-united with Edouard, for whom he did some engravings, to illustrate the latter's books.[50]

In December 1841, just after having been successful at his third year medical examination, Edouard passed the Concours de l'externat des hôpitaux. The new year, 1842, saw him serving as an **Externe** at the **Hôtel-Dieu** Hospital, in the service of Armand Trousseau. This hospital is, probably, the oldest medical institution in the world. It was founded in 651 by Landericus (Saint Landry), Bishop of Paris. It also boasted the longest serving religious order, the **Augustine Sisters of the Hôtel-Dieu,** who worked there from the foundation of the hospital through to the first decade of the twentieth century. This amounted to over 1,250 years of continuing service.[51]

The top ten successful candidates to the Concours de l'externat were permitted to choose the service and the hospital they would attend. Thus, coming fifth out of 300 candidates,[52] Edouard chose to serve under Armand Trousseau, the most renowned clinician of the nineteenth century. He was the first to perform a

---

[47] *Ibid.*

[48] *Ibid.*

[49] Brown C (1840) Letter to Augustine Maisonneuve. GMcCC, Ms 975/3. 21st Apr.

[50] Brown-Séquard CE (1873) Letter to his second wife, Maria. GMcCC, Ms 978/15, 15th Apr.

[51] Meyer A (1878) Les religieuses Augustines de l'Hôtel Dieu et leur passage à l'hôpital Boucicaut (1897–1975). Hist Sci Méd (Paris) 12: 277–281.

[52] Brown-Séquard, *op. cit.*, note 8, above.

tracheotomy in France; though not the first in the world, for it is said that Alexander the Great used to do it with the point of his sword! Trousseau also generalised the use of intubation. His name is familiar to generations of French medical students, due to his famous three-volume **Clinique médicale de l'Hôtel-Dieu**. Its descriptive literary style is unsurpassed in French medical literature; not to mention the minutest details with which every ailment is described.

It was in Trousseau's service that Edouard met Charles Robin, another Externe. It was the start of a lifelong friendship. Robin, in later years, was to distinguish himself as one of the pioneers of Histology, ranking with Louis Antoine Ranvier, the German Rudolph Albert von Kölliker, the Italian Camillo Golgi and the Spaniard Santiago Ramón y Cajal. He discovered Candida albicans, a parasitic fungus and identified it as the causative agent of thrush (candidiasis), an infection of the mouth in infants and of the vagina in women.

Edouard now dreamt of achieving the ambition that all Externes have in common: success in the Concours de l'internat des hôpitaux, leading to a hospital career. No small achievement. As there were often ten times more candidates to the Concours, than there were posts available in the hospitals. As early as 1839, he had written:

> I aspire with all my mind to the internat in the hospitals. I wish I could reach this top grade as soon as possible.[53]

The more so that

> I would have 500 francs per year and I would easily earn a thousand to 1,500 francs above that by giving lessons, for an interne always finds pupils.[54]

The year 1842, which had started so well for him with his brilliant success in the Concours de l'externat, the previous December, was to end in a disastrous manner. In the early part of the year, his studies and teaching activities were interrupted by pricking his finger in the dissecting room. It appears that an infection set in and spread, causing permanent damage to the phalangeal articulations of two fingers of his left hand. Inconvenient as this was, it was a mere setback compared to the events of later that year.

He was still recovering from his finger infection, when his mother died. Despite the fact that he had been nursing her through an illness, her death was still an unexpected blow.[55] She died at the fairly early age of 54 on July 10, 1842.

It was a prostrating blow for Edouard. He was now alone in the world, bereft of his mother who had been the centre of his emotional life for 25 years. Despite his own earnings, there would be no financial support for the rest of his student years. The strength of their bond can be seen in the following tribute to his mother, written 10 years after her death:

[53] Brown-Séquard, *op. cit.*, note 46, above.

[54] *Ibid.*

[55] Lantour Mme. (1852) Letter to Brown-Séquard. GMcCC, Ms 980/4, 21st Apr.

> Her love for me gave her strength and she succeeded in earning enough money to enable me to be given as complete an education as possible in a country like mine, and to accompany me to France and to enable me to do my first studies in medicine.[56]

For months, he was grief stricken. He went into an acute depressive state which, eventually, led to social isolation and an inability to function in a normal manner. He wandered all over France, penniless, sleeping rough and begging in the streets. He must have had some quite unpleasant experiences and, despite his state of confusion, those disturbing memories lingered with him for years. He was in the habit of "confessing" about this period of his life to his American cousin, Henry J Feltus, who later, recalled in a letter one such experience:

> It is not necessary to assure you of my sympathy for your feelings in visiting Dijon. The distress that you, once, endured there is too well remembered by me to be recalled by any allusion to the scene of it without pain.[57]

Even when he was in his late fifties, he was prone to intense grief if anything or anyone, reminded him of his mother's death. The quotation, which follows, is a passage from a letter he wrote, in 1876, to his future wife, Emma Doherty:

> Here I am, crying like a child my dearest. I happen to find among papers that I am putting in order the enclosed. I do feel now, as deeply as ever before, the loss of that most kind and loving mother, whose tomb is spoken of in that paper.[58]

He later gave his own account of the aftermath of his mother's death, revealing how completely his personality had been shattered:

> At this moment, I very nearly went mad, and I was at times, and my career was interrupted. I gave up everything and I tried, by travel, to restore a little of the love of life, that I had completely lost. After having wandered I know not where in France, I left for my native country.[59]

Indeed, on the insistence of his Mauritian friends based in Paris, who were filled with apprehension about his state of mind, he set sail from Le Havre for Mauritius, accompanied by Dr. Alexandre Bonnefin, who had been his mother's lodger.[60] His presence was a great comfort to Edouard,[61] who was extremely depressed and in an awful physical state, complaining of constant headaches, stomach pains and loss of appetite. The violent grief, resulting from the loss of his mother, had triggered the first symptoms of a latent mental illness. Henceforth, bouts of depression, sometimes verging on suicide, alternating with bouts of elation, restlessness and physical and mental hyperactivities, were to plague him remorselessly for the rest of his life. These depressive spells were to appear at more or less

56 Brown-Séquard, *op. cit.*, note 8, above.

57 Feltus HJ (1865) Letter to Brown-Séquard. GMcCC, Ms 981/162, 18th Aug.

58 Brown-Séquard CE (n.d.) Letter to Emma Doherty. GMcCC, Ms 978/9.

59 Brown-Séquard, *op. cit.*, note 8, above.

60 *Ibid.*

61 *Ibid.*

regular intervals, lasting for varying lengths of time, exacerbated by a stubborn insomnia, tenacious headaches, hypochondriac obsessions, anxiety paroxysms and panic reactions. This disturbing mental state, moreover, co-existed with symptoms of a seasonal affective disorder: frequent mood swings on dull and wet autumn and winter days.

The two friends arrived at Port Louis on March 24, 1843, and by June, Edouard who had been cared for by Emile Gausseran, his godfather and the many friends of his mother, had recovered his composure and was in a fairly normal state of mind. On the first day of June, he presented his very first academic paper to the local **Natural History Society**, later known as **The Royal Society of Arts and Science of Mauritius**. It was a report on a water-spout that he had observed at sea on February 21, 1863.[62] Before presenting his paper, he had applied for membership of this Society and had been unanimously elected a member.

He left Mauritius some time in August, after having settled his mother's affairs. She had some investments in local companies. He also carried out a study of the hibernation of the tanrec, a small insectivorous mammal, not unlike the hedgehog. He was back in Paris in November 1843, in time for the new academic year.[63]

In Paris, he went to live at 5, rue Neuve-des-Beaux-Arts.[64] Anyway, for the next 3 years, he does not seem to have suffered greatly from any financial inconvenience, living on the money he had inherited from his mother. At the beginning of 1844, during his fourth academic year, he served as an **Externe** at **La Charité** Hospital in the service of Pierre Rayer,[65] and resumed his work as an assistant in Martin-Magron's laboratory.

That same year, he used himself as a subject for experiment. It was the first of many he was to carry out on himself. At that time, he was interested in the physiology of digestion and inspired by the work of René Antoine Ferchault, Seigneur de Réamur who, in 1752, was the first to carry out experiments to determine the exact nature of digestion in birds. Experiments which were the subject of further researches by Lazzaro Spallanzani in 1780. Edouard therefore began collecting specimens of his own gastric juice or partly digested and liquefied content of his stomach for study.

> Thus he repeated on himself the studies of Spallanzani, carried out on ravens, by collecting gastric juice by means of a sponge which he swallowed attached to a piece of string, so as to remove it afterwards from his stomach, soaked with the precious liquid.[66]

---

62 Rouget FA (1930) Brown-Séquard et son oeuvre. Esquisse biographique. General Printing & Stationary Cy, Port Louis, Mauritius. p. 7–8.

63 Role A (1977) La Vie étrange d'un grand savant: le professeur Brown-Séquard. Plon, Paris, p. 42. According to this author, Brown-Séquard was not allowed to resume his medical studies prior to March 1844. There is no proof to substantiate this statement.

64 *Ibid.*

65 Olmstead JMD (1946) Charles-Edouard Brown-Séquard. A nineteenth century neurologist and endocrinologist. The John Hopkins Press, Baltimore, p. 14.

66 Berthelot MPE (1898) Notice sur la vie et les travaux de M. Brown-Séquard. Typographie Firmin-Didot et Cie. Paris, p. 17.

This continuous experimentation on his digestive system effectively turned him into "an animal that chews the curd". It caused a few complications in his social life. He felt ill at ease in society, especially at the dinner table, because of constant eructations and regurgitations of food. The effect of these experiments was so great, that he was able to throw up the whole content of his stomach with no great effort, a capacity he was later to make use of in other experiments. Thus, in 1858, after consuming large amounts of starchy food, he carried out a series of experiments, by vomiting the content of his stomach, to study the transformation of starch into glucose.[67] Years later, after giving him a medical check-up in The United States, Dr. Samuel Ward Francis reported that:

> His general health had been very good, being exempt from many of the affections that flesh is heir to. But, a desire to investigate the contents of his own stomach, under different circumstances, by means of which he could examine the gastric juice or partially digested food, has brought on a rare affection, which is sometimes seen in man, namely a persistent merycism or rumination, when one is forced to chew a second time what had been swallowed.[68]

During 1844, he studied for the **Concours de l'internat**, which he sat in December of that year. He failed to make the grade that would have secured him an **Interne's** position in a hospital. Two years later, on January 3, 1846, he successfully defended and upheld his thesis for the Doctorate of Medecine in front of a panel of examiners of the Medical Faculty, presided over by Professor Pierre Eloy Fouquier. The title of his thesis was **Recherches et Expériences sur la Physiologie** de la **Moelle Epinière** (Researches and Experiments on the Physiology of the Spinal Cord).[69] It was inscribed to his mother. It was written under the guidance of Martin-Magron to whom he paid the following tribute in the introduction

> To my most excellent master and friend, to whom I am happy to pay a public tribute of my gratitude for the liberality with which he has always gracefully opened to me the treasures of his heart and mind.

His thesis was divided into two distinct parts. In the first one, all the experiments, carried out on batrachians, had been done in collaboration with Martin-Magron. It was the study of the reflex activity of the spinal cord after it had been separated from the brain. The general conclusion was a marked diminution in reflex activity, immediately after separation of the cord from the brain, followed later by a net increase in that activity. This finding was, in itself, "the first

---

[67] Brown-Séquard CE (1858) Expérience sur la transformation de l'amidon en glucose dans l'estomac. J Physiol (Paris) 1: 158–160.

[68] Quoted in Major RH. (1943) Charles Edouard Brown-Séquard. In: Essays in honour of Herbert M. Evans. University of California Press, Los Angeles, p. 375.

[69] Thèse pour le Doctorat en médecine de Paris par Charles-Edouard Brown, né au Port Louis, Ile Maurice (Isle de France), Docteur en médecine. Rignoux, Imprimerie de la Faculte de Médecine, rue Monsieur-le-Prince, 29bis, Paris.

FACULTÉ DE MÉDECINE DE PARIS.

# THÈSE

POUR

## LE DOCTORAT EN MÉDECINE,

*Présentée et soutenue le 3 janvier* 1846,

Par CHARLES-ÉDOUARD BROWN,

né au Port-Louis, Ile Maurice (Ile de France),

DOCTEUR EN MÉDECINE.

RECHERCHES ET EXPÉRIENCES

SUR LA

## PHYSIOLOGIE DE LA MOELLE ÉPINIÈRE.

Le Candidat répondra aux questions qui lui seront faites sur les diverses parties de l'enseignement médical.

PARIS.

RIGNOUX, IMPRIMEUR DE LA FACULTÉ DE MÉDECINE,
rue Monsieur-le-Prince, 29 *bis*.

1846

1846. — *Brown*.

TITLE PAGE OF EDOUARD BROWN'S DOCTORATE THESIS, 1846

**Fig. 5.1** Faculté de médecine © Celestin

unmistakable description of spinal shock,"[70] and this was 4 years before Marshall Hall gave this phenomenon its name. This neurophysiologist considered the spinal cord, separated from the encephalon, as an independent organ able to lead its own existence. He had reached such a conclusion given the persistency of spinal reflexes, after the decapitation of criminals. This state of shock is referred to, in clinical medicine, as spinal shock syndrome, characterised by a period of areflexia, followed by one of hyperreflexia, consecutive to a spinal cord injury.

The second part of his thesis was done independently of Martin-Magron. It was, basically, a study of the spinal cord as a means of transmitting sensory and motor impulses. This was a problem that appeared to have been solved by the discovery of two types of nerve roots originating in the spinal cord: sensitive roots and motor roots. Charles Bell had extended this distinction to the columns of the spinal cord: the posterior or dorsal columns concerned with sensation and the anterior or ventral columns with movement. It was a simple straight-forward doctrine, which Edouard challenged by his experiments, showing that "there is in the spinal cord, another pathway than the posterior columns which conduct sensation."

This thesis was an important landmark in his scientific career. He was now moving into his chosen field of research: the nervous system. It showed that he had the strength of character not to be afraid of challenging the prevailing doctrine of his day. (Fig. 5.1)

Furthermore, even if his thesis did not, actually, demonstrate a now well established fact: that the sensory pathways cross from one side to the other of the spinal cord, he did, however, end by stating:

> I must draw attention to another important fact, demonstrated by my experiments, it is the ease with which sensitive impressions are transmitted from one side to the other of the cord.[71]

It was this penultimate paragraph of his thesis which contained the germ of his discovery: the decussation of the sensory pathways in the spinal cord, which led to his elaboration and description of the clinical syndrome which bears his name.

---

[70] Ruch TC (1946) Yale Journal of Biology and Medicine. Quoted by Olmsted, *op. cit.*, note 65, above.

[71] Brown-Séquard, *op. cit.*, note 69, above.

# Chapter 6
# The Lone Experimenter: 1846–1851

In October 1846, a communication from Edouard Brown appeared in the **Comptes-rendus de l'Academie des sciences** signed Brown-Léquard.[1] For a while this double-barrelled name was spelt in different ways in various publications, appearing as Brown-Léquart, Brown-Séguard or Brown-Séquart, before being finally, properly spelt: Brown-Séquard. Adding his mother's maiden name to his patronymic was, no doubt, the ultimate compliment to the woman who had stood by him for 25 years. He even reversed the usual order of double-barrelled surnames, choosing to be known as Brown-Séquard instead of Séquard-Brown. In public, he was reluctant to admit that this was a sentimental gesture in honour of his mother's memory and would give various reasons to explain this change of name; namely that it was to avoid confusion between him and other persons bearing the name Brown,[2] or that it was a common Mauritian custom to add the mother's maiden name to the patronymic.[3] The change was never made legal for he never applied, officially, for a change of identity. In January of the same year, when he submitted his doctoral thesis, he not only had inverted his forenames, but hyphenated them as well: Edouard Charles became Charles-Edouard.[4]

As a fully qualified physician, he did not set himself up in practice, deciding instead, to carry out original researches from 1846 to early 1852. Furthermore, following a trend that he had started in 1843,[5] he used thousands of laboratory animals to check and recheck the experiments that had been carried out by European physiologists. When carrying out his own researches, he experimented "in a roundabout way, seeking anything by intuition, without any leading hypothesis."[6] Thus, he studied the pathways of sensitive impulses in the spinal cord, animal heat, rigor mortis, digestion, blood circulation, etc. To quote him:

---

[1] C R Acad Sci (Paris) (1846). 23: 719.

[2] Affidavit, 12th Dec. 1859. GMcCC, Ms 987/4.

[3] This is not a current custom in Mauritius.

[4] The forenames on his thesis were Charles Edouard. His birth certificate bears Edouard Charles.

[5] Brown-Séquard (n.d.) Autobiographical letter. In: Notebook in the hand writing of Charlotte McCausland. GMcCC, Ms 999/7.

[6] Le Gendre P (1924) Un Médecin philosophe. Charles Bouchard. Son Oeuvre et son temps (1837–1915). Mason et Cie., Paris, p. 491.


DOI: 10.1007/978-3-319-03020-3_6, 

> From 1843 to 1852 (February), I consecrated nearly all my time to original researches and to courses in Experimental Physiology. (The courses were given at the Practical School of Medicine, Paris.)[7]

These were public courses run independently of the Medical School curriculum. While the practice of medicine was of little concern to him, it was his wish to demonstrate to his auditors the importance of Physiology in the day to day life of organisms.

On February 23, 1848, a revolution broke out. Following the outbreak of fighting between demonstrators and troops in Paris, Louis-Philippe abdicated as the mob ransacked the Palais Royal and the National Guards turned against the king. A provisional government was formed, which proclaimed a republic. Promising work for all, the government created national workshops for that purpose. A constituent assembly was elected, in which the moderate republicans were in the majority. The benefits that the Revolution gave the unemployed were short-lived. The workshops were closed on June 24, provoking another revolt. The workers took to the barricades but, after 4 days of bloody fighting, General Louis Cavaignac crushed the uprising.

Brown-Séquard took part in that Revolution of February, either in the ranks of the National Guards or at the head of one of their companies.[8] It is also possible that he was, at one stage, fighting at the barricades in the Latin Quarter, where one of his Paris-based American friends, William Birney, a member of the Republican Student Movement, was in charge of a barricade in the rue Saint-Jacques.[9] Birney was a freelance correspondent for American newspapers, who eventually returned to The States. He was a strong advocate for the liberation of slaves and, serving as a Union officer in 1863, he was responsible for the recruitment of Blacks into the Unionist army. He finished the American Civil War as a major-general.[10]:

Brown-Séquard's enthusiasm for the Revolution was fuelled by his republicanism and by his conviction that a republic would abolish slavery in the French colonies. Despite constant pressure from the Left, Louis-Philippe's Government had hesitated too long on the abolition issue, with the result that, on the eve of the Revolution, abolition remained the foremost request of the Left. The subsequent victory of the revolutionary forces was a personal triumph for Brown-Séquard, because slavery was definitely abolished by decree, on March 4, 1849 and entered into the Constitution of the Second Republic.

Although his forebears and his mother had been slave-owners, Brown-Séquard loathed slavery. He shared this loathing with his mother. In the Isle de France, as in all French colonies where slavery existed, slaves represented not only a capital for their masters, but also a social status symbol. Any family which did not own slaves

---

7 Brown-Séquard, op. cit., note 5, above.

8 Dupuy E (n.d.) Letter to Charlotte McCausland. GMcCC, Ms 997/7, p. 48.

9 Macdonald W (1929) William Birney. In: Dictionary of American Biography, vol 2. Oxford University Press, Oxford.

10 *Ibid.*

was considered not only poor but proletarian. Brown-Séquard deplored the way that his great grandmother had been treated: a young Indian woman, bought or seized by force on the Malabar Coast and carried away to the Isle Bourbon to be sold as a "servant" and who was the concubine or common-law wife of Wilhelm Leichnig.[11]

Brown-Séquard's part in the Revolution was not just an isolated manifestation of republicanism. The majority of France's physicians were ardent republicans. For too long, the medical profession had been the impotent witness of the inefficacy of Louis-Philippe's government, which had failed to carry out reforms to improve the living conditions of the working classes, who lived in abject poverty. Ill-treated by their employers, living and working amid rampant diseases. These conditions had been the subject of many damning reports by physicians such as René Villermé and Jules Auguste Béclard.[12]

As soon as the fighting broke out, the medical press: **La Gazette des Hôpitaux, L'Union Médicale** and La **Gazette Médicale de Paris**, openly declared their republicanism. Léon Louis Rostan, professor at the School of Medicine, started his regular lecture on clinical medicine by extolling the virtues of the Republic[13] and hailing Freedom which had made itself heard at last.[14] At the **Val-de-Grâce** Hospital, a tree of Liberty was planted while the Marseillaise was sung.[15] The physicians of Paris, headed by Jean-Baptiste Bouillaud and Etienne René Antoine Serres, collected among their colleagues, a sum of 3,000 francs to help the setting up of the Second Republic.[16] Physicians and surgeons were, everywhere, in the thick of the disturbances. Dozens of them were wounded, including Rémy Lucien Corvisart, the nephew of Napoléon's famous physician, who introduced the term tetany in the medical language.[17]

Several physicians were in command of revolutionary forces. Thus, Louis Rémy Aubert Roche persuaded the duke of Nemours to withdraw his troops from the Palais Royal. He was the first to read Louis-Philippe's declaration of abdication to the crowd.[18] Philippe Joseph Buchez, who was to form the provisional government which included his colleagues Adrien Recurt and Ulysses Trélat, entered the Tuileries, leading a detachment of the National Guards.[19] Louis Pasteur and Emile Littré fought at the barricades. Many physicians did not have the right to vote or to

---

[11] Scherer (1990) La Réunion. Presses Universitaries de France. Paris, p. 18.

[12] Laffort L (1949) Médecins devant la Révolution de 1848. Librairie Le François, Paris, p. 101. Also Astuc P (1946) 1848 et la Médecine. Progrès medical N°12: 268–281 and N°13: 297–302.

[13] Rostan LL (1848) Les Bienfaits de la République et les devoirs qu'elle impose. Gaz des Hop, 15th Apr.

[14] *Ibid.*

[15] Gomez M (1932) Trousseau (1801–1867). Librairie médicale et scientifique., Marcel Vigné. Paris, p. 55.

[16] *Ibid.*

[17] Corvisart FRL (1852) De la Contraction des extrémités ou tétanie. Thèse N°223, Paris.

[18] Laffort, op. cit., note 12, above.

[19] *Ibid.*

stand as candidates for the Chambre des députés, but in the election of the constituent assembly, 34 physicians were elected, Armand Trousseau was among them.[20]

A direct result of the Revolution was the impetus it gave to science. **The Société de biologie** was created by young republican physicians and surgeons influenced by the Positivism of the philosopher, Auguste Comte, whose doctrine was the recognition of only that which can be scientifically verified or which can be proved logically or mathematically, thereby rejecting theism and metaphysics. As the Hebraic scholar, Ernest Renan wrote: "This Revolution was for the young and energetic intellectuals, the fall of a curtain of clouds that concealed the horizon." In May 1848, Brown-Séquard joined this Society, which was founded by three young physicians, François Anthelme Eugène Follin, Charles Nicole Houel and Charles Robin. Their respective ages were 25, 33 and 37. Welcoming the membership of anatomists, chemists, naturalists, physicians, physicists, physiologists and surgeons, the Society aimed to understand all the phenomena of life. The founder-members invited Pierre Rayer to become President for life. He accepted and duly held the presidency until his death in 1864. It was on his initiative that this Society was recognised as a public utility by an imperial decree in 1864.[21] The vice-presidents were Claude Bernard and Charles Robin, who were then, respectively, substitute professor of medicine at the Collège de France and professor of Natural History at the Paris Medical School. The treasurer was Huette and at first there were two secretaries: François Follin and Lebert, but after a few months, the Society found that it needed two more and Brown-Séquard and Louis Auguste Segond were appointed. The members met every Saturday in Robin's rooms at the Practical School of the Faculty of Medicine.[22]

The Société de biologie was an innovative one, which turned out to be the most prestigious one in France. To maximise attendance, it imposed a one franc fine for any absence without a valid reason.[23] Brown-Séquard submitted 35 reports for discussion during the Society's first year. He was immensely stimulated by all the debates and there can be no doubt that the Society had a fundamental influence on his future research work.

His passion for Experimental Physiology knew no bounds. Having turned his room at 5, rue Neuve-des-Beaux-Arts into a laboratory, he was devoting as much as 18–20 h a day to experimentation. He was forced to use all his savings to support his work. There was very little official interest in Experimental Physiology in the 1840s and 1850s, and no establishment would have offered him any assistance. In his book, **Physiologie générale**, Claude Bernard made these comments about the attitude that was then prevalent:

[20] Gomez, op. cit., note 15, above.

[21] Cavaribert R (1931) La Vie et l'oeuvre de Rayer (1793–1867). Thèse pour le Doctorat en médecine. Librairie médicale et scientifique, Paris, p. 14.

[22] Gley E (1899) Cinquantenaire de la Société de biologie. C R Soc Biol (Paris) 51: 1011–1080.

[23] *Ibid.*

> How sad was the fate of beginners in Experimental Physiology when, …they had not been able to be hidden or tolerated in some public establishment. I have known some who, despite their love for physiological studies, have retreated in front of such obstacles, have been defeated in the struggle, and have been compelled to change course or to leave France.[24]

So engrossed was Brown-Séquard in his research work that, by the middle of 1848, he had nothing left of the money from his mother's inheritance. By October of that year, his situation was very grim indeed. In poor physical and mental health and living on a meagre daily ration of dry bread, water and strong coffee, he started looking for work and for friends who could help him.

Aghast at his plight, two of his Fourierist friends, Jean Auguste Barral, a chemist, and Désiré Laverdant sought to use their influences on his behalf. Both asked their very good friend and Fourierist sympathizer, Jacques Alexandre Bixio, a physician, the Minister of Agriculture and Commerce, to back Brown-Séquard's candidature for an academic post, vacant at the time. Bixio told Laverdant to ask Brown-Séquard to send him a résumé of his qualification. The following letter from him, written on October 6, 1848, reveals the extent of his plight:

> Sir,
>
> I am providing you with a résumé of my qualifications in support of my application for the position about which I have spoken to you in the last few days.
>
> Allow me to add a few words regarding the frightful situation I am in.
>
> For a number of years, science has been my sole occupation. I have made the greatest sacrifice for it.
>
> The purchase of several thousands of living animals, which have served for experiments, ever increasing expenses for instruments, chemicals and toxic substances have, totally, wiped out my small fortune, while surfeit of work, a pitiful diet and a near constant sojourn in a seedy room full of foetid animal smells, have destroyed my health.
>
> I beg you, therefore, Sir, come to my help, should the rights of my rivals not indisputably prevail upon mine.
>
> Brown-Séquard D.M.P.[25]

Bixio, immediately approached Alexandre Pierre Freslon, the Minister of Public Education, writing also to Brown-Séquard to promise his conditional support:

> I cannot tell you in advance that I shall be the advocate of your candidature. To do so, I need to know exactly who are the candidates who will present themselves; but what I can tell you is that my support and my vote will be in your favour and that, in the circumstances, I will consider myself happy at being useful to a man who has made so many sacrifices for science.[26]

Unfortunately, Bixio's help was to no avail. All that he could do, was suggested in his letter to Désiré Laverdant, written on October 12, 1848

---

[24] Bernard C (1872) De la Physiologie générale. Hachette, Paris.

[25] Brown-Séquard CE (1894) Lettre inédite à Bixio, Published by Le Figaro, 5th April.

[26] Bixio A (1848) Lettre à Brown-Séquard. GMcCC, Ms 981/106. 6th Oct.

> I am sorry, …that the hope we had entertained for your poor friend Brown-Séquard is indefinitely postponed. There are, at the Ministry of Public Education, funds intended to help men of letters and scholars not comfortably well off. Do you want me to ask a portion of that fund for M. Brown? If so, tell me, as soon as possible, what is the sum which is essential for him.[27]

Another person to come to his help was Pierre Rayer. He lent him an induction machine to treat the former's private patients who could benefit from the application of galvanic current. This was the stimulation of nerves by an electric current, a common treatment of nervous ailments at that time, which had been made popular by François Magendie. Rayer was a kind and caring man who, through his own efforts, had acquired wealth and an enviable professional status. He had been a victim of religious intolerance during the Restoration—the period from 1814 to 1830 which marks the return to power of the Bourbon dynasty after the fall of the First Empire—and barred from pursuing an academic career, because he had married a Protestant.[28] For that reason, he was always ready to help younger scholars, making use of the considerable influence which he wielded through "medical services rendered to the mighty of this world."[29] He had been the physician of Louis-Philippe and he held the same office for Napoléon III, for Charles, duke of Morny, Napoléon Ill's half brother, for Princess Mathilda Bonaparte and for the financial aristocrats of the capital. Brown-Séquard was one of the many scholars to whom Rayer gave assistance. Among them were Claude Bernard, Marcelin Berthelot, Charles Jacques Bouchard, Jean-Martin Charcot, and Emile Littré.

Despite his poor health, Brown-Séquard never shunned his duty. Early, in 1849, a cholera epidemic broke out in Paris and he immediately, on April 13, enrolled as an Auxiliary Physician in the 1st Military Division of the fortified town of Paris.[30] He was attached to the Royal Guards' Gros Caillou Hospital, near the Invalides, where he distinguished himself throughout the duration of the epidemic. There, he helped Baron Félix Hippolyte Larrey, the son of the legendary surgeon-in-chief of the Grande Armée, who had opened a reception centre for the victims of cholera.

During these years of poverty which Brown-Séquard endured, between 1848 and 1852, some amusing and true anecdotes have still emerged. One day, he received a small and unexpected sum of money from the Ministry of Public Education. He was so thrilled that he spent all of it on the purchase of a dog—which was to serve as experimental subject—and a tail coat. He was to wear this coat on the following day, to be officially introduced to an eminent medical man who was looking for a prosector in anatomy. He shut the dog inside his room, left the tail coat on the back of a chair and went out. He returned, later, to find the coat

---

[27] Bixio A (1848) Lettre à Laverdant. GMcCC, Ms 981/107. 12th Oct.

[28] Cavaribert, op. cit., note 21, above.

[29] Berthelot MPE (1896) Notice sur la vie et les travaux de M. Brown-Séquard. Typographie Firmin-Didot et Cie, Paris, p. 12.

[30] Ordre de rattachment militaire à la lère Division Militaire, Place de Paris en date du 3 avril 1849. Brown-Séquard comme médecin auxiliaire à l'Hopital Gros Caillou. GMcCC, Ms 984/1.

in shreds. The dog it seems, instinctively aware of its fate, had avenged itself in anticipation. Needless to say that, the next day, the prospective candidate improperly dressed was not employed![31]

Another story concerns his good Fourierist friend, César Daly, who reared guinea-pigs, animals he was particularly fond of. Whenever Brown-Séquard could not afford to purchase a laboratory animal, he would pay a visit to Daly and, invariably, use the same trick to acquire a guinea-pig. He would take hold of one of the animals, feel its belly and express doubts about its chances of survival. He would hint that the animal would stand a better chance of recovery if he took care of it. All the animals that were entrusted to his care duly perished. After a while, Daly realised what was going on and bought more guinea-pigs to replace those that had died, so he could enjoy his friend's elaborate charade.[32]

Perhaps, it was a sense of altruism that inspired Daly to sacrifice his guinea-pigs to Science. Brown-Séquard published over 100 original articles on the results of his experiments from 1846 to 1851. These publications deal with a great variety of subjects, namely rigor mortis, blood perfusion of limbs of dead humans and animals, organ implantation, regeneration of nervous tissues, artificially induced epilepsy and electrical stimulation of the vagus nerve.

His studies on rigor mortis were first undertaken on guinea-pigs and rabbits. He took note of the time of this rigid stiffening after death.[33] It was not known then that this phenomenon was due to the anaerobic transformation of glucose into lactic acid in the muscles. This discovery was made, in 1906, by Frederick Gowland Hopkins. Brown-Séquard showed that rigor mortis was reversible by perfusion of defibrinated oxygenated blood. In an experiment on a decapitated dog's head, which he perfused through the vertebral and carotid arteries, he obtained some muscular movements, winking of the eyes and alterations of facial expression through muscular contractions and relaxations. This experiment was at the root of macabre tales going around Paris at that time, like this one:

> the severed head recovering some sort of life under the influence of warm blood; the eyes recovered their brightness and even followed the movements of a light ... A progress on Claude Bernard's dog, whose decapitated head moved its eyes at the sound of its master's voice.[34]

In 1851, Brown-Séquard together with his pupil and compatriot, Frédéric Bonnefin, the brother of Alexandre, who had accompanied him to Mauritius in 1842, injected his own blood into the radial artery of a severed arm of a criminal,

---

[31] The St James's Gazette (1894) The late Professor Brown-Séquard. Anecdotes of a great physician, 4th Apr. Also, l'Eclair (1894) Brown-Séquard. Quelques notes intimes sur le célèbre physiologist. Paris, 4th Apr.

[32] Paris (1894) Brown-Séquard. Une grande figure scientifique. La carrière du célèbre physiologiste. Sa jeunesse. Paris, 4th Apr.

[33] Brown-Séquard CE (1851) Persistance de la vie dans les members atteints de rigidité cadavérique. C R Acad Sci (Paris) 32: 855–856.

[34] Joly C (1894) Statues à élever. Le Moniteur du Puy du Dôme, Clermont-Ferrand, 6th Apr.

who had been decapitated 13 h previously and recorded flickers of movements in most of the muscles of that limb.[35] The **Journal des débats** reported this experiment in an altogether more sinister way after Brown-Séquard had made known his findings to the **Académie des sciences**:

> A horrible drama, so sad, that in normal times not only a gathering of academicians, but a meeting of executioners would have fled horror stricken.[36]

Whatever the tone of the reactions of the press, Brown-Séquard did not let them deflect him from his researches. In a similar experiment on a second criminal's decapitated body, he substituted the blood of a dog for his own. In this case, the injection was made in the brachial artery of a severed arm and the results were, somewhat, surprising: the skin regained its elasticity and softness, there was erection of hair on the arm and the alternative increase and decrease in the flow of the injected blood produced beatings of the pulse in the radial artery.[37] Years later, Alfred Vulpian, in the course of one of his lectures on the physiology of the nervous system, delivered at the **Muséum national d'histoire naturelle**, said that he had suggested to Brown-Séquard to perfuse the head of a freshly executed criminal and try to read his lips, to learn of his thoughts after death![38]

His perfusion of dead tissues with blood, led him to try implanting a young cat's tail to a cock's comb. This was done "by stitching the cut end of the cat's tail to the cut surface of the cock's comb."[39] After a week or so, the cat's tail bled when pricked, indicating some sort of circulation within the implanted part. Eleven days after the operation, however, the cat's tail was torn off by another cock, presumably jealous of his rival's prominent appendage! What was interesting to Brown-Séquard was that the tail bled and that its tissues were alive. His experiments were still fuelling journalistic imagination. One newspaper reported that he excelled in grafting tails on rats' back and showing you salamanders which lived happily with a head reduced to one third—or one half.[40]

---

[35] Brown-Séquard CE (1851) Recherches sur le rétablissement de l'irritabilité musculaire chez un supplicié, treize heures après décapitation. C R Acad Sci (Paris) 32: 897–902.

[36] Janin L (1851) La Semaine dramatique. Monstrueusse entreprise d'une docteur en médecine. Feuilleton du Journal des débats, 7th July.

[37] Brown-Séquard CE (1851) Recherches sur le rétablissement de l'irritabilité musculaire, chez un second supplicié, plus de quatorze heures après la mort. C R Soc Biol (Pairs) 3: 103–107.

[38] Vulpian EPA (1866) Leçons sur la physiologie générale et comparée du système nerveux, faites au Muséum d'histoire naturelle. Baillière, Paris, p. 459.

[39] Brown-Séquard CE (1853) On a singular case of animal graft. In: Experimental Researches applied to physiology and pathology. Baillière, New York.

[40] Joly, *op cit.*, note 34, above.

He was also experimenting on the regeneration of nervous tissues. He found that in birds, after a complete or partial section of the spinal cord, the reuniting of the two separated surfaces takes place with return of the lost function to the normal state.[41]

> Thus, in a pigeon, the entire spinal cord was divided transversely, at the level of the fifth and sixth vertebra. Complete paralysis, both of motion and sensibility, was at once produced in the whole of the posterior or lower half of the body ... Not only had sensibility and voluntary movements completely returned fifteen months after the operation, but also the function of the generative (male) organs had been completely restored, and females were fecundated.[42]
>
> In cases of partial division of the spinal cord, reunion takes place in dogs, cats, as well as in guinea-pigs, especially in young animals. Many facts seem to show that the same thing can take place in man.[43]
>
> In a guinea-pig, there was complete fusion of a divided sciatic nerve, 11 months after its section, and the restoration was so complete that no indication of the division could be discovered at post-mortem.[44]

The goal that he was pursuing in his experiments on rigor mortis, on the irrigation of dead tissues with blood, the implantation of organs of and the regeneration of nervous tissues, was never made quite clear. All too often, he did not carry his experiments to their logical ends. Whether he had some vision of the possibilities of organ transplantation or the replantation of limbs, we will never know.

He was fascinated by epilepsy. He had induced it in guinea-pigs by injuring the spinal cord. In August 1850, while staying at Trouville-sur-Mer, in the Calvados department of Normandy, he wrote to Pierre Rayer, the president of the **Société de biologie**, to announce that he had triggered epileptic fits in guinea-pigs. This is what he wrote:

> As you are aware, I have found that after section of the lateral half of the spinal cord in guinea-pigs, it is possible to trigger convulsions in three non-paralysed limbs by pinching a sensitive area, especially the face. I wanted to see if convulsions occurred in the non-paralysed parts in guinea-pigs whose spinal cord had been totally severed transversely at the level of the 10th and 11th dorsal vertebrae. They did occur, I have just seen them in two guinea-pigs I had operated on in Paris and which I had brought here: very strong convulsions of the muscles of the face, of the neck and of the anterior limbs, following the pinching of the face.[45]

---

[41] Brown-Séquard CE (1851) Sur plusieurs cas de cicatrisation de plaies faites à la moelle épinière avec retour des fonctions perdues. C R Soc Biol (Paris) 3: 77–79.

[42] Brown-Séquard CE (1859) Possibility of repair and of return of function after a partial or complete division of the spinal cord in man and animals. Lancet 1: 96–97. In this article, he quotes experiments that he had carried out in 1849–1850.

[43] *Ibid.*

[44] *Ibid.*

[45] Brown-Séquard CE (1850) Letter to Pierre Rayer. GMcCC, MS 995/2, 23rd Aug.

He was greatly interested by the vagus nerve. In 1850, he studied its influence on the heart beat.[46] Five years previously, the brothers Eduard and Ernst Weber had shown that the electrical stimulation of the peripheral end of that nerve causes the heart to stop He repeated this experiment in the frog. What interested him most was, that this discovery of the Webers was the first description of the inhibitory action of a nerve. In 1873, he was the first to draw attention to the importance of inhibition in the normal and pathological activities of the central nervous system.[47]

Of all the discoveries he made, during this period of febrile activity, the one which ensured him a permanent place in the medical Pantheon, was the crossing-over of the sensory pathways in the spinal cord. It was the culmination of the research that he had began in the second part of his doctoral thesis. At that time, the prevailing doctrine was that of Charles Bell, upheld in France by François Achille Longet; namely that the sensory pathways in the spinal cord ascended uncrossed to the cerebellum. In his 1850 report to the Académie des sciences, Brown-Séquard challenged this doctrine in the following words:

> Everyone agrees, to this day, that the transmission of the sensory impressions, received by a lateral half of the body, arises from the corresponding lateral half of the spinal cord. We have found that this transmission takes place, mainly, in a crossed manner.[48]

He had thus established that the sensory nerve fibres crossed in the grey matter of the spinal cord and not as believed then, that this decussation takes place somewhere in the brain. He had reached this conclusion by hemisecting the spinal cords of guinea-pigs and rabbits.

He showed that a lesion affecting one lateral half of the spinal cord is characterised by a spastic paralysis on the side of the lesion and a loss of pain and thermal sensation on the opposite side, while light touch is little disturbed. This clinical picture is known as the Brown-Séquard syndrome. It is pathognomonic of lateral cord disorders due to various causes: lateral fracture of one or several vertebrae or penetrating injuries; a compression of the cord by an epidural abscess, a haemorrhage, a tumour or a plaque of demyelinating disease. This syndrome is often referred to by other names, such as spinal **hemiparaplegia** or **hemiparaplegia or hemisection syndrome** (Fig. 6.1).

The existence of such a syndrome, prior to the advent of radiography, computer-assisted myelographies, magnetic resonance imaging (MRI) or computerised tomography (CT), made it possible to identify the level of the spinal cord lesion and, to some degree, assess its extent.

---

[46] Brown-Séquard CE (1850) De l'influence des nerfs vagues sur les battements du coeur. C R Soc Biol (Paris) 2: 45–46.

[47] Brown-Séquard (1873) On the mechanism of production of symptoms of diseases of the brain. Arch Sci Pract Med (New York) 1: 117–122.

[48] Brown-Séquard CE (1850) Mémoire sur la transmission des impressions sensitives dans la moelle épinière. C R Acad Sci (Paris) 31: 700–701.

**Fig. 6.1** Brown-Sequard's syndrome or hemisection syndrome © Celestin

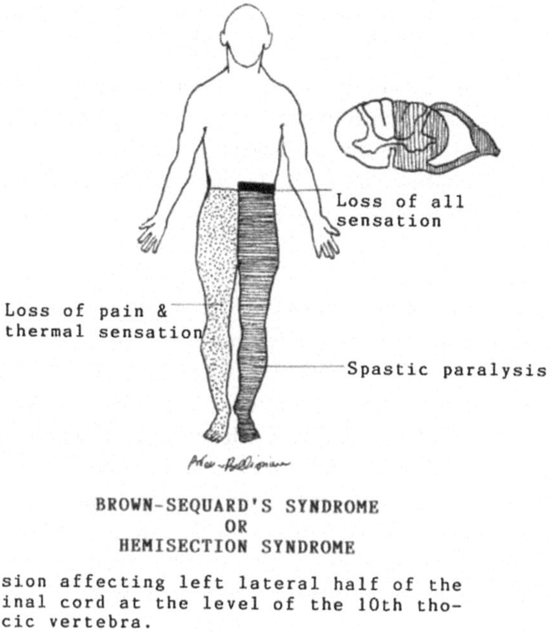


There were many other researches of secondary importance that he undertook at that time, such as the hibernation of the tenrec. The contractility of the iris of vertebrates and the negative role of the encephalon in the act of suckling in newborn animals.

In 1849, he published the results of a study, undertaken in 1843, while staying in Mauritius, on the hibernation of the tenrec or tanrec (**Tenrec ecaudatus).** This is a small, insectivorous mammal, not unlike the European hedgehog **(Erinaceus europaeus**), tailless and covered with spines. The female gives birth to litters of 20 or more, the highest number of young for any mammal. It is a native of Mauritius, having been introduced from Madagascar and the Comoros. The well-known palaeontologist, George Cuvier, had said that cold weather was not a pre-requisite for hibernation as tenrecs did so in summer. Brown-Séquard proved him wrong. Tenrecs do not aestivate but hibernate from June to November, which are the winter months in Mauritius.[49]

His work on the iris of vertebrates dated back to 1846. However, in August 1850, while staying at the seaside, he studied the fish's iris. He reported his findings by letter to the Société de biologie:

> You know that I have discovered, a few years ago, that direct light excites the iris of some animals. Moreover, I have found that the iris of fish is mobile, contrary to the studies

[49] Brown-Séquard CE (1853) On the causes of the torpidity of the Tenrec (*Erinaceus ecaudatis*). In: Experimental Researches applied to physiology and pathology. Baillière, New York.

of Muck and Loemmering. I have noticed that the animal whose iris is the most reactive, under the influence of light is a fish, the eel.[50]

He studied the iris of sea-water fish and concluded that it reacted like that of fresh-water ones. In the calamari, he noticed that the veil-like folds which serve as iris, react to the direct influence of light.[51]

In new-born animals, he showed that the act of suckling is a mechanism independent of the brain's influence, since the complete ablation of the latter does not affect it.[52] It is likely that this act is a motor activity under the control of a genetic factor.

His numerous reports to the Société de biologic and to the **Académie des sciences** did not go totally unnoticed. He won some official recognition. In 1847, he was awarded an honourable mention for the **Montyon** Prize in Experimental Physiology of the Académie des sciences. On December 29, 1849, he was elected a member of the **Société Philomatique de Paris,** rejoining there Claude Bernard, who had been elected three years previously. At that time, this Society was the most prestigious one next to the Académie des sciences.[53] In 1851, he won a second honourable mention for the Montyon Prize, when he submitted the results of his research work on the sensory pathways in the spinal cord. This award is named after Jean-Baptiste Auget de Montyon, who created several prizes awarded annually by the **Institut de France**.

In 1851, Brown-Séguard directed the theses of two medical students. One was Jean-Baptiste Coste whose thesis, presented on August 1st, was concerned with experimental researches on the role of the encephalon and pons Varoli on respiration.[54] He collaborated with Coste on the experimental work, eventually challenging the views of Pierre Marie Flourens that the respiratory centre, the noeud vital, is located in the medulla oblongata. The other student was his compatriot, Frédéric Bonnefin, whose thesis, presented on 29th August, dealt with the mode and site of action of convulsive poisons such as strychnine, brucine, morphine, cyanide and nicotine.[55] Brown-Séquard had shown, previously, that strychnine had an excitatory effect on the spinal cord.[56]

Soon after helping Bonnefin with his thesis, Brown-Séquard suffered, what was said to be a "severe physical and mental fatigue" exacerbated by lack of money, lack

---

50 Brown-Séquard, *op cit.,* note 45, above.

51 *Ibid.*

52 Brown-Séquard (1849) L'action de têter est indépendante du cerveau. C R Soc Biol (Paris) 1: 60.

53 Brown-Séquard CE (1852) Letter to Lady Blanche. GMcCC, Ms 997/1, 17th Dec.

54 Coste B (1851) Recherches expérimentales et observations cliniques sur le rôle de l'encéphale et particulièrement de la protubérance annulaire dans la respiration. Thèse pour le Doctorate em médecine. Paris, 1st Aug.

55 Bonnefin E (1851) Recherches expérimentales sur l'action convulsive des principaux poisons. Thèse pour le Doctorat en médecie. Paris, 29th Aug.

56 Brown-Séquard CE (1848) Recherches sur l'action de la strychnine. C R Soc Biol (Paris) 1: 119–121.

of food, lack of comfort, lack of sleep and lack of distractions. His Mauritian friends, Désiré Laverdant, Joseph Désiré Tholozan, Henri Lolliot and the brothers Frédéric and Camille Bonnefin took him to the seaside and paid for his stay there. More than 20 years after, he wrote about this illness in an article entitled: "On a new treatment of functional dyspepsia, anaemia and chlorosis,"[57] which appeared in the first number of his English language journal, Archives of Scientific and Practical Medicine. In this article, he refers to himself as a patient whom he had cared for:

> In 1851, I had to treat a very bad case of dyspepsia, and succeeded in curing the patient by a plan of treatment which, I think, deserves attention.
>
> The first patient I submitted to this plan was a scientific man, thirty-four years old, of strong constitution, but reduced from several causes to a lamentable state of health. For eight years, he had been working very hard, taking no exercise, and living almost all the time in a vitiated atmosphere. He slept very little, and usually passed 18 to 19 h a day writing, reading or experimenting. His diet was miserable and, with the object of avoiding the need of much food, he took a great deal of coffee. He gradually, though slowly, became exceedingly weak. His digestion which had been very good all his life, before he began to work so much, had gradually become bad. He suffered greatly from pyrosis, and a feeling of great distress, and gastric distension after every meal. Acid eructations and gas were frequently thrown up in his mouth and, when he did not vomit, he found that his food remained in his stomach so long that, in the morning he frequently rejected things eaten the previous day. At last, he had to give up work and stay in bed. But no improvement occurred from the rest he then had, nor from various modes of treatment. His emaciation and weakness and dyspeptic condition increased, and his friends decided to have him removed to the country. He was so weak that he had to be carried in a litter to the railway station.
>
> After a few days, feeling that he had not improved, I decided to try a radical change of his alimentation, as regards the quantity of food to be taken at a time. Instead of three meals a day, I made him take sixty or more. Every 12 to 15 min, he took two or three mouthful of solid food, chiefly meat and bread. He drank a little less than a wine glass of Bordeaux wine and water very thirty or forty minutes…

This pitiful physical condition was the culmination of a five-year period of ceaseless mental hyperactivity in his home laboratory, alternating with periods of depression, tinged with anxiety. When his general health improved, he moved to another sea resort: Trouville-sur-Mer. His stay there was also paid for by his Mauritian friends.

His life-style, which had brought about this "severe physical and mental fatigue" baffled his colleagues. It was, three years later, in 1854, that this alternation of episodes of elation and depression was recognized as a morbid mental disorder and described, almost at the same time, by Jules Baillarger, under the name of folie à double forme and by Jean Pierre Falret, who called it **folie circulaire** (circular insanity). In 1899. Emil Kraepelin gave this disorder the name of manic-depressive psychosis, nowadays often referred to as bipolar psychosis.

While Brown-Séquard was resting in Trouville-sur-Mer, political events were slowly coming to a head. In November 1848, a new constitution had come into force, providing for a single assembly of 750 representatives elected for 3 years by

[57] Arch Sci Pract Med (New York) (1873) 1: 30–38.

universal suffrage, and for a president elected for a single 4-year term. On December 10, 1848, Louis Napoléon had been elected president by an overwhelming majority. Three years later, on December 2, 1851, he seized overall power of France. It was a **coup d'Etat** which led to fighting in the streets and was followed by a harsh repression. It was, however, ratified by a referendum and the Constitution of January 14, 1852, gave extensive powers to Louis Napoléon for a period of 10 years. These were the events that preceded France's transformation from a democratic republic into a imperial monarchy.

Brown-Séquard was, no doubt, a staunch republican, but he was not vehemently opposed to Napoléon's coup d'Etat. Three years previously, he had taken part in the events that had helped to bring this Prince to power. There has been much confusion about this period of his life and particularly, about the reasons for his departure for America, in the months that followed this coup d'Etat. Even he in his letters, is vague in explaining it. For instance: "After the coup d'Etat, compelled to flee France, I went to The United States."[58] Such statements have, merely, been repeated by people who were unaware of the real circumstances. The first person to state outright that Brown-Séquard had been forced to take refuge in The United States was Marcel Eugène Emile Gley, who wrote in 1894:

> Ardent republican, he had taken up arms to defend liberty against the coup d'Etat; he feared justifiably to be troubled and left for America.[59]

Gley's inaccuracy is probably due to the fact that he was not yet born at the time of these events. He had known Brown-Séquard in later years, because of the latter's interest in his researches on the thyroid and parathyroid glands; but he was not as intimate with him as the Mauritian-born physician, Eugène Dupuy, who was quite unequivocal about his departure for America: "It is not true that he fled because of his revolutionary ideas."[60]

From two letters of Brown-Séquard's American friend, William Birney, it is apparent that the former used the fall of the Second Republic as an excuse to try to obtain an academic position in The United States. Birney's letters, written from Paris, on February 6, 1852, explain Brown-Séquard's decision to settle in America, as a consequence of his republican convictions and his dislike of Napoléon III's imperial monarchy. The first letter is addressed to Alexander Cummings of Philadelphia, the editor of the Evening Bulletin, and says:

> This letter will be handed to you by Dr Edouard Brown-Séquard who emigrates to America because he is republican for the present regime in France.[61]

The second is addressed to Louis Tappan of New York, one of the founders of the American Anti- Slavery Society and reads:

---

[58] Brown-Séquard, *op cit.,* note 5, above, p. 32b.

[59] Gley E (1894) La Vie et l'oeuvre de C.E. Brown-Séquard. Arch Physiol norm pathol, 76: 501–516.

[60] Dupuy, *op cit.,* note 8, above.

[61] Birney W (1852) Letter to Alexander Cummings. GMcCC, Ms 986/1, 6th Feb.

> He being a foreigner, for he is American by birth, has prevented him from competing for some of the Professional chairs. This and his republican opinion, subjecting him to the momentary dread of expulsion from France, has led him to abandon his position here and emigrate to New York.[62]

Brown-Séquard's decision to go to The United States was born out of the coup d'Etat, but was not a direct consequence of this event. His departure for America, ten weeks after the coup was, far from being a flight, a well-orchestrated venture. It is true that he, like his Fourierist friends, Barral, Laverdant and Daly and many others were very apprehensive about their freedom. Some of their republican, socialist and Fourierist acquaintances, among members of the **Chambre des députés** had been arrested and incarcerated. One of them was Alexandre Bixio, the ex-minister of Agriculture and Commerce, who had tried to back Brown-Séquard's candidature to an academic post in 1848. On the night of the coup d'Etat, he and a group of deputies drafted and signed a declaration calling for the deposition of Louis Napoléon. The next morning, when it was obvious that the Prince had triumphed, Bixio fearing that he might be charged with treason if he fled, gave himself up.

Brown-Séquard's Fourierist activities arose suspicion. Since 1840, he had been an active member of a Paris Fourierist society and since 1848, one of the editors of the review La Phalange, which its founder, Victor Considérant, had made into the organ of Fourierism. The official proof of Brown-Séquard's involvement in the editorship of this periodical is contained in an authorization granted to him by François Arago, the permanent secretary of the Académie des sciences, which reads:

> Paris, 7th February 1848
> The Permanent Secretary of The Academy authorizes M. Brown-Sequard, editor of the review La Phalange, to become acquainted at the Secretariat of the Institute [of France], with the works, memoirs and correspondence presented to the Académie des sciences.[63]

Immediately after the coup d'Etat, Brown-Séquard was warned by a friend, in high position, most likely a police superintendent, that he could face expulsion from France, because of his relationship with deputies opposed to the coup; of his friendship with the exiled Fourierist apostle, Victor Considérant and of his editorship of the radical review **La Phalange**. Moreover, that his status as a foreigner meddling in French internal politics had not escaped the attention of the Ministry of the Interior. There are some circumstantial evidences available that, in the days that followed the coup, he fled to England, staying in London until the end of December 1851, before returning to Paris, in January 1852. At the time of his death, in 1894, the medical periodical, **The Lancet** made a passing reference to a visit of his in London, prior to 1852.[64] Furthermore, a passage in a letter he wrote

---

[62] Birney W (1852) Letter to Lewis Tappan. GMcCC, Ms 986/2, 6th Feb.

[63] Arago E (1848) Authorisation given to Brown-Séquard. GMcCC, Ms 981/1, 7th Feb.

[64] Lancet (1894) Death of Professeur Brown-Séquard. 1: 906–907.

from Boston, to an American woman friend, in 1852, appears to allude to his having visited London.[65] He says:

> It is cold here and the sky is grey like that of London.... The women, here, are somehow more beautiful than those in New York. They look like the English women without being as stiff. I think that the streets here are more irregular than those of London.

His association with the Fourierist movement might have inconvenienced him in the political climate which followed the coup d'Etat, but there is ample evidence to suggest that his active participation in that movement was of considerable advantage to him. Désiré Laverdant, as an apostle of Fourierism, had doors to open for him on both sides of the Atlantic. The following passage, from a letter, written in 1912, by Eugène Dupuy and addressed to Charlotte McCausland, Brown-Séquard's daughter, bears witness to this fact:

> He was intimately attached to Désiré Laverdant, who was one of the apostles of 'Fourierism'. Mr. Brisbane was an American who had come over to become an apostle also, he belonged to a branch of the creed that had founded a 'phalanstere'... in which all the members lived together and worked for the common good.... Dana, Horace Greeley, and others, who became eminent afterwards in American history, also belonged to the phalanstere.[66]

Indeed, Désiré Laverdant introduced Brown-Séquard to two of his American Fourierist colleagues: Albert Brisbane, and Charles Anderson Dana, who became his lifelong friends.

Albert Brisbane had studied under the personal guidance of Charles Fourier, in France, from 1831 to 1833. In 1848, he published an exposition of Fourierism in America under the title The Social Destiny of Man. Horace Greeley, the founder and editor of the **New York Daily Tribune** was so impressed by Brisbane's book that he allowed him to use his newspaper as an outlet for his views. Brisbane's exposition of Fourierism led to the creation of some 40 phalansteries in The United States, the best known of which were Brooke Farm in Roxbury, Massachusetts and the **North American Phalanx** at Red Banks. New Jersey.

Charles Anderson Dana was, without doubt, the most influential figure in American journalism in the second half of the nineteenth century. He spent five years at Brooke Farm, starting in 1843, when this phalanstery had just been established by George Ripley. On leaving Brooke Farm, he became the city editor of Horace Greeley's New York Daily Tribune, where he remained for 16 years. Laverdant introduced him to Brown-Séquard, in Paris, in February 1848, during the Revolution.

As disciples of Fourier, Brisbane, Dana, Greeley and Ripley made connections with a great many influential and distinguished people in American society, in the

---

[65] Brown-Séquard CE (1852) Letter to an American woman friend. GMcCC, Ms 981/3, Nov or Dec.

[66] Dupuy, *op cit.,* note 8, above.

cities of New York, Philadelphia, Charleston, Boston and Richmond. What better prospects could there have been for Brown-Sequard, on the eve of his first visit to The United States. There, he would receive help and hospitality from many Americans, Fourierists in particular, who were already aware, or would soon be made aware of his visit.

# Chapter 7
# The Visitor to America: 1852–1853

Early in 1852, Brown-Séquard started preparing for a visit to The United States. His intention was to settle there where, he hoped, he would be offered an academic post. He asked his friends, colleagues and acquaintances for testimonials and letters of recommendation, with which he hoped to meet people who would introduce him to members of centres of learning and medical schools in Boston, New York, Philadelphia and Richmond. Thus, the Maison Goupil, Editors and Printers, gave him a letter for their agent, asking the latter "to do everything in your power to be useful to him."[1] The banking firm of Donan, Aubry and Gautier, wrote to their New York correspondent that Brown-Séquard is "a man who has worked hard and who knows everything. To succeed, all he needs is to be known. Please help him to reach his objectives."[2]

The historical and portrait painter, William Powell, who was working on The Discovery of the Mississippi River by De Soto—a painting commissioned to hang in the Capitol—from his studio at 17 Quai Voltaire, wrote to Valentine Mott, the vascular surgeon of world-wide reputation that, as Brown-Séquard

> will make the object of his visit to the United States known to you, I do not deem it necessary to say anything about it. But feel assured that you will do all in your power to facilitate his visit.[3]

Brown-Séquard had, with much publicity, made it known that he would establish himself, anywhere in The States, where a position as a research physiologist or as a professor of physiology was vacant. Newspaper coverage and mention of his visit in the medical and lay press were vital, and he had a reliable friend in the person of Charles Anderson Dana, in New York, who was the city editor of the New York Daily Tribune. In Philadelphia, Alexander Cummings, the editor of the Evening Bulletin, had been approached by William Birney. The following passage is from the latter's letter dated February 6, 1852:

---

[1] Goupil & Co (1852) Letter to their agent, Mr Schaus. GMcCC, Ms 986/8, 12th Feb.
[2] Donan, Aubry, Gautier & Co (n.d. probably Feb 1852). GMcCC, Ms 986/1.
[3] Powell WH (1852) Letter to Valentine Mott. GMcCC, Ms 986/3, 10th Feb.

L.-C. Celestin, *Charles-Edouard Brown-Séquard*,

DOI: 10.1007/978-3-319-03020-3_7, 

> He [Brown-Séquard] will be, I think, as valuable an acquisition to us as Professor Agassiz. His reputation as a man of science being already European. … Such a man should find a place in some of our medical schools. Could you make him acquainted with gentlemen connected with the Philadelphia Medical College?[4]

We can reasonably assume that a newspaper editor was approached in Boston as well—perhaps the editor of the Boston News Letter—as Boston's proximity to Harvard College would not have escaped Brown-Séquard's attention.

The most interesting of these introductory letters was written by Pierre Paul Broca and addressed to Professor George Bacon Wood of the University of Pennsylvania. His letter is strikingly verbose and portrays a remarkable picture of Brown-Séquard's academic plight:

> M. Brown-Sequard is one of the most eminent of the physiologists of our day. His remarkable researches on the nervous system are well known in France. Still very young, he has enriched Science with a great number of new and important facts. I like to believe that the fame of his work has already crossed the seas and that the one I am introducing to you is not unknown to you.
>
> Such beginnings promised a great future for him in Science. We were proud to number among us a man who had given so many proofs of progress; we anticipated far more still. We hoped that this obstinate worker, this young scholar full of courage, of self-denial and endowed with high moral standards, would reap a reward worthy of himself and worthy of the science to which he had dedicated his life.
>
> Unfortunately, science today, in the old world is a cruel mother who does not feed her children. France, shaken by political struggles, has ceased to protect her artists and scholars. Intrigue prevails over merit and, to earn favours, one must serve material interests. The cult of Science is no more possible for he who is not in possession of a personal fortune. During the last eight years, M. Brown has used up all his resources, and has imposed upon himself unbelievable hardships in order to carry out expensive researches in experimental physiology. Today, all he is left with is an honourable name, a profound knowledge and published articles that everyone can appreciate.
>
> In this state of affairs, M. Brown leaves an ungrateful country and is looking for patronage and support in America, which France has denied to his invaluable intelligence.[5]

So, with these letters, in the second half of February 1852, Brown-Séquard left France for The United States. His Mauritian friends feeling that he had not fully recovered from his "severe mental and physical fatigue," insisted that he be accompanied by one of them, and it was Henri Lolliot[6] who volunteered. He was a friend from their adolescent years in Mauritius and now a final year medical student. They set sail for New York from Le Havre.

There is an apocryphal story that, with scant knowledge of English, Brown-Séquard "chose a slow sailing vessel in which to cross the Atlantic in order to have time to acquire at least the rudiments of the language."[7] The confusion was

---

4 Birney W (1852) Letter to Alexander Cummings. GMcCC, Ms 986/1, 6th Feb.

5 Broca PP (1852) Letter to Professor Wood. GMcCC, Ms 986/4, 15th Feb.

6 Brown-Séquard CE (1852) Letter to Lady Blanche. GMcCC, Ms 977/1, 17th Dec.

7 Olmsted JMD (1946) Charles-Edouard Brown-Séquard. A nineteenth century neurologist and endocrinologist. The John Hopkins Press, Baltimore, pp. 34–35.

probably caused by his financial embarrassment. He might well have made a casual remark to this effect, namely that "this mode of travel will give me time to learn English before I get there."[8] But this was to cover the real reason for taking a slow ship: that he could not afford the price of a quicker passage.

Moreover, a slow ship to New York in the 1850s would have taken less than three weeks to cross the Atlantic. Even for someone of Brown-Séquard's intellectual capability, this is not much time to get to grip with the rudiments of the English language! The fact is that his knowledge of that language is not in doubt. He had spoken English throughout his childhood and adolescence and, not only was he now keeping up to date with Anglo-Saxon medical literature, but he was associating with his American contemporaries in Paris: William Birney and William Powell, to name but two. Besides, he and César Daly were in the habit of carrying out their conversation in English. The latter, a talented architect, was the son of an English officer, who had married in France. Daly, however, was educated in England, where he spent his childhood and teens.

Far from cramming his English, Brown-Séquard spent most of his time, during the voyage, measuring the temperature of his urine and that of "ten strong sailors, ... in the Atlantic Ocean, between the 43rd and 45th deg. of north latitude."[9] It must be said that, at that time, the exact temperature of human urine at micturition was not known.

There are many apocryphal stories about Brown-Séquard's lack of knowledge of the English language. One author wrote that as he was approaching "Philadelphia, his father's birthplace, he picked it up by instinct and soon spoke fluent English"!

The aim of his visit to The States was to inform the American medical profession about the level that Physiology had reached in Europe, with particular regard to the nervous system and also, to introduce his own researches, backed by practical demonstrations. He travelled from town to town, paying visits to physicians, especially those who had been pupils of Andral, Bouillaud, Chomel, Louis and Magendie. He sought their help to promote courses, which he hoped to give in Philadelphia, New York, Richmond and Boston. In the course of his journeys across The United States, he carried with him various species of animals, ready for demonstrations. Thus in December 1852, after travelling by night from New York to Boston, he wrote:

> Thank God, my frogs and pigeons have had a peaceful journey. They behaved like real Gentlemen and deserve the noble fate which awaits them, that of promoting the progress of Science.[10]

---

[8] Damrau F (1937) Brown-Séquard. In: Pioneers in Neurology. Dios Chemical, St Louis, Missouri, p. 12.

[9] Brown-Séquard CE (1853) On the normal degree of temperature of man. In: Experimental Researches applied to physiology and pathology. H Baillière, New York, pp. 30–31.

[10] Brown-Séquard CE. Letter to an American woman friend (n.d. probably Nov or Dec 1852). GMcCC, Ms 980/3.

That same day, having arrived in Boston at five o'clock in the morning, he wrote in the afternoon:

> I have already paid more than 20 visits, and seen 8 to 10 Physicians. They all anticipate a great success for me. But every rose has its thorn: an old Professor accused me of being cruel towards animals.[11]

He was well aware that Physiology and Experimental Physiology in particular, was in its infancy in The States. As a science, its scope was rather limited and taught as part of Anatomy. The only American physiologist of note was the aged William Beaumont, who had undertaken a prolonged study of digestion on a human being. As an army surgeon, stationed in Michigan, in 1822, he had treated a young French Canadian trapper, Alexis St Martin, who had been severely and accidentally wounded on the left side of his chest by a shotgun fired at near point blank range. St Martin recovered after a year, but developed a gastric fistula, between the stomach and the outer chest wall. Beaumont took the young trapper home and collected his gastric juice through the fistula, at various times in the day, for a period of 8 years. His findings were published in 1833: Experiments and Observations on the Gastric Juice and the Physiology of Digestion.[12]

In May 1852, Brown-Séquard attended the Medical Convention in Richmond, where he made the acquaintance of many physicians, including members of the Medical School of the Hampden-Sidney College of Richmond. A month later, he began his first series of lectures in Philadelphia, which was so successful that an additional series was planned for the next year. In September and October, he delivered lectures in New York, then in Boston in November and December. Each was well attended by students and physicians alike. In Boston, when he gave a one-hour lecture, three times a week, there were 60 physicians in an audience of 100.

He received praise from all quarters in the three cities were he lectured. His audience, the medical press, as well as the daily newspapers all applauded. In anticipation of his visit, the Boston Medical & Surgical Journal wrote:

> His lectures will demonstrate points especially connected with his own discoveries. ... The appreciation which the fame and labours of Dr Séquard have secured him in this city, is being manifested in the active interest which some of our well-known physicians are taking in the forthcoming lectures.[13]

In New York, on the initiative of Dana, The New York Daily Tribune reported that the students of the Medical Department of the University unanimously passed a resolution which stated that

> Dr Brown-Séquard of Paris, in his experiments and investigations for the advancement of Physiological science, has arrived at conclusions, and rendered truths demonstrable, which have been, hitherto, unknown or conjectural.[14]

---

[11] *Ibid.*

[12] Published in Plattsburg in 1833.

[13] Boston Medical & Surgical Journal (1852) 47: 336–339.

[14] *Ibid.* Quoting the New York Daily Tribune (1852), 10th Oct.

In Philadelphia, at the end of his second lecture tour, on April 25, 1853, held at the Medical College of the Pennsylvanian University, those attending his course of lectures passed a resolution of gratitude. It stated that they were

> under the greatest obligation to the learned and able lecturer for his admirable series of experiments so happily explained and illustrated. ...That we hail his visit to this country and the delivery of the various and brilliant and successful courses on his favourite subject in the cities of Boston, New York and Philadelphia as likely to mark a new era in the progress of biological research in the United States.[15]

Despite the success of his lecture tours and his busy programme during his 16-month stay in The States, there is a persistent story that he had to resort to other forms of work to supplement his income. He was reduced to giving lessons in French and to delivering babies at five dollars a case. This was especially so at the beginning of his visit and, later on, as a result of inadequately remunerated lectures. In November 1852, he was staying with a family in New York, and it becomes apparent, from a letter of thanks to the lady of the house, that he helped her with her French.[16] It may well be, that he exchanged lessons in French for board and lodging. However, if he did have to teach French to make a living, he is, by no means unique in the annals of French medicine. Georges Clémenceau, the statesman, who led France to victory in the First World War, did exactly the same from 1865 to 1869.

A story, which appears to be apocryphal, has it that he produced a text-book on obstetrics, in association with another physician, as another way of boosting his earnings. The book is not listed among the publications in his own records of his work. As the information comes from the reliable source of Dr Eugène Dupuy, his most intimate friend, it cannot be ignored. This is what Dupuy wrote about this book:

> He applied himself to collaborating in a treatise on obstetrics, the only one of its day where are to be found physiological explanations of the phenomena of gestation, of the breathing of the newborn, etc., and the names of physiologists such as Claude Bernard, himself, Robin, etc. This work has been translated into French and has had several American editions. This collaboration was a godsend for Brown-Séquard - it allowed him to live and to work.[17]

From August 1852 to June 1853, he published a monthly series of memoirs in the Medical Examiner of Philadelphia. These were brought together with his lectures in a book entitled: Experimental Researches applied to Physiology and Pathology,[18] which was published in 1853. In a review of this book, the Virginia Medical & Surgical Journal commented that it "presents the results of a most careful experimenter, whose contributions to physiological science are most valuable."[19]

---

[15] Medical Examiner Philadelphia (1853) May issue.

[16] Brown-Séquard, *op cit.,* note 10, above.

[17] Dupuy E (1894) Notice sur M. Le professeur Brown-Séquard, ancient Président de la Société de biologie. Revue Scient (Paris) 737–743.

[18] Published in 1853 by H Baillière.

[19] Virginia Medical & Surgical Journal (1854) 2: 842.

The memoir of August 1852, entitled: "Researches on the influence of the nervous system upon the functions of organic life,"[20] contains an account of his remarkable discovery of the vasomotor functions of the sympathetic nerve, which he had alluded to in his June lecture, in Philadelphia. There is some speculation, as to the date on which this experimental work, leading to that discovery, had been carried out. According to Claude Bernard, Brown-Séquard had done the work in America.[21]

This vasomotor function of the sympathetic nerve is its ability to affect the calibre of the blood vessels. Vaso-constriction being the contraction of the blood vessels, through the narrowing of their calibre. Vaso-dilatation, the expansion of the blood vessels, through the widening of their calibre. This control of the blood vessels by the nerves, was not an entirely new notion. Friedrich Gustave Jacob Henle, in 1840, had stated that nerve fibres, going to the muscles fibres in the walls of arteries, exerted an action on the latter, and the term nervus vasomotorious had, already, been coined by the anatomist-surgeon, Benedict Stilling.

In October 1851, eight months prior to Brown-Séquard's report of his discovery, Claude Bernard had made known his findings, on the section of the sympathetic nerve in the neck of rabbits, to the Société de biologie. The main manifestation of that section was that the face and particularly the ear became warmer on the side where the sympathetic had been cut. Brown-Séquard decided to stimulate the sympathetic by applying an electric (galvanic) current to it, with the following result:

> If galvanism is applied to the superior portion of the sympathetic nerve, after it has been cut in the neck, the vessels of the face and of the ear after a certain time, begin to contract; this contraction increases slowly, but at last it is evident that they resume their normal condition if they are not even smaller. The temperature and the sensibility diminish in the face and ear, … when the galvanic current ceases to act, the vessels begin to dilate again, and all the phenomena described by Dr Bernard reappear.[22]

He went on to give a clear explanation, and the first one of the mechanisms which follow the section in the neck and the electrical stimulation of the sympathetic nerve, in the following terms:

> The section of the sympathetic nerve in the neck is followed by a paralysis of the blood vessels of the head. As a consequence of this paralysis, the blood vessels, under the blood impulsion, … become distended, while the temperature and sensibility of the skin is increased through increase of blood in the vessels.
>
> Stimulation of the sympathetic nerve determines a contraction of the blood vessels of the head and, in consequence of this contraction, a decrease of the quantity of blood, or of the temperature and of the sensibility.[23]

---

[20] Brown-Séquard CE (1853). Experimental Researches applied to physiology and pathology. H Baillière, New York, pp. 6–16.

[21] Bernard C (1852) Recherches expérimentales sur le grand sympathique et spécialement sur l'influence que la section de ce nerf exerce sur la chaleur animale. Mem Soc Biol (Paris) 5: 77–87.

[22] Brown-Séquard, *op cit.*, note 20, above.

[23] *Ibid.*

The discovery of the vasomotor properties of the sympathetic nerve, the second of Brown-Séquard's major discoveries is one which, for some medical historians, he shares with Claude Bernard. Others dispute this statement, because the latter's first report associates the sympathetic nerve with a role in the production of animal heat,[24] and not to its action in altering the calibre of the blood vessels; whereas, Brown-Séquard's report stresses this property. In Anglo-Saxon countries, where Claude Bernard enjoys an immense prestige, the tendency is to attribute this discovery to Brown-Séquard for it was, six months after him, in November 1852, that Claude Bernard, in a second report to the Société de biologie, mentions the action of the sympathetic nerve on the calibre of the blood vessels.[25]

However, it is fair to add that, soon after Claude Bernard's first report to the Société de biologie, in October 1851, the studies of Brown-Séquard in The United States, of Auguste Volnay Waller in England and of Julius Budge in Germany, on the vasomotor properties of the sympathetic nerve, were corollaries of Claude Bernard's experiment; but this does not, in anyway, diminish the value of Brown-Séqaurd's work. He was the first to link the phenomena he had observed with a vasomotor property of the sympathetic nerve. However, none of the aforementioned scientists was the first to carry out experiments on the sympathetic nerve. In 1727, François Pourfour du Petit had reported the contraction of the pupil of the eye, following the section of the sympathetic nerve in the neck.

Brown-Séquard's discovery did not result from an isolated research on the sympathetic nerve or on the functions of various components of the Autonomous Nervous System. He had traced the origin of the sympathetic nerve fibres back to the spinal cord. He had studied the ganglionic innervation of the stomach, the reflex control of mammary glands and of the secretion of digestive cells, for which he provided the following explanation:

> The consensus between various digestive organs affords the most positive demonstrations of reflex secretions. For instance, we find saliva secreted when the mucous membrane of the stomach is irritated by food. … The reverse takes place also; the excitation of the nerves of taste produces an abundant reflex secretion of gastric juice, and also a flow of bile and pancreatic juice in the bowels.[26]

Moreover, in 1851, as a result of a collaboration with his childhood friend, another distinguished Mauritian physician, Joseph Désiré Tholozan, he was the first to describe a vasomotor reflex; that which occurs when one hand is plunged into icy water: a thermometer held in the other hand, registers a fall in temperature, whereas a thermometer in the mouth shows no variation of temperature. What is remarkable, is the conclusion that these two collaborators reached (Fig. 7.1):

---

[24] Bernard C (1852) Expérience sur la fonction de la partie céphalique du grand sympathetique. C R Soc Biol (Paris) 4: 155–156.

[25] C R Soc Biol (Paris) (1852) 4: 168–170.

[26] Brown-Séquard CE (1858) Course of lectures on the physiology and pathology of the nervous system. Lecture 10. Lancet 2: 467–468.

**Fig. 7.1** Illustration of a vasomotor reflex © Celestin

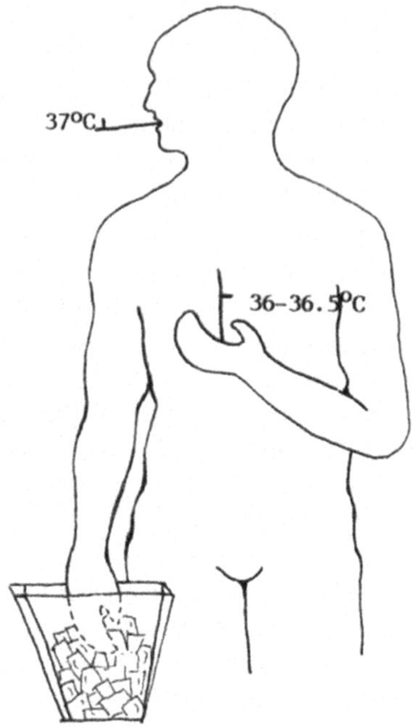


**ILLUSTRATION OF A VASOMOTOR REFLEX**
When one hand is plunged into icy water: a thermometer, held in the other hand, registers a fall in temperature, whereas a thermometer in the mouth shows no variation of temperature. In 1851, Brown-Sequard, collaborating with his colleague and compatriot, Joseph D Tholozan, was the first to describe such a reflex.

> We are induced to admit that the hand's blood vessels are contracted. But now, what is the cause of that contraction? We will try to show that it is an action of the nervous system. The nervous system in consequence of that sensation, …acts upon the blood vessels and excites them to contract. The calibre of the visible vessels is sensibly diminished.[27]

Brown-Séquard's visit to The States was an occasion for him to make contact with the descendants of his relative, Canon Henry Feltus, who had been the husband of his paternal great aunt, née Ryan. Long before his visit to America, he had been

> anxious to discover if he had kindred in this country. He had applied to Mr Brisbane of the Fourierist Society in Paris and through him had obtained the names of Dr Feltus's descendants in New York.[28]

---

27 Medical Examiner Philadelphia (1852) 8: 486. Also Brown-Séquard (1858) Recherches expérimentales sur quelques-uns des effets du froid sur l'homme. J Physiol (Paris) 1: 479–481.

28 Dupuy E (n.d, probably 1912) Letter to Charlotte McCausland. GMcCC, Ms 999/7.

His search was greatly helped by the fact that Dr Feltus's son, Henry J Feltus, had closed links with the American Fourierist movement.[29]

Brown-Séquard had been provided with letters of introduction to several members of various branches of the movement in America, from the Fourierist Society of Paris, as revealed by the following letter of James T Friedlin of Boston, bearing a Fourierist logo and the motto Unité Universelle addressed to Alex Harrison of Philadelphia:

> Permit me to introduce to you my friend and a good phalansterian Dr Brown-Séquard of Paris. Dr Séquard is a very distinguished physiologist in France and visits this country for the purpose of giving lectures before the physicians in our cities upon this branch of the nervous system in which he has acquired a high reputation.
>
> Any attention which it will be in your power to show him while in Philadelphia will confer a great favor and oblige you.[30]

Three months after his arrival in America, when Brown-Séquard called at Henry J Feltus's workplace in Philadelphia, in May 1852, his cousin was away in New York. He did, however, see there Paul Laying, an associate of his cousin, who gave him a letter of introduction to the latter, which reads as follows:

> Allow me to make you acquainted with Dr Brown-Séquard of Mauritius. This gentleman has come from Paris strongly recommended as an Experimental Physiologist. I have learned today from him that he is related to you, his Grandmother and your Mother having been Sisters. He tried to see you here but, having learned that you were in New York having business there himself, he proposes calling to see you at Mr Campbell's. Mr Brown talks English very well - he has already made friends here, at the Medical Convention at Richmond and I hope will impress you personally.[31]

Brown-Séquard eventually met his American relatives in New York at the home of Mr. Campbell, where he saw Henry J Feltus, his father's first cousin, along with relatives of the late Canon Feltus: the Gassners, the Coes and the Campbells.[32] The memory of this visit was still vivid, sixty years after, for some of the younger members of these families. One of those he met that day, was a small girl, who later became Mrs Townsend, née Coe, the grand-daughter of Martha Feltus, Canon Feltus's daughter, who was the wife of Peter Gassner. Mrs Townsend wrote the following recollection of Brown-Séquard's visit to his daughter, Charlotte McCausland:

> I distinctly remember your father, to me as a child - he was foreign. His bright, vivacious manner and restless eyes, being so different from the men I was accustomed to see. When he met the family he not only kissed the women, but kissed my grandfather [Peter Gassner] and Father [Charles Coe] on both cheeks.[33]

---

[29] Olmsted, *op cit.,* note 7, above.

[30] Friedlin J (1853) Letter to Alex Harrison (1853). GMcCC, Ms 986/8, 11th Feb.

[31] Laying P (1852) Letter to Henry J. Feltus. GMcCC, Ms 981/128, 14th May.

[32] McCausland C. Notebook in her handwriting. GMcCC, Ms 999/7, pp. 48–50.

[33] *Ibid.*

Charles Campbell, Mrs Townsend's cousin adds:

> It was late one afternoon, ... that I first saw him. I remember distinctly Uncle Peter [Gassner] and my Father in close conference with a mysterious stranger who had fierce eyes like a hawk and a stock of black hair.[34]

This visit to his American relatives resulted in a lasting friendship with Henry J Feltus, his senior by probably a good 20 years. He was a cousin who acquired the status of a father figure for Brown-Séquard. He was the latter's confident and, more than anyone else, was well aware of his mental instability, but greatly respected his intelligence and had an immense affection for him.[35] There was a regular exchange of letters between both of them over a period of 15 years, which ended with the death of the older man. Feltus came to his cousin's help financially, on more than one occasion. In the late 1860s, when Brown-Séquard heard that Feltus had suffered a financial setback as a result of a bad business deal, he made available to him, all the money he had in a bank, in The States.[36]

So, on both sides of the Atlantic, he had made contact with his grand-parents' relatives. In France, he met and befriended Alexandre Séquard,[37] a man of about his age, the grand-nephew of Pierre Paul Séquard, his maternal grandfather. Alexandre had two sons, one having the same forename as himself[38] and another, Aristide, born in 1850, who was, later, an employee of the Banque de France.[39]

Not only did Brown-Séquard meet his American cousins, but he also met his wife. In March 1853, he married Ellen Fletcher in Boston. He was 36 years old and probably 15–17 years older than his wife.[40] The couple must have met some time before December 1852, perhaps at the start of his Boston lectures in November. This much is clear as there is an extant autobiographical letter that he wrote to Ellen, addressing her as Lady Blanche, which is dated December 17, 1852.[41]

Ellen was from Portland, Maine. She was a descendant of Robert Fletcher, a Yorkshire man who emigrated from England in 1630 and settled in Concord, Massachusetts. Ellen was the eighth generation of the Fletchers of America. The family was distinguished through several generations. Six of its members are listed in the Dictionary of American Biography.[42] Ellen was related, by marriage, to the

---

34 *Ibid.*

35 Feltus HJ (1861–1869) Letters to Brown-Séquard. GMcCC, Ms 981/129-144, 981/129-144.

36 Feltus HJ (1869) Letters to Endicott. GMcCC, Ms 981/145, 18th Feb.

37 Brown-Séquard CE (1881). Letter to a lady, née Blaize. Wellcome Institute for the History of Medicine. Department of Western Manuscript, 7th Dec.

38 *Ibid.*

39 Huguet F (1991) Les professeurs de la faculté de médecine de Paris.Dictionnaire biographique 1794–1939. Editions du CRNS, Paris, p 534.

40 Role A (1977) La Vie étrange d'un grand savant: le professeur Brown-Séquard. Plon, Paris, pp. 76–77.

41 Brown-Séquard, *op cit.,* note 6, above.

42 Johnson A, Malone D (eds) (1931) Dictionary of American Biography, vol 6. Oxford University Press, Oxford, pp. 464–465, 466–467, 469–470.

statesman and abolitionist, Daniel Webster, whose first wife, Grace Fletcher from Hopkington, New Hampshire, was her aunt.

After the wedding, the couple went to live at 17 University Place, New York. Brown-Séguard had decided to practise medicine in America. He had told Ellen that:

> Up to now having only to care for myself, I have not given a thought to money. Now, I am determined to act otherwise. I am in a country far different from France. It is not admissible to be poor here, and truly, it is so easy, given some intelligence not to be, that I do understand why those that do not make a fortune are blamed. ... It is easy for me to earn a lot, if not immediately, at least in a few years' time.[43]

However, in a bout of depression, he suddenly gave up the idea of practising medicine in New York and left for Paris, accompanied by Ellen.

His sojourn in The States had not borne fruit. When he had left Paris for America, in February 1852, he was convinced that Philadelphia, his father's birthplace, would have welcomed him with open arms. It was not to be so. He found there, that nepotism was ripe when it came to creating a new post, or when choosing a candidate for a vacant academic one. At Richmond, he had a vague promise of a teaching post in a medical school, which was to be opened in the foreseeable future.

---

[43] Brown-Séquard, *op cit.*, note 6, above.

# Chapter 8
# The Cholera Physician: 1854

On his return to Paris, in August 1853, Brown-Séquard mistakenly believed that he would earn enough money to live, by giving lectures in Experimental Physiology.[1] He was convinced that he would be "in a position to earn far more than was needed for two persons."[2] Even as his misjudgement became clear to him, he did not make any attempt to shove off impecuniosity through practising medicine. As the money ran out, his anxiety reached a pathological level, culminating into a state of self-recrimination, combined with feelings of unworthiness and guilt. He wished to die, for he had behaved badly towards his wife, by having her to share his poverty.

His irrational behaviour and his poor physical condition caused by anorexia, insomnia, persistent headaches and digestive troubles, alarmed his friends. His conversation was an incessant repetition of his grievances and regrets. He was constantly pacing up and down the streets and, in the course of a visit to Frédéric Bonnefin,

> he rushed in like a whirlwind, refused to sit down; he was restless, and had scarcely arrived before he was in a hurry to be away again.[3]

He wanted to move to London, to open a practice. Although hesitant and undecided, his friends had difficulties in dissuading him. They advised him to go to Mauritius in company of Henri Lolliot and Frédéric Bonnefin, on their three-month journey back there, where they were returning, after completing their medical studies. Penniless, Brown-Séquard finally agreed to go. Désiré Laverdant, Joseph Tholozan, Henri Lolliot and the brothers Frédéric and Camille Bonnefin contributed towards the cost of travel for him and Ellen. Years later, recollecting on that period of his life, he wrote:

---

[1] Brown-Séquard CE (n.d.) Autobiographical letter. In: Notebook in the handwriting of Charlotte McCausland. GMcCC, Ms 99/7, p. 42.

[2] Brown-Séquard CE (1852) Letter to Lady Blanche. GMcCC, Ms 977/1, 17th Dec.

[3] Olmsted JMD (1946) Charles-Edouard Brown-Séquard. A nineteenth century neurologist and endocrinologist. The John Hopkins Press, Baltimore, p. 66.


DOI: 10.1007/978-3-319-03020-3_8, 

> After having gone through the little money that I had earned in giving lectures in America, and 1,500 francs which I received from the Royal Society of London and 1,200 francs from the Académie des sciences of Paris, I left dispirited and sick for my country in February 1854.[4]

His depressive mood and lack of money had affected Ellen's health. She was disappointed that he had done nothing to overcome their financial difficulties. When she had met him in Boston, she was earning her living by giving private lessons in French. He had told her then, that he was prepared to give up scientific research work for the practice of medicine, in the same way that he had given up a career as a writer for his mother's sake. He had written to Ellen:

> There is no sacrifice that I am not willing to make for you. If, I had to give up what I gave up for my mother, I will do the same for you.[5]

During the voyage to Mauritius, Ellen, wrote a letter to her mother, which reveals her predicament:

> Both of us in better health than when we left France. Dr. S., though not perfectly well, is yet so much better, that he has no more anxiety about himself. When we were in Nantes, many of his friends said to me "pauvre dame". I thought they pitied me because I was so mentally fatigued and because I was to be seasick—but now, I know many of our friends feared Dr. S. would not live to reach Mauritius and that is why in Paris they dreaded his going to England.[6]

The Brown-Séquards finally left France from Nantes with their two Mauritian friends and three other passengers on February 19, 1854. They travelled in a 350-ton sailing vessel, carrying a cargo of mules and a few dairy cattle. Ellen recorded her impressions of the three-month voyage and eventually published them as a series of letters in the New York Daily Tribune[7] in 1858.

The voyage was intended to be therapeutic for Brown-Séquard. Lolliot and Bonnefin hoped that he would open a practice in Port Louis. He spent his time, at sea, carrying out a study of animal heat, by recording temperatures of both humans and birds at different latitudes in the Atlantic and Indian Oceans.[8] Thus far, everything had gone to plan, but on their arrival in Port Louis, on May 12, 1854, they were forced into a hasty rethink of their future plans, as they learnt to their dismay, that a cholera epidemic was raging on the island and especially in Port Louis.

Cholera is caused by the Vibrio cholerae or comma-bacillus, which enters the body through the mouth, usually by ingesting contaminated food or water.

---

[4] Brown-Séquard, *op cit.,* note 1, above.

[5] Brown-Séquard, *op cit.,* note 2, above.

[6] Brown-Séquard Ellen (1854) Letter to her mother. GMcCC, Ms 999/6, 30th Apr.

[7] The articles appeared as from 27th June, 1857.

[8] Brown-Séquard CE (1858) Note sur la température de quelques palmipèdes longipennes. J Physiol (Paris) 1: 497–499. Also Dupuy E (1894) Notice sur M. Le professeur Brown-Séquard, ancient Président de la Société de biologie. Revue Scient (Paris) 2: 737–743.

The bacillus is present in the stools and vomits of the victims. Since Antiquity until the end of the nineteenth century, the mortality in the course of epidemics has been as high as 80 %. Nowadays, the death rate has been cut to single percentage figures by modern fluid-and-electrolyte replacement therapy and the use of antibiotic drugs to eradicate the infectious organisms.

The ship's passengers were advised not to stay in Port Louis, the focal point of the epidemic, but to go to the outlying districts. The Brown-Séquards went to stay in the country house of Emile Gausseran, Brown-Séquard's godfather. He was a wealthy man who had business interests in Port Louis, and he had given refuge to some 30 relatives and friends fleeing the epidemic in the capital.[9]

Anxious to help fight this scourge, Brown-Séquard immediately applied to the Authorities for permission to practise medicine locally. On May 30, 1854, he received the following authorization from George Clerihew, the Chief Medical Officer of the island:

> I have the honour to acquaint you that the Honourable the Officer, administering the Government, in the absence of the Governor, has been pleased to grant you permission to practise your profession in the Colony.
>
> It will be necessary that you should address Her Majesty's Attorney-General to be permitted to take the usual oath according to the Laws of the Colony.[10]

Within days of receiving this authorization, Brown-Séquard swore the required oath, though he had already been visiting patients for fifteen days.

Cholera was not new to Mauritius, having first occurred in 1775 and striking again in 1819–1820. What made the present epidemic such a disaster was its scale. In the space of 10 weeks, it was to strike down 5 % of the island's population and as much as twice that percentage of the inhabitants of Port Louis and its surroundings. The death toll was such that a great number of dead were hastily buried outside of cemeteries, and a great many deaths were not registered. In the last days of May, weeks before the epidemic peaked, it had claimed the lives of 65 % of its victims. Anywhere in the civilised world, such high incidence and death rate would have been an unprecedented catastrophe, still more so in Mauritius with its limited hospital facilities. The weekly medical journal, The Lancet, which heard of the epidemic in July, by despatches brought by the vessel Aringo, which had left Mauritius late in May, commented:

> Port Louis was never less prepared than at the present for this dreadful disease, and should it break out there with any violence the effect will be terrific. The number of cases to the 30th May was 276, and the deaths, 170.[11]

At that time, two-thirds of the island's population was living in appalling conditions, in shanty bush villages, on the outskirts of Port Louis, especially in the Pamplemousses district. Fifteen years previously, 80,000 slaves had been liberated

---

9 Brown-Séquard Ellen (1854) Letter to her mother. GMcCC, Ms 999/6, 2nd June.

10 Clerihew G (1854) Letter to Brown-Séquard. GMcCC, Ms 980/6, 30th May.

11 Lancet (1854) Cholera in Mauritius, 2: 96.

and were now reduced to living in these bush bidonvilles. These ex-slaves were, inevitably, the worst hit section of Mauritian society.

The Port Louis Municipal Council, responsible for the public health of the town and its surroundings, had the unenviable task of caring for this vast population of liberated slaves, which became progressively more difficult as the means to help them ran out. Most of the physicians of the outlying districts were kept busy by fee-paying patients, who were being cared for in their homes. Several of the most dedicated of them had already paid the ultimate price for their devotion to duty. Indeed, "many talented and brave men had been the victims of their courage."[12] Physicians were so busy at the peak of the epidemic, that none were available to care for the new cases of cholera. No doubt some refused[13] or were reluctant to venture into the bush villages to attend to victims living in shacks, in squalid conditions. The Municipal Council was obliged to appoint physicians for the task,[14] but there were too few of them.

Added to this lack of medical facilities was the element of panic which seizes a population at the sheer toll of death and sickness. People fled Port Louis, to stay with relatives or friends outside the capital. Those who had nowhere to go, confined themselves to their homes. Shops closed, not because of a shortage of products, but because shopkeepers would not serve anyone likely to have been in contact with a diseased person.

Another facet of the chaos was the moral panic which ensued. Most of the islanders, regardless of ethnic background, shared the view that cholera resulted either from breathing in an evil air or from God venting his wrath on sinners. This latter view was widely prevalent in Europe.

There were certain measures that the islanders could take in their efforts to avoid the spread of infection. To prevent the evil air entering their homes, they kept bonfires burning in their gardens, feeding them constantly with leaves, branches and trunks of aromatic trees. Indoors, charcoal stoves were kept alight day and night, burning incense. To purify the air, garlands of scented plants and flowers were hung in houses, across the streets and in places of worship. Other measures that the multi-denominational Mauritians took were less pragmatic but, nonetheless, deeply felt as necessary: Roman Catholics, Muslims and Hindus organised processions to holy places to implore the mercy of their deities.

Although there were, no doubt, some pockets of superstitious beliefs on the island, the general consensus accorded to the view of physicians of the day. It was widely accepted in European medical circles that some diseases, particularly those of an epidemic nature, were caused by miasma, which is foul vapours emanating from decaying matter, excrement, mud, cesspools, refuse, etc. This miasmatic or phytogenic theory held that cholera was caused by breathing in these vapours.

---

[12] E de P (1854) Leçon de physiologie de M. Le docteur Brown-Séquard. Le Mauricien, Mauritius, 10th Oct.

[13] Brown-Séquard, *op cit.*, note 9, above.

[14] *Ibid.*

Amid the turmoil of the epidemic, Brown-Séquard distinguished himself, from his very first day in practice, by caring for the great number of destitute living on the outskirts of Port Louis. He toiled relentlessly for the poor people,[15] interspacing visits to their shacks with calls to fee-paying patients. He was spending the money he was receiving from his well-to-do patients on buying the medicines he was prescribing to the poor. He was seeing as many as fifty cholera victims a day.[16] This selfless attitude won him widespread admiration and came to the attention of several members of the Municipal Council, such as the Councillors, Frédéric de Chazal, Georges de Courson and the Mayor, Gabriel Fropier.

On June 1st, Brown-Séquard approached Gabriel Fropier with a request for a hospital exclusively for the cholera victims "where the poor could be taken as it is impossible to cure them in their miserable habitations."[17] The Municipal Council immediately provided a large empty town house, known as **La Maison Hugon** in Valonville street, off Labourdonnais street, which subsequently came to be known as **l'Hospice Sainte Marie** (St Mary's Poorhouse). Georges de Courson was appointed as director of the project and, on Brown-Séquard's advice, he had the whole house equipped with all the facilities of a makeshift hospital.

In this Poorhouse, Brown-Séquard worked with an ex-army surgeon, named Macpherson, who came from Cluny in Scotland and a nursing staff of nuns from the **Order of the Sisters of Charity**. The first patients were admitted within 2 days of Brown-Séquard's request to the mayor. As well as cholera victims, the Poorhouse received other extremely sick persons, as both out- and in-patients, through the months of June to late September.

The two physicians, in charge at the Hospice, favoured different treatments for cholera. Macpherson believed in the ancient **Doctrine of the Four Humours**, expounded in Antiquity, which attributed all diseases to alterations in four basic fluids: choler associated with yellow bile, the source of bad temper; phlegm, a watery humour which made someone calm and phlegmatic; black bile or melancholia which was the source of sadness and blood which made a person cheerful and sanguine. His cholera treatment, therefore, involved repeated and daily cold water-baths and showers and the occasional blood-letting. This elaborate application of remedies was supposed to stimulate breathing and to cleanse the blood. Brown-Séquard's treatment, on the other hand, maintained the precepts of François Magendie, conceived during the Parisian cholera epidemic of 1832. This involved the administration of high doses of laudanum (tincture of opium) up to the threshold of intoxication and, should it be necessary, reviving the patient thereafter with strong coffee. The purpose of this treatment was to sedate the patient and to soothe the diarrhoea, giving the body time to overcome the infection.

---

[15] *Ibid.*

[16] *Ibid.*

[17] *Ibid.*

By the last week of August, the epidemic was on the wane, and the local newspapers acknowledged the population's debt of gratitude "to all the young physicians who had given such dazzling proofs of their talent and of their zeal during the furies of the epidemy [sic]."[18] Brown-Séquard, however, was singled out for special praises by the **Commercial Gazette of Port Louis** for his unmitigated devotion, thus reflecting the feeling of the majority of the inhabitants of Port Louis:

> The services rendered by Dr Séquard to the poorer inhabitants of Port Louis, during the prevalence of cholera, were of such nature as to have secured for him the lasting gratitude of those who came under his treatment, and the esteem of all who witnessed his absolute forgetfulness of every selfish consideration in his ardour for the cause of humanity.[19]

There was, however, another unsung hero of this epidemic who, according to local traditions, Brown-Séquard met in the shanty bush villages; this was Jacques Désiré Laval, a Roman Catholic missionary priest who, prior to taking holy orders, had practiced as a doctor in his native Normandy. A graduate of the Paris Medical School, he had presented, in 1830, his doctoral thesis, entitled **Essai sur le rhumatisme articulaire** (Essay on articular rheumatism).[20] After years of private practice, he felt the call to the priesthood and was ordained in 1838. Three years later, he was sent to Mauritius to care to the spiritual needs of the slaves who had been set free, after a period of four years compulsory labour, following the 1835 Decree of Abolition of Slavery. He was entrusted with the spiritual welfare of 80,000 emancipated slaves, who had been denied equal rights with the rest of the population. He lived in a wooden shack outside of Port Louis, and was viewed with great suspicion by the non-Black population. He became an object of their derision and on several occasions was beaten up. Laval, throughout the whole of the epidemic, toiled day and night, with little sleep, bringing consolation to the sick and dying in both his capacities of priest and physician.

He comforted over 1,500 victims. Unacknowledged and scorned during his lifetime, it was after death that this man of God outshone his atheistic colleague, Brown-Séquard. He is now recognised as one of the founding fathers of the Mauritian nation. The day of his death, 9th September, has been proclaimed a national public holiday. He is venerated as a saint by Mauritians of all creeds.

During the epidemic, Brown-Séquard's scientific curiosity got the better of him. Unable to resist the temptation of experimenting on himself, he ended up putting his own life at risk, by swallowing his patients' vomits.[21] When he showed the first symptoms of the disease, he took such a high dose of laudanum that he poisoned

---

[18] Le Cernéen (1854), Port Louis, Mauritius, 16th July.

[19] The Commercial Gazette of Port Louis (1854). Mauritius, 28th Aug. Quoting an article which appeared in French in Le Cernéen.

[20] Grandrille M & MS (1979) Le père Jacques Laval, médecin et prêtre normand, missionnaire à l'île Maurice. His Sci Méd (Paris) 13:219–225.

[21] La Patrie (1894) Brown-Séquard. Mort de l'illustre savant, Paris, 4th Apr. Also La Gazette de France (1894) Brown-Séquard. Paris, 4th April.

himself and had to be revived. Locally, some say that this incident happened at his home, which seems to be borne out by Ellen's letter to her sister, in which she wrote: "... in my house one night, Edouard had an attack of cholera."[22] Others believe, however, that this happened at the Hospice Sainte Marie, where he was found, by one of the Sisters of Charity, in a semi-comatose state.[23] Until the 1930s, a rumour was rife in Mauritius that he had tried to commit suicide during his 1854-stay on the island.[24] However, this rumour was not attributed to his involuntary poisoning by laudanum. Given the severity of the depressive state, which motivated his journey to Mauritius, it is difficult not to exclude the possibility of such a self-destructive attempt.

His vomit swallowing experiment does suggest that he was thinking along the lines that cholera was a transmittable disease, or that he had read John Snow's essay **On the Mode of Communication of Cholera**.[25] This was published in England, in 1849, and received an award of £1,200 from the **Institut de France.** Snow, whose fame rests on his use of ether as an anaesthetic, and his administration of chloroform to Queen Victoria for the birth of one of her children, had cared for the cholera victims of Killingsworth colliery, near Sunderland, where the first English outbreak of cholera occurred in 1831. He believed that cholera was transmitted by water polluted by faecal matter and probably caused by a water-borne **animacule.** His ideas were ahead of his time. It was 35 years before Robert Koch isolated the comma-bacillus and long before Pasteur's work on bacteria. He advocated the boiling of drinking water, the washing of hands and the decontamination of soiled linens. Furthermore, he recommended that cholera be treated with saline solutions administered intravenously.

At the beginning of September, as the epidemic petered out, the Acting Governor, Major-General Sutherland, appointed Brown-Séquard a member of a committee which was to investigate the origin of the cholera outbreak. Even though this committee was made up of a chairman and five other physicians, one of which was George Clerihew, the Chief Medical Officer of Health, Brown-Séquard seemed to be regarded as the most prominent member. Thus, the local papers urged the public

> to put at the disposal of Brown-Séquard all the information which he might require to trace the history of the cholera which raged at Port Louis during the months of May and June.[26]

In October, however, Brown-Séquard had to abandon his investigations as he was about to leave the island to take up a post in The United States. He did,

[22] Brown-Séquard, Ellen (1854) Letter to her sister. GMcCC, Ms 999/6, 6th July.

[23] William H (1949) The Healing Touch. Charles Edouard Brown-Séquard. Jonathan Cape, London, p. 262.

[24] Rouget FA (1930) Brown-Séquard et son oeuvre. Esquisse biographique. General Printing & Stationary Cy, Port Louis, Mauritius. p. 19.

[25] Published in 1849 by John Churchill, London.

[26] Le Cernéen, *op cit.*, note 18, above.

however, report his results at the Hospice Sainte Marie. He had personally treated 201 patients and the mortality rate had been 28 % compared with an overall rate of 71 % for the whole epidemic. He modestly attributed such good results to the zeal and devotion of the **Sisters of Charity** and of the project manager, Georges de Courson.

It was later established that the disease had been brought to the island by a ship from Calcutta, which had reached Mauritius on March 24, 1854. Thirty immigrant Indian labourers had died during the ten-day voyage. The crew of 80 men and the remaining 345 migrant workers were confined to the Ile Plate (Flat Island), which was the quarantine station, situated a few miles north of the northern tip of the main island. Despite this precautionary measure, a few isolated cases of cholera had been reported by mid-April. By May, the epidemic was in full flow. The peak came in June, when three-quarters of the deaths occurred: 6,000 out of 8,500 victims. The epidemic started to decline in July and was over by the end of August, having claimed the lives of 6 % of the population.[27]

With the epidemic practically over, Brown-Séquard immersed himself in research work for the last two months of his stay, carrying out experiments on the domestic fowls from his godfather's poultry-yard. His work caught the imagination of the public and aroused the suspicion of many local people. He implanted rats' tails to cocks' combs and it was alleged that the hens wore fish fins instead of wings![28] Some regarded him as an able but eccentric scientist. To others, especially the Black population, his ability to cure cholera and other diseases was attributed to his power as a medicine man and he came to be feared.

However, among the most informed elements of the Mauritian society, his reputation as an outstanding physician had reached unprecedented height. He was asked to see many patients for all sorts of ailments, but mostly for incurable diseases.[29] Had he stayed in the island, he would have been the most sought after and the most respected physician of his native country, but to a mind like his, the place was too restrictive for his aspirations. In the words of the Mauritian novelist, Arthur Martial: "Mauritius as delightful, as maternal as she can be, is a cage whose bars bruise wings that are too large to be contained!"[30]

As early as July, when the epidemic was declining, the newspaper **Le Cernéen** suggested that the public should present Brown-Séquard with a medal as a token of the people's gratitude. Other papers soon followed the lead of Le Cernéen. Thus, **The Commercial Gazette of Port Louis** printed this appeal:

---

27 Bedingfell E (18540 Report of the Committee appointed by the Government to investigate the history and particular of the cholera epidemic of 1854. Also, Anderson DE (1918) The Epidemics of Mauritius, with a descriptive and historical account of the island. HK Lewis, London.

28 Hardy J (1894) l'Actualité. La Séquardine. Le Petit Clermentois, Clermont Ferrand, 6th Apr.

29 Chazal F de (1854) Letter to Brown-Séquard. GMcCC, Ms 980/20, 18th Sept.

30 Martial A (1939) Conférence de M. Arthur Martial. L'Essor, Port Louis, Mauritius, N°220, May–June, p. 64.

> We call upon our fellow citizens, before this medical gentleman leaves our shores, to present him with a Medal as a remembrance of his services that, on returning to his adopted country, he may contemplate it by his domestic hearth or show it to his numerous friends.[31]

At a public ceremony, shortly before his departure from the island, the Mayor, Gabriel Fropier, presented Brown-Séquard with a gold medal, which was especially struck for the occasion and inscribed with the words:

> The inhabitants of Mauritius to their compatriot Dr Brown-Sequard as a token of their esteem and gratitude for services rendered during the cholera of 1854.

As well as the medal, he was given a silver cup and Ellen a cashmere shawl. In his address, at the ceremony, the mayor stressed that Brown-Séquard

> had been especially in charge of l'Hospice Sainte Marie opened on purpose for the poor, where many recovered their health and where all the others found a relief in their last suffering.[32]

Brown-Séquard had been, repeatedly, asked to lecture on the principles of physiology. He obliged on the 6th of October, lecturing in a large hall, in Port Louis. There was an entrance fee of one shilling and all the proceeds were given to the poor. It was an enthusiastic audience, made up of the elite of Mauritian society. The last paragraph of his lecture reveals how much he had been overcome by the esteem of his fellow countrymen. He concluded:

> I am certainly far from claiming to prophesy; but should I ever have such a pretension, I will remember rightly that my compatriots have, in my regard, given the lie to the saying: "no prophet is ever recognized in his own country."[33]

These words were echoed by his wife, when she wrote about the tremendous welcome they had received in Mauritius: "If the Dr had been Solomon and I the Queen of Sheba, we could not have received more attention."[34]

---

[31] The Commercial Gazette of Port Louis (1854). Mauritius, 28th Aug.

[32] Rouget, *op cit.*, note 24, above.

[33] Mauritius Sentinel (1854) Leçon physiologique. Port Louis, Mauritius, 9th Oct.

[34] Brown-Séquard Ellen (1854) Letter to her friend. GMcCC, Ms 999/6, 28th Aug.

# Chapter 9
# The Richmond Professor: 1854–1855

The Brown-Séquards left Mauritius for The United States in late October 1854. Brown-Séquard was going to take a professorship in the Medical College of Virginia in Richmond. The post had been the subject of much correspondence and of a number of newspapers' stories prior to the departure of the couple from the island. As early as August 22, 1854, the Mauritius Sentinel wrote:

> We are peculiarly happy to be able to announce that during his absence [Brown-Séquard's] from his adopted country, his professional character is held in such high regard there that he has been unanimously invited by the Board of Directors of the Medical College of Virginia to occupy the professorship of the vacant chair of Physiology and Medical Jurisprudence. It is, therefore, another illustration which thus furnish us of the truth of the proverb, nul n'est prophète dans son pays.[1]

The newspapers also leaked a letter from the President of the Board of the Medical College of Virginia, which had been sent to Brown-Séquard in Paris. It was probably written in May 1854 and ran as follows:

> At a meeting of the Board of Visitors of the "Medical College of' Virginia" held at this city on the 26th instant, you were appointed to fill the chair of the vacant professorship of "Physiology and Medical Jurisprudence".
>
> The high esteem in which the Board have been of your eminent attainments in medical science, and especially those branches of it which you are called on to teach in this institution overcame all consideration of local pride and personal performance, in tendering this Chair to you, although a stranger and a foreigner.[2]

In the absence of Brown-Séquard from Paris, Pierre Paul Broca immediately replied to the Medical College of Virginia, while Brown-Séquard was being contacted in Mauritius. This is Broca's reply:

> Your young and great nation throws aside the prejudice which oppresses old Europe. The narrow question of boundaries occupy you much less than the true merits of the man How long will it be before we dare to follow your example? … M. Sequard himself, is he

[1] Mauritius Sentinel (1854). Port Louis, Mauritius, 22nd Aug.
[2] *Ibid.*

L.-C. Celestin, *Charles-Edouard Brown-Séquard*,
DOI: 10.1007/978-3-319-03020-3_9, © Springer International Publishing Switzerland 2014

> not an instance of what I have said? … He is not a Frenchman, although educated in Paris and speaking the language like one of us; although acknowledged to be possessed of eminent talent, he has nevertheless been unable to hold any official position, only because he is a foreigner.[3]

Brown-Séquard was joining a new establishment. The Medical College of Virginia was founded in 1854, having previously been the Medical School of the Hampden-Sidney College.[4] He was not, however, totally unknown to some of the members of its governing body, as he had previously addressed the Richmond Medical and Chirurgical Society on the subject of epilepsy.[5] Wishing to establish a Professorship of the Institute of Medicine and Medical Jurisprudence, the Board of Visitors had voted to elect a candidate on May 26, 1854. Brown-Séquard's name was among those of seven other candidates that were proposed for the new chair. In the first ballot, he received 11 out of 13 votes. Then, the voters, whose opinion differed, transferred their votes to render the final decision unanimous.

The positive feeling for Brown-Séquard's candidature was expressed in a letter by Thomas Hudson Bache,[6] written prior to the Board's decision:

> I hear with much pleasure of the probability that my friend, Brown-Séquard, will be a candidate for the professorship at the Richmond school not merely because he will advance the interests of the institution, but because the medical profession in this country will enrol amongst them one who has, by personal experience, done much for Physiology. Dr Brown-Séquard belongs to a class of men of whom we have but few in this country. I mean those who personally experiment with a view of discovering or establishing physiological facts.
>
> Too many of our Professors here content themselves with merely culling from abroad and elsewhere, hence I have, with delight, the hope of having amongst us a professor who will teach facts as observed by himself.
>
> From the estimation in which Dr Brown-Séquard is held by Broca, Robin , Bernard and others in Paris (the two former having often conversed with me of his ability and untiring industry) together with the reputation he gained in this country during his stay among us, I doubt not that he will give satisfaction should the place be offered to him.[7]

Brown-Séquard's appointment was warmly welcomed by the Virginia Medical & Surgical Journal, which wrote:

> M. Brown-Séquard is probably not well known to medical men of our State: but we are well satisfied that there is not one of the candidates for the physiological chair who can dispute the propriety of the appointment. In the great field of experimental physiology , M. Sequard and his celebrated co-labourer and rival, M. Claude Bernard , have gained

---

[3] Virginia Medical & Surgical Journal (1854) Editorial & Miscellaneous. 3: 276–278.

[4] Carmichael E (1972) Charles Edouard Brown-Séquard, physician, endocrinologist, neurologist, physiologist. Alabama Journal of Medical Sciences, 9: 224–227.

[5] Blanton WB (1933) Medicine in Virginia in the nineteenth century. Garrett & Massie Incorporated, Richmond, p. 51.

[6] This physician bears the name of a distinguished American family—the Baches were descendants of Benjamin Franklin—all attempts at identifying him have failed.

[7] Bache Hudson TH (1854) Letter to an unidentified colleague. GMcCC, Ms 986/9, 22nd May.

> equal reputation. M. Bernard , in reward of his investigations, has recently been appointed to the new chair of general physiology in the Faculty of Sciences at Paris. What more fitting compliment could one pay Dr. Séquard, American as he is, ... and desirous of giving this country the fruit of his future researches, than to select him for this position.[8]

This was an opinion which did not meet with universal accord and the Journal replied tersely to its critics:

> We are striving to build a great College in Virginia, not to make fat offices to put our friends in. We look round for the best man to fill a professorship, and we take him, whoever he is.[9]

The Brown-Séquards arrived in Virginia in the late autumn of 1854, ready for Brown-Séquard to start his course of lectures at the College in the new year. But he was greatly disappointed from the very first day of his professorship. No provisions had been made for laboratory animals, either for demonstrations to the students or for the professor's own research work. He had to fall back on:

> assiduous assistants among the students who had gathered together for him an innumerable caravan of dogs and cats and racoons and terrapins and specimens of nearly every other variety of the inferior forms of animal life which roamed the fields or the waters or the streets or the house tops of Richmond and Henrico County.[10]

Apart from the shortage of animals, there was no set place for such menagerie to be kept and the animals had to be housed in the Medical College's cellar, fed exclusively by the students. This non-provision of laboratory animals might have been an administrative oversight, but it could be interpreted as a deliberate measure, taken by the College, to limit the professor's teaching to mere facts which the students needed to get through their examinations. As it was, the noise that came from the cellar disturbed the students during the lectures and even gave the caretaker and his wife some sleepless nights.[11]

The reports of the students' reactions to Brown-Séquard's courses are mixed. Writing in 1913, William H Taylor, a student at the time, spoke of a language problem. He says that Brown-Séquard's "discourse was not very unlike an attack of spasmodic asthma,"[12] a rather surprising remark when viewed in the light of the latter's recent history of lecturing in America. He had drawn enthusiastic and

---

[8] Virginia Medical & Surgical Journal (1854). Richmond, 3: 174.

[9] *Ibid.* Also quoted by Olmsted JMD (1946) Charles-Edouard Brown-Séquard. A nineteenth century neurologist and endocrinologist. The John Hopkins Press, Baltimore, p. 80.

[10] Taylor WH (1913) Old days at the Old college. Old Dominion Journal of Medicine and Surgery 17: 57–100.

[11] Tucker KR (1937) Charles-Edouard Brown-Séquard (Read as the Chairman address of the historical section of the Richmond Academy of Medicine, April 13, 1937 at Richmond, Virginia) Enlarged from an article in the Bulletin of the Richmond Academy of Medicine, June 1937.

[12] Taylor, *op cit.*, note 10, above.

distinguished audiences in Boston, New York and Philadelphia. Furthermore, letters of that period, written by him, leave us in no doubt of his command of the English language.[13]

Another factor in this mixed reception was the level of his lectures, which was far above the knowledge that the students had attained. They were fascinated by his demonstrations, though they did not always understand what they were about. It appears that his agony in trying to make himself understood was, if anything, greater than theirs in trying to understand him.[14]

A teaching post such as this one was always going to compromise his real aspirations: the pursuit of scientific investigations. Added to this, was the unhappy situation that he did not get on with some of the other professors. Some were openly opposed to his experiments on animals, while others were bored by his constant preoccupation with medical matters. Most of his colleagues were more concerned with their fees and American current affairs than with the progress of medical science.

The social circles of Richmond depicted in Margaret Mitchell's Gone With The Wind were another cause of discomfort for him. He made a point of never going out of his way to attend social events. There is a story that he did not attend an evening party given in his honour by some friends, he was staying with in Baltimore. Dismayed by his absence, his hosts, eventually, found that he had gone to bed, in order to wake up early for work, and that is where he stayed despite repeated exhortations for him to make a short appearance.[15]

Added to these irritations, was a more insuperable barrier between him and the people he met in Richmond: the issue of slavery. Although it had been illegal in the North since 1846, it was still flourishing in the Southern States, and the cotton and tobacco industries of the Old Dominion were totally dependent on slave labour. Brown-Séquard was "passionately opposed to slavery, he was saddened by what he saw around him,"[16] and constantly reminded his listeners that the continued existence of such a wretched institution made a mockery of the wordings of the Declaration of Independence of July 4, 1776. He was in the habit of quoting extensively from it, namely the following lengthy passage:

> We hold these truths to be self-evident, that all men are created equal, that they are endowed by their Creator with certain unalienable Rights, that among these are Life, Liberty and the pursuit of Happiness. That to secure these rights, Government are instituted among Men, deriving their just powers from the consent of the governed. That whenever any Form of Government becomes destructive of these ends, it is the Right of the People to alter or to abolish it, and to institute new Governments, laying its foundation

[13] Brown-Séquard CE (1852) Letter to an American woman friend (1852, Nov or Dec). GMcCC, Ms 980/3. Also, Laying P (1852) Letter to Henry J Feltus. GMcCC, Ms 981/128, 14th May.

[14] Taylor *op cit.*, note 10, above.

[15] William H (1949) The Healing Touch. Jonathan Cape, London, p 265. Also, Olmsted, *op cit.*, note 9, above.

[16] Dupuy E (1894) Notice sur M. Le professeur Brown-Séquard, ancien Président de la Société de biologie. Revue Scient (Paris) 737–743.

on such principles and organizing its powers in such form, as to them shall seem most likely to effect their Safety and Happiness.

It was a time when The United States were moving slowly towards the War of Secession, a fact which exacerbated the hostile reception to this "dago's opinions". The previous year, at the annual convention of the Anti-Slavery Society, bitter divisions had surfaced. There were talks of America splitting into two: the pro-slavery Southern States going their way. The possibility of a fratricidal war was in the air. No doubt, many of Brown-Séquard's arguments were quite erudite: quoting Thomas Jefferson's condemnation of slavery in the original draft of the Declaration of Independence, as a "cruel war against human nature itself, violating its most sacred rights of Life and Liberty," or referring to Harriet Beecher Stowe's recent novel, Uncle Tom's Cabin, which stirred the conscience of all America and was acclaimed as the greatest abolitionist novel. It presented the story of a devoutly religious Black slave who had rescued a White child from death. He was sold to a sadistic master, who was incapable of comprehending the goodness of this slave and had him flogged to death.

The situation was further complicated, as many of his listeners failed to grasp that behind his sincere revulsion for slavery, he was often driven by the desire for intellectual combat. Ellen shared his loathing for slavery wholeheartedly. She was, by marriage, the niece of Daniel Webster, an anti-slavery man. Moreover, she had introduced her husband to Charles Sumner, a disciple of the great champion of the slaves, William Lloyd Garrison.

Brown-Séquard's frankness had unfortunate consequences. His detractors started to pay malicious attention to his features: his flaming black and restless eyes, his wavy jet-black hair and his dark skin. It was rumoured that he was a mulatto and had, therefore, mixed blood in his family line and it began to be whispered that, coming from Mauritius and having a dark complexion, he must himself have negro blood. In Virginia, there could be no surer way of discrediting a man than to hint that he had tinted blood.[17]

The accumulative effect of all these obstacles was that Brown-Séquard suffered from recurrent bouts of depression. This was readily apparent to his wife, who did her best to keep "up his spirit which sometimes was low."[18] She resented the fact that there was "no sympathy and little politeness shown to her husband."[19] Eventually, coming to despise their life in Richmond, she wished that they had remained in Mauritius, where they had a great number of sincere and genuine friends, where they were constantly invited out and where they have had a better house and more devoted servants.[20]

---

[17] Olmsted, *op cit.*, note 9, above.

[18] Brown-Séquard CE (n.d.) Letter to a friend. In: Notebook in the handwriting of Charlotte McCausland. GMcCC, Ms 999/36, pp. 27–28.

[19] *Ibid.*

[20] Brown-Séquard, Ellen. (1854) Letter to her family. GMcCC, Ms 967/9, 1st March.

Not surprisingly, Brown-Séquard's sojourn in Richmond was a comparatively sterile period of his scientific career, with perhaps the exception of the work he carried out on a "comparison between the drug opium and the newer bromides, chloral and that class of remedies."[21] Nevertheless, it requires some real effort of the imagination to believe William H Taylor's claim that Brown-Séquard was a clumsy vivisectionist. His story goes that he was asked to hold cats, which were spitting, biting and scratching, while Brown-Séquard "worked his way into their interior."[22] Dr James McCaw, who later became the Dean of the Medical College of Virginia, and worked with Brown-Séquard in many of his vivisections had quite another view of his colleague's skill. He wrote that:

> He was the most expert operator on the living subject I ever saw, and his dogs, rabbits and guinea-pigs were cauterized and handled in the most artistic way.[23]

The same William H Taylor reported a bizarre story of one of Brown-Séquard's experiments in the article he wrote in 1913, entitled "Old Days at the Old College".[24] He says that the latter covered the whole of his body, including his face, with thick varnish and was found unconscious in the cellar where the animals were kept. The student who found him, revived him and removed the varnish with alcohol. Writing in 1937, however, Dr Beverley Tucker said that it was Taylor himself who claimed to have found Brown-Séquard in that state, adding that the former, at that time "thought that he had saved a crank but lived to find out that he had saved a world famous figure."[25] Tucker confirmed his version of the event, in 1939, in a reply to a letter from Brown-Séquard's daughter, Charlotte McCausland.[26]

William H Taylor's account of this event is pure fabrication and not based on any real story. Brown-Séguard, who kept himself abreast of reports to the Académie des sciences, was aware of Alexandre Fourcault's 1843-communication to this Academy, in which he reported the dire consequences which follow the covering of mammals' bodies with a layer of water-proof varnish, namely "a cutaneous asphyxia, a gradual fall in body temperature, leading to death."[27]

Despite the many setbacks he suffered during his time in Richmond, Brown-Séquard was not entirely friendless. Notably, he became very close to the previously mentioned James McCaw , who complimented him in the following terms

21 Ott I (1896) quoting JB McCaw The Medical Bulletin 18: 361–366.

22 Taylor, *op cit.,* note 10, above.

23 Ott, *op cit.,* note 21, above.

24 Taylor, *op cit.,* note 10, above.

25 Tucker, *op cit.,* note 11, above.

26 Tucker B (1939) Letter to Charlotte McCausland. GMcCC, Ms 938/8, 18th March.

27 Bernard C (1965) Cahier de notes 1850–1860. Edition intégrale du "Cahier Rouge", presentée et commentée par Mirko Drazen Grmeth. Gallimard, Paris, p. 226, note 81.

> The enthusiastic nature of Brown-Séquard shows us his whole life and bearing. Simple-minded and guileless, he was truth itself as he saw it. His most affective nature made dear friends wherever he was.[28]

Brown-Séquard resigned his appointment at the end of his first term in office, having delivered 65 lectures during his professorship. He had also addressed the Medical Society of Virginia with a paper on galvanism.[29] His resignation was formally accepted on March 30, 1855. The record book of the Medical Faculty mentions that he attended several Faculty meetings, and that he was appointed as one of the delegates to the American Medical Association Meeting in Philadelphia, starting on May 1, 1855.[30] After this official function was over, the Brown-Séquards spent a short time in New York, before setting sail for France.

[28] Ott, *op cit.,* note 21, above.

[29] Blanton, *op cit.,* note 5, above.

[30] Haag HB (1959) Charles Edouard Brown-Séquard: his Richmond sojourn. Virginia Med Monthly 86: 311–313.

# Chapter 10
# The Paris Practitioner: 1856–1857

On his return to Paris from Richmond in May 1855, Brown-Séquard opened a general practice which seemed to be moderately successful. In addition to what he had earned in Richmond, he was awarded a sum of money as a prize by the Académie des sciences. This enabled him to set up a small physiological laboratory in the rue Saint-Jacques in conjunction with Charles Robin, who had been his friend since his days as an Externe in Trousseau's service at the Hôtel-Dieu Hospital. Apart from pursuing their own researches, they both took as pupil-assistants, several post-graduate students who were later to make their mark in several of Europe's capital cities. Among them: Johann Nepomuk Czermak, who became professor of physiology at Budapest; Jean Joseph Alexandre Laboulbène, who was to occupy the Chair of History of Medicine and Surgery in Paris; Isidore Rosenthal, who was to become the professor of neuropathology in Vienna, and the most illustrious of them all, Karl Otto Westphal, the first professor of neurology and psychiatry in Berlin, whose pupils acquired a world-wide reputation, such as Herman Oppenheim, Karl Wernicke and Arnold Pick. Westphal and William Heinrich Erb, were the first to draw attention to the disappearance of the patellar tendon reflex or Westphal's sign in tabes dorsalis.[1]

During the months of May and June 1855, Brown-Séquard attended regularly, the meetings of the **Société de biologie**, where his main objective was to force the Society to decide "on the most fundamental question of physiology of the nervous system;"[2] namely, the pathway of sensory impulses in the spinal cord. Up to that point, his work in this area, which dated back to 1850,[3] had been "greeted with some mistrust and had attracted but passing interest."[4] At the Society's meeting of June 23, he carried out a demonstration on two rabbits. There were considerable

---

[1] Not to be mistaken for Alexander Karl Otto Westphal (1863–1941) who described the Westphal-Plitz pupil's reaction and the Westphal-Strumpbell pseudo-sclerosis.

[2] Gley E (1894) Brown-Séquard (1817–1894). Arch Physiol norm pathol 26: 501–516.

[3] Brown-Séquard CE (1850) Mémoire sur la transmission des impressions sensitives dans la moelle épinière. C R Acad Sci (Paris) 31: 700–702. Also: De la transmission croisée des impressions sensitives dans la moelle épinière. C R Soc Biol (Paris) 2: 33–34.

[4] Broca PP (1855) Rapport sur les expériences de M. Brown-Séquard relatives aux proprietes de la moelle épinière. Mém Soc Biol (Paris) 7: 25–50.


DOI: 10.1007/978-3-319-03020-3_10, © Springer International Publishing Switzerland 2014

objections to his experimental procedure, especially from Paul Broca. Given the size of the rabbits' spinal cords, it was difficult to ascertain whether the dorsal columns—which were considered to be the pathways of sensitive impulses—had been completely severed.

In the light of this uncertainty, Pierre Rayer, the President of the Society, appointed a commission to supervise experiments which would be carried out on a horse and a sheep, at the Veterinary School of Alfort. The commission was chaired by Broca and included Claude Bernard, Henri Marie Boulay, the best known veterinary surgeon of his day, the surgeon Joachim Albin Cardazo Cazado Giraldès, the veterinary surgeon Armand Charles Goubaux and Alfred Vulpian. The results of the investigations were crowned with success. Broca's report to the **Société de biologie**, on June 25, 1855, confirmed Brown-Séquard's earlier findings in guinea-pigs and rabbits.[5] Broca stated:

> The commission is convinced that it is sufficiently enlightened on the truthfulness of M. Brown-Séquard's statements, however painful it is to disprove what was acknowledged as a fact. It has no hesitation whatsoever to state that Charles Bell's doctrine on the functions of the spinal cord contradicts the most unchallengeable facts. Perhaps, in entrusting me with the drafting of this report, it [the Society] wished to punish me for having displayed, at the start of this debate, so little inclination to believe. If that was the Society's purpose, I willingly submit, preferring the triumph of truth to any other consideration.[6]

Furthermore, Broca reminded the Society that the contradictions were so numerous that they

> made the physiology of the spinal cord an inextricable maze and many observers, despairing of unravelling these thorny questions, had ended by rejecting the localization of sensitivity and movement, to believe, like in the olden days, that these properties were uniformly distributed throughout the columns of the spinal cord.[7]

For Brown-Séquard, this vindication of the results of his researches, 5 years after their discovery, was a triumph. He had proved, as anticipated in his doctoral thesis, that Charles Bell was at fault, and likewise François Achille Longet who, in France, had upheld Bell's doctrine. He had confirmed the existence, beyond any doubt of his hemiparaplegic syndrome. To quote Broca:

> The remarkable experiments of M. Brown-Séquard have overthrown forever this edifice so securely cemented together, whose foundations had been laid by Charles Bell and whose capstone had been set by M. Longet.[8]

Broca's part in this vindication of his colleague's work was a deliberate move to help the latter. By contradicting him during the Society's debates and acting as

---

[5] Brown-Séquard, *op cit.*, note 3, above.

[6] Broca, *op cit.*, note 4, above.

[7] *Ibid.*

[8] *Ibid.*

an agent provocateur, he had compelled Rayer to appoint an investigating committee. This is clear from Broca's letter to his parents on August 11, 1855:

> This morning, I saw M. and Mme Coste who have been kind enough to take to you a bundle of papers. It is an off-print of my report on the functions of the spinal cord. Report which produced quite a commotion in the scientific world; the ancients have not replied yet. I know that they do not lack the desire to do so. This revolution should have taken place 5 years ago, but Brown was an unfortunate fellow of a poor republican, unknown, awkward in his speech and writing, whose sole merit was simply of being the foremost physiologist of our time. He was too much or not much enough. A conspiracy of silence had been organised around him, and the poor man, without bread or support, had been forced to leave France and to seek a living in America. Two months ago, he came back with some savings. I considered that this joke had lasted too long and that it was time to put an end to it. So, when Brown came back to the Société de biologie to speak about his experiments, I started to wage a vigorous campaign against him, which occupied the Société during several sittings. Therefore the president, although an ancient, had to make up his mind, and pursue the matter by appointing a commission. So, I made my report, not for the physiologists who would have shelved it, but for the general medical public, who is indifferent to scientific questions only because it is not available. Public opinion has favoured Brown-Séquard, who suddenly has acquired the importance he deserves. It is even murmured that the Institut [de France] will have to award him the grand prize of physiology. This is how one gets the ancients on the move, and I do not regret having put aside surgical work for a few days to concern myself with this important physiological question.[9]

Indeed, Broca's report established Brown-Séquard's reputation as the leading neurophysiologist of his day and earned him a permanent place in the medical Pantheon. His reputation, as a physiologist, was so great in scientific circles that Alfred Vulpian commented that there were not more than ten practitioners in the whole of Paris who knew that Brown-Sequard, the physiologist, was also a qualified physician.[10] According to the weekly medical journal The Lancet, he was awarded the Magendie Prize for Physiology.[11]

In the United Kingdom, Broca's report was treated with scepticism. Many felt that Brown-Séquard's discovery had not overthrown Bell's doctrine. This prompted a letter from the former to the Editor of The Lancet, on April 26, 1856,[12] in reply to an anonymous article published by this periodical on April 15, in which the author argued that Brown-Séquard's experiments were "confirmatory instead of being in opposition with the views of Charles Bell."[13] In his letter, Brown-Séquard affirmed that there was no concordance between his doctrine and that of Bell's as the latter's was flawed (Fig. 10.1).

In October 1855, François Magendie, the Professor of Medicine of the Collège de France died, leaving vacant the Chair he had held since 1831, when he

[9] Broca PP (1886) Correspondence [de Paul Broca]: 1848–1857. Vol 2. Letter to his parents, 11th Aug 1855. Typographie Paul Schmidt, pp. 377–378.

[10] McCausland C (n.d.) Notebook in her handwriting. GMcCC, Ms 999/7, p. 51.

[11] Lancet (1856) 1: 349.

[12] Lancet (1856) 1: 348–349, 377–378.

[13] Lancet (1856) Correspondence. The discoveries of Sir Char. Bell and M. Brown-Séquard on the nervous system. Letter from Brown-Séquard. 1: 456–457.

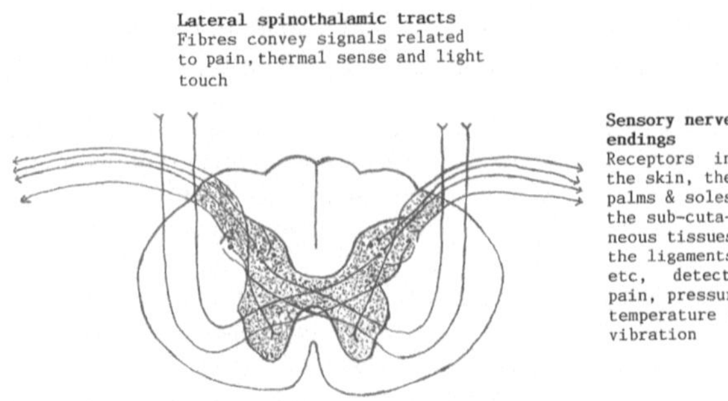


**Fig. 10.1** Schematic representation of decussation of some sensory pathways in the spinal cord © Celestin

succeeded Joseph Claude Récamier. There was not the slightest doubt that Claude Bernard, who had been Magendie's assistant for years and had acted as his substitute in the last 4 years, would succeed to his Chair. Brown-Séquard immediately applied for the post. On November 17, 1855, he sent his application to the Administrator of the College, together with a printed list of all his published work to that date.[14]

On December 9 1855, the Assembly of the Professors of the Collège de France voted to choose two candidates to be recommended to the Minister of Public Education. The candidates were Claude Bernard, François Achille Longet, Alexandre Albert Daremberg and Brown-Séquard. The first ballot for the choice of the first candidate gave 15 votes to Claude Bernard and one to Daremberg. The second ballot for the choice of the second best applicant gave 13 votes to Longet and 3 to Brown-Sequard.[15] Claude Bernard was duly appointed to the Chair.

However, Brown-Séquard was rewarded in another way. Ever since 1847, he had competed for the **Montyon Prize in Experimental Physiology** of the **Académie des sciences**. Twice he had to settle for an honourable mention while, on two occasions, Claude Bernard walked away with the Prize. In 1855, the latter chaired the committee which examined the papers submitted for the Prize and in January 1856, Brown-Séquard was, at last, honoured for his work on the pathway of sensory impulses in the spinal cord.[16]

The early months of 1856 gave cause for another celebration. On February 19, Ellen gave birth to a son at their home at 30, rue Monsieur-le-Prince.[17] He was named Arthur Désiré Jules Charles Edouard, thus bearing the forenames of three of his father's best friends: Joseph Désiré Tholozan, Jules Chauvin and Désiré Laverdant.

---

[14] Brown-Séquard CE (1855) Notice sur les travaux de M. Brown-Séquard. Imprimerie Masticot. Paris.

[15] Procés-verbal de l'assemblée des Professeurs du Collège de France. Assemblée du 8 décembre 1855. Copy made available to the author by M. Le Professeur Yves Laporte, Professeur de neurophysiologie et Administrateur du Collège de France.

[16] Egli N (1970) Der "Prix de physiologie expérimentale" in 19 Jahrhundert. Juris Druck Verlag, Zurich, p. 24.

[17] Birth certificate of Arthur Désiré Jules Charles Edouard Brown-Séquard. GMcCC, Ms 937/2.

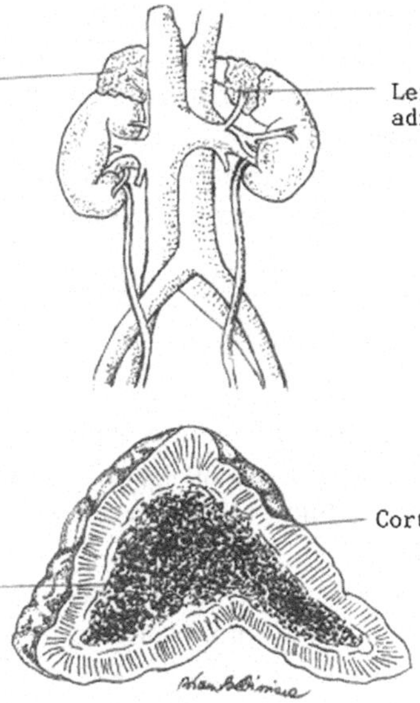


**Fig. 10.2** Adrenal glands two small triangular endocrine glands bilaterally attached to the *top* of the kidneys. Each gland comprising two distinct parts: the outer adrenal cortex which secretes the hormones aldosterone and hydrocortisone; the inner adrenal medulla which secretes adrenaline and noradrenaline. In August 1856, Brown-Sequard showed that laboratory animals did not survive bilateral adrenalectomy © Celestin

Later that year, on August 25, Brown-Séquard reported to the Académie des sciences on the effect of removing the adrenal glands from various laboratory animals.[18] These glands which are small, triangular organs, bilaterally attached to the top of the kidneys, had been discovered in the sixteenth century by the Italian anatomist, **Bartolomeo Eustachio**. They were referred to as the suprarenal capsules until the last decade of the nineteenth century. In humans, they weigh between 8 and 12 g and were thought to be vestigial organs, that is structures of an embryonic nature, of reduced size and functionless. They had attracted little attention, apart from the anatomical studies of Alexander Ecker and the anatomico-pathological ones of Pierre Rayer (Fig. 10.2).

In 1849, Thomas Addison, a physician at Guy's Hospital in London, had presented a paper to the **South London Medical Society** entitled: "Anaemia: disease of the suprarenal capsules."[19] He reported that in three cases of anaemia, in which autopsies were performed, he had noted pathological changes in the suprarenal capsules, concluding that these changes and the anaemia were probably correlated. Six years later, he extended the scope of his original observations in a monograph

[18] Brown-Séquard CE (1856) Recherches expérimentales sur la physiologie et la pathologie des capsules surrénales. C R Acad Sci (Paris) 43: 422–425.

[19] Addison T (1849) London Medical Gazette 49: 517–518.

entitled **On the Constitutional and Local Effects of Diseases of the Supra-renal Capsules.**[20] Here, Addison described the symptoms of the anaemia which later came to be known as pernicious or **Addisonian** anaemia. Significantly, he added that while looking for other instances of that anaemia, he had stumbled on another disorder affecting the suprarenal capsules, to which he gave the name of bronzed disease. The symptoms of this morbid condition were, in his own words:

> Anaemia, general languor or debility, remarkable feebleness of the heart's action, irritability of the stomach, and a peculiar change of colour in the skin; namely a bronze-blue pigmentation of the latter and of the mucous membranes and, always, in those days, a fatal outcome.

Brown-Séquard read Addison's monograph and commented that "it was a remarkable book,… which has recently drawn attention to the suprarenal capsules."[21] This work inspired him to research on the importance of these capsules in experiments on animals.

As early as 1851, he had studied the adrenal glands. He had noted that in mammals, the hemisection of the spinal cord resulted in congestion, haemorrhages and an increase in size of these glands.[22] Moreover, he has observed that rabbits suffered from an acute inflammation of the adrenal glands, which caused death.[23] His present report to the Académie des sciences was

> that the suprarenal capsules appear to be organs essential to life, at least in dogs, cats, rabbits and guinea-pigs; that the ablation of these organs leads, in general, to death more rapidly than the ablation of the kidneys; that the suprarenal capsules have numerous important inter-relationship with the cerebro-spinal centre.[24]

His experiments showed that, in the above-mentioned animals, including mice, survival after the removal of the adrenal glands was "for the five species of animals, an average of 11 1/2 h."[25] But, he was quick to point out that

> Maybe some of the animals, whose suprarenal capsules I have removed, survived for a longer period. Indeed, I took into account…only the animals whose death I witnessed; as for others, whose time of death I do not know, I have seen life last as long as the maximum indicated above; they may probably have lived longer than the maximum.[26]

He described the symptoms that he had noticed after total adrenalectomy, namely that they were "more or less the same for animals of different species."[27] The clinical picture was

---

20 Published by S. Highley in London in 1855.

21 Brown-Séquard, *op cit.,* note 18, above.

22 Brown-Séquard (1851) Influence de la moelle épinière sur les capsules surrénales. C R Soc Biol (Paris) 3: 146–148.

23 Brown-Séquard, *op cit.,* note 18, above.

24 *Ibid.*

25 *Ibid.*

26 *Ibid.*

27 *Ibid.*

> a marked weakening, various disturbances in respiration and blood circulation and finally convulsions, spinning, delirium and coma.[28]

He had not been content with performing bilateral adrenalectomy; he had studied the consequences of unilateral ablations. The results, in these cases, were rather negative. He registered a maximum survival time of 55 h in cats and dogs, of 40 h in rabbits and 33 h in guinea-pigs.[29] He added, however, that

> although I have not seen up to now, any animal survive for good the ablation of one suprarenal capsule, I believe that probably in multiplying the experiments, definite survival will follow this operation.[30]

It appeared to him that "the blood of animals deprived of their suprarenal capsules seemed charged with a toxic substance,"[31] because "this blood (taken from dying rabbits) considerably hastened the death of rabbits which had been deprived of one capsule for several hours."[32] He went to great length to prove that, though adrenalectomy is a traumatic operation, given the deep location of the glands, death was not due to

> a haemorrhage, nor to peritonitis, nor to an injury of the viscera adjoining the capsules. On the one hand, these causes of death did not exist in the experiments that I have taken into account; on the other hand, in the numerous experiments in which I lacerated the peritoneum in several places and injured the visceral organs adjacent to the capsules, without removing these small organs, I have seen the animals generally survive much longer than after ablation of the capsules and I have seen some recovering completely.[33]

Armand Trousseau, the eminent clinician, supported Brown-Séquard, arguing first of all, that the adrenal glands could not be vestigial organs, since—as stated by the latter—they "gain weight, nearly as much as the kidneys, from birth to adulthood, in Man, in cats, in dogs, in rabbits and above all in guinea-pigs."[34] He then suggested that instead of a toxic substance, present in the blood, which accounted for the death of adrenalectomized animals, it could be that the adrenals themselves supply the blood with a vital substance. Finally, he reported that in the case of one of his patients, who had died of bronzed disease, the adrenals removed at autopsy showed complete destruction by tuberculosis. To Trousseau, this clinical observation was conclusive evidence of the applicability to humans of findings in adrenalectomized animals.

However, the criticism of Brown-Séquard's report and his experimental procedure was sharp and protracted. Louis Gratiolet pointed out to an experimental bias: the fact that Brown-Séquard had only taken into consideration those animals whose

---

28 *Ibid.*

29 *Ibid.*

30 *Ibid.*

31 *Ibid.*

32 *Ibid.*

33 *Ibid.*

34 *Ibid.*

death he had witnessed. In the course of another session of the Académie des sciences, Gratiolet reported the results of his own experiments, attributing the deaths after adrenalectomies to the closeness of the liver to the right adrenal gland, which on ablation results in hepatitis or peritonitis followed soon after by death.[35] Brown-Séquard in replying, stressed that there had been neither hepatitis nor peritonitis after total adrenalectomy, and that the ablation of only the right adrenal gland was not for sure fatal. He asserted that "death is, above all, due to the absence of the suprarenal capsules, that is to the absence of their functions."[36] Jean-Marie Philipaux reported that not only did albino rats (Mus retus) survive the ablation of both adrenals,[37] but they even survived the combined ablation of these glands and of the spleen.[38] However, in some of the reports, the rats' survival was attributed to a fact that became known later: that they had supernumary adrenal glands.

The fiercest of Brown-Séquard's critics was the renowned Jean-Baptiste Bouillaud who, at the **Académie de médecine** referred to the former's experiments as "a physiological recreation."[39] To which Brown-Séquard retorted that "removal of organs was a grand method of scientific investigation."[40] Bouillaud deplored the latter's experimental method, namely extirpation of an organ to prove its use or importance. Claude Bernard also did not share Brown-Séquard's conclusion: that the adrenals are essential to life.[41] For him, total adrenalectomy reveals neither the process causing death, nor the physiological malfunctions which brought about this death. He was used to studying organs in vivo, because of the possibility that they had more than one function, or that they shared their function or functions with other organs. He wrote that the ablation of an organ, to prove its vital importance, was the most primitive of all experimental procedures.[42] In one of his unpublished notes, he stated:

> Ablation of organs—one gets nothing or gets false results. Ex. suprarenal capsules, spleen, vessels, nerves. Ablation of organs misleads. Brown-Séquard removes the suprarenal capsules. The very error of experimentation.[43]

---

[35] Gratiolet LP (1856) Notes sur les effets qui suivent l'ablation des capsules surrénales. C R Acad Sci (Paris) 43: 904–906.

[36] Brown-Séquard CE (1856) Recherches expérimentales sur la physiologie et la pathologie des capsules surrénales. C R Acad Sci (Paris) 43: 542–546.

[37] Philipaux JM (1856) Sur l'extirpation des capsules surrénales chez les rats albinos (*Mus retus*) C R Acad Sci (Paris) 43: 1155–1156.

[38] Philipaux JM (18570 Ablation successive des capsules surrénales, de la rate et du corps thyroïde sur des animaux qui survivent à l'opération. C R Acad Sci (Paris) 44: 396–398.

[39] Bouillaud J-B (1856) Academy of Medicine, Session of 26th Aug. Bull Acad Méd (Paris) 21: 1054–1056.

[40] Brown-Séquard (1856) Academy of Medicine, Session of 2nd Sept. Bull Acad Méd (Paris) 21: 1067–1070.

[41] Brown-Séquard, *op cit.,* note 18, above.

[42] Schiller J (1966) Claude Bernard and Brown-Séquard. The Chair of general physiology and the experimental method. J His Med 21: 260–269.

[43] *Ibid.* Quoting Archives, Collège de France, Fonds Claude Bernard, Mss 24d.

To this day, there are those who dispute Brown-Séquard's claim to the discovery of the adrenals' vital importance. Indeed, bilateral adrenalectomy does not reveal the mechanism by which these glands control physiological processes; but, if his subsequent researches on the endocrine glands, on organ extracts as well as on internal secretion are taken into account, it has to be acknowledged that he ranks among the founders of the science of Endocrinology.

A few months after Brown-Séquard's report, Alfred Vulpian confirmed Trousseau's hypothesis that the adrenals supply a substance to the blood. He noticed that the emerald-green stain which appears when perchloride of iron is placed in contact with histological sections of the adrenal medulla also appears when it is mixed with the blood in the adrenal veins, but not in other organs or in the blood from elsewhere in the body. He stressed that this perchloride reaction applied to the adrenals of man, sheep, dog and other animals, and that the substance stained must be linked to the function of these glands. This is what he wrote:

> Therefore, a special substance does exist unknown till now, endowed with remarkable chemical properties, which is to be found exclusively in the medulla of the suprarenal capsules and which consequently constitute the specific property of these organs.[44]

After these studies of Brown-Séquard and Vulpian, very little work was carried out on the adrenals. In 1892, Jean Paul Lucien Langlois confirmed and completed Brown-Séquard's work. The breakthrough came in 1894, the year of the latter's death, when Edward Sharpey-Schafer and George Oliver reported that intravenous injections of a liquid extract of adrenal glands cause a sudden, sharp rise in blood pressure, adding that these extracts came from the medulla and not the cortex of these glands.[45] This was the discovery with which Endocrinology came to age. It led to the isolation of adrenaline from the adrenal medulla by Jokichi Takamine and Thomas Aldrich in 1901.[46] In 1928, Rogoff and Stewart were among the first to use, with marked success, extracts of the adrenal cortex in adrenalectomized animals[47] and in the treatment of **bronzed disease** (**Addison's disease**).[48] In 1936 and in the following years, Edward Calvin Kendall isolated the main hormones of the adrenal cortex and described their main physiological properties.

In Brown-Séquard's time, the destruction of the adrenals was caused mainly by tuberculosis. Nowadays, Addison's disease is a fairly rare condition known to be

---

44 Vulpian A (1856) Note sur quelques réactions propes à la substance des capsules surrénales. C R Acad Sci (Paris) 43: 663–665.

45 Oliver G, Schafer EA (1895) The physiological effects of extracts of the suprarenal capsules. Journal of Physiology 18: 230–275.

46 Aldrich TBA (1901) A preliminary report on the active principle of the suprarenal gland. Amer J Physiol 5: 457–461.

47 Rogoff JM, Stewart GN (1928) Studies on adrenal insufficiency in dogs; influence of adrenal extracts on survival period of adrenalectomized dogs. Amer J Physiol 84: 660.

48 Rogoff JM, Stewart GN (1928) Suprarenal cortical extracts in suprarenal insufficiency. JAMA 92: 1569–1571.

due to a deficiency of the hormones hydrocortisone and aldosterone caused by an auto-immune disorder in the course of which antibodies produced by the immune system attack the adrenals. Moreover, the increase in secretion of another hormone: **menalocyte stimulating hormone (MSH)** leads to the production of the pigment melanin which is manifested by the appearance of the bronze-blue pigmentation of the skin.

The discovery of the vital importance of the adrenals that Brown-Séquard made in this period of his life did not come without its price. By spending most of his time experimenting in the rue Saint-Jacques Laboratory, he neglected his medical practice. His patients drifted away in search of practitioners who were not constantly unavailable.

One patient, however, was luckier: the American senator, Charles Sumner. He had travelled to Paris with the sole purpose of consulting Brown-Séquard. He was then suffering from the post-traumatic consequences of having been badly beaten on the head, with a heavy walking stick, by Preston Brooks, a relative of senator Butler, whom he had criticized in a speech at the Senate for his pro-slavery opinions. Brown-Séquard submitted him to several sessions of the application of moxas to the back of the neck, and confessed to his patient that it was "the greatest suffering that could be inflicted on a mortal man."[49] The application of **moxas** is a disused medical treatment, whereby pieces of cotton wool soaked in potassium nitrate solution—or the pith of the sunflower which contains this salt—were burnt on the skin so as to produce an eschar. Sumner was cured. From that visit on, until his death in 1874, he corresponded with Brown-Séquard on matters pertaining to his health and private life.[50] He introduced the latter to many of his American friends, notably the palaeontologist of world-wide reputation, Jean Louis Rodolphe Agassiz and Jacob Bigelow, Professor of Materia Medica at the Harvard Medical School. Moreover, Sumner proved an excellent publicist for Brown-Séquard's medical art. Three years after consulting him, he referred to him, the historian, Francis Parkman who authored The Oregon Trail.

The natural outcome of the lack of patients was that Brown-Séquard was, once more, perilously short of money. Finally, in November 1856, he gave up his practice and his research work in the rue Saint-Jacques laboratory, and left Paris for America accompanied by his wife and son. He hoped to be able to support himself through lecturing to colleagues and students despite the fact, as he had found before, that the life of an itinerant lecturer was far from lucrative.

---

49 Pierce EL (1877–1893) Memoirs and letters of Charles Sumner, vol 3. pp. 564–565.

50 Sumner C (1864–1874) Letters to Brown-Séquard. GMcCC, Ms 981/187–197.

# Chapter 11
# The Itinerant Lecturer: 1856–1859

Shortage of money was the main motivation that decided Brown-Séquard to take his family to America in November 1856. This visit was, for Ellen, an occasion to present her first-born to her family. On their arrival in The States, they headed for Ellen's parents' house in Boston. It was Brown-Séquard's third visit to America, and somehow, his origins were the subject of some published remarks in either a local newspaper or more likely in a medical journal. He promptly wrote to the Editor of the Boston Medical and Surgical Journal, declaring:

> I was not born in Europe, I am not in any way a European. I am an American citizen not by naturalization, as you might think, but by the right of birth, according to the United States law, that wherever a man is born, if he is the son of an American, he is himself an American. I might add that my Father's family in the last century settled in New York and Philadelphia, and my Father, who was born in Philadelphia, served several years when young, as a midshipman in The United States Navy, I am therefore—and I am proud to be able to call myself—an American.[1]

Soon after his arrival in The States, Brown-Séquard embarked on a lecture tour without delay, which took him from Boston to Philadelphia, New York, Baltimore and Charleston. His Boston lecture centred on epilepsy in man, taking in the modes of producing it in guinea-pigs and its inference on the treatment of this condition in humans. It was a subject he had been studying since 1850, when he first artificially induced epileptogenic fits in guinea-pigs to which he had inflicted injuries to the spinal cord. He was among the first physicians to recommend the treatment of that disorder with compounds of bromine. These were first used by Charles Locock in 1837. Prior to that year, treatment consisted in the use of Indian hemp (Cannabis sativa), alkaloids of various plants and salts of tin and zinc. Treatment with bromides held sway for a long time, before being replaced by barbiturates in the twentieth century. In 1912, phenobarbitone, a synthetic product, was used as a therapeutic agent of grand mal, characterised by tonic–clonic seizures involving involuntary muscles and lack of respiration with a somewhat prolonged loss of consciousness.

---

[1] 55: 254, 1856.

L.-C. Celestin, *Charles-Edouard Brown-Séquard*,

DOI: 10.1007/978-3-319-03020-3_11, 

At the end of November 1856, the Boston Medical and Surgical Journal began publishing his lectures. A year later, the whole series of lectures were brought out in book form under the title: **Research in Epilepsy, its Artificial Production in Animals, its Etiology, its Nature and its Treatment in Man.**[2]

After his Boston lectures, he went to New York, where he lectured at the Academy of Medicine and from there he moved to Philadelphia in December. There, his cousin, Henry J Feltus had made the preliminary arrangement for his appearance in a hired theatre and also at the Pennsylvanian Medical College. A letter to his wife gives us some information about the lectures in that town:

> I have begun my courses yesterday in a hired theatre. I do not know how many tickets have been sold, but there were from 150 to 200 persons, and perhaps more (240 according to Mr Feltus), many have paid for the lecture last night, 50 cents. I will deliver two lectures at the Pennsylvanian Med[ical] Col[lege], admission 50 cents.[3]

In the new year of 1857, he lectured in Baltimore and then in Charleston, but he was disheartened by the small number of auditors who attended his courses, confiding to Ellen:

> I have begun my lectures yesterday, there were about 25 persons present, and I have already received $65. That is very little for the trouble and the expenses. I have no hope of being successful anywhere now and I truly would not go to Charleston if I had not positively promised to do so.[4]

The lecture tour was a financial disaster for him. Nothing could convey better the sense of utter dejection that he felt, than a letter that he wrote to his wife from Baltimore:

> I must try other means of gaining money than to lecture, because lecturing as I do, does not pay and cannot pay. In Boston, I gained about $160 for five lectures in three weeks. In New York, in one place I gained about $145 and in another $85: in all $230 for six lectures in two weeks. In Philadelphia in all $130 for 5 lectures in 2 weeks. Here, it will be about $80 in a week.... We have spent $670 in two months! More than I have gained.... I cannot, therefore, continue to live so. There is no profit in it.... I have been losing my time almost for nothing since I have been in this country, and I cannot continue to lose it. What I will do in the future I don't know, but I certainly must do some other thing than what I am doing now.[5]

These desperate tones have to be contrasted with what he wrote years later: something approaching a triumphant tour of America:

> I had to leave for The United States in order to earn enough to live. I came back soon after having obtained a great financial success from my lectures in Boston, New York, Philadelphia, Baltimore and Charleston.[6]

---

[2] Published by Clapp in Boston in 1857.

[3] Brown-Séquard CE (1856) letter to his wife, Ellen. GMcCC, Ms 977/5, 19th Dec.

[4] Brown-Séquard CE (1857) letter to his wife, Ellen. GMcCC, Ms 977/7, 7th Jan.

[5] *Ibid.*

[6] Brown-Séquard CE (n.d.) Autobiographical letter. GMcCC, Ms 874/2.

Acute shortage of money forced him to look for an academic post and to seek financial help from his cousin, Henry J Feltus and his American Fourierist friends. At the end of July 1857, the **Boston Medical and Surgical Journal** reported that he would be returning in the autumn to occupy a chair as professor of physiology at the Cooper Institute in New York.[7] There is not much evidence as to whether he had been offered the position, though there had, undoubtedly, been some talk of it. He even appears to refer to it in a letter to Ellen from Philadelphia, written in December 1856:

> Mr Feltus has sent you yesterday an article of the Daily Tribune of N.Y. certainly written by Dana and you will easily find out how important this may be for me to help Physicians and Surgeons who are trying to get a situation for me in New York.[8]

The Cooper Institute was in the course of being founded by Peter Cooper for the advancement of the Arts and Sciences. He was a philanthropist who, in 1830, was the first to build a steam locomotive in The United States: **Tom Thumb**.

Brown-Séquard was so short of money that, in January 1857, in Charleston, he sold a pocket microscope to make ends meet, telling his wife that he had made a profit of 8 dollars: "I have sold for $36 the little microscope which I have here & which is worth $28 in France;"[9] but help arrived in the form of Charles Anderson Dana, his Fourierist friend and the city editor of the New York Daily Tribune. Not only did Dana buy the articles which Ellen wrote, when she visited Mauritius in 1854, but he had her husband prepare lengthy entries for an encyclopaedia which he and the phalansterian, George Ripley were co-editing. This was a monumental work for which Brown-Séquard supplied a number of articles on medical and medically-related subjects. Two of Dana's letters to the latter are worth quoting from. In June 1857, he wrote from Cyclopaedia Office at 17, Appleton Buildings, New York:

> A thousand thanks for your excellent articles on blood and brain which have both arrived, and also for your kindness in speaking to Daly. I have written to him today.
>
> All the articles you want shall be given to you, except Diet, which has already been written by McCready under the title, Aliment. We have not been able to publish all of Madame Séquard's letters on the Mauritius. Two of them wait for more room in our columns.[10]

His other letter, dated June 4, 1858, after Brown-Séquard had left America and was just completing a course of lectures in London, reads:

> Your letter of last autumn with regard to the article Brain…It is true we do not use engravings as a general thing; but any you might have thought necessary would have been inserted. It is now too late, however, to request what cannot be remedied, and this article will have to be written by another hand…. But there are certain subjects connected with

---

[7] Boston Medical and Surgical Journal (1857) Honor to Science, 56:525.

[8] Brown-Séquard CE (1856) letter to his wife, Ellen. GMcCC, Ms 977/6, 20th Dec.

[9] Brown-Séquard CE (1867) letter to his wife, Ellen. GMcCC, Ms 977/9, January.

[10] Dana CA (1857) Letter to Brown-Séquard. GMcCC, Ms 980/9, 6th Oct.

> the article on Blood which is already in print, and these subjects are **Circulation, Nutrition, Respiration**, etc. If you will kindly undertake them, I will see that you are paid at such rate as you yourself may think just. I dare say too, there are other topics which have been matters of special study with you, which ought to be written by you on the same terms and I shall like to have you undertake them, also (Fig. 11.1).
>
> You are perhaps not aware that though the articles are not signed by their authors, we publish the names on a separate sheet which goes out with the volume. Thus, Animal Electricity has been the means of making your name known to the American public and I am confident that your remarkable essay on Blood will be even more highly appreciated.[11]

The Cyclopaedia appeared in 16 volumes, each volume containing 750 two-column pages. The first volume came out in 1857. The work took six years and two editions sold over 3 million copies at 3 dollars per volume.

By July 1857, the Brown-Séquards were back in Paris. Brown-Séquard resumed his research work in the rue Saint-Jacques laboratory. He did not practice medicine regularly during this period, though he saw a few patients who were referred to him, mostly American and English visitors to Paris, as it had been the case for Charles Sumner in the past, and was to be so now for Francis Parkman, who came to Paris to consult him. Parkman was the grandson of Samuel, the richest merchant in Boston. He had married in 1850, Catherine Scollay Bigelow, the daughter of Jacob, Professor of Materia Medica at the Harvard Medical School. Parkman suffered for quite a long period of his life from some sort of nervous disorder as well as a chronic effusion on the knee. After seeing Brown-Séquard, he wrote back home:

> I have seen Dr Brown-Séquard who fixed Sumner's head. He says he can cure the lameness, but the head is quite another matter. He says, however, that it will not kill me, and that at some remote period may possibly become better. He has two other cases of this kind, but says they are very rare. I am still unable to walk for more than five minutes at a time.[12]

A month later, he was much better and wrote:

> In one respect, I have gained greatly from Brown-Séquard's treatment. The muscles, which ever since my first lameness, have been very much reduced and weakened, are restored wholly to their initial size and strength, so that when the neuralgic pain subsides, I shall be in a much better condition than before.[13]

In 1850, Brown-Séquard had treated an Englishman, a friend of the British surgeon, James Paget. He wrote to the latter and from that moment on, they became friends.[14] In December 1855, Paget had written to him, advising him to apply for a grant from the Royal Society of London, to further his scientific research, which he did. Soon after, he received a £100-award from this Society.[15]

---

[11] Dana CA (1858) Letter to Brown-Séquard. GMcCC, Ms 980/12, 3rd June.

[12] Atwater EC (1967). The lifelong sickness of Francis Parkman (1823–1893). Bull Hist Med 41:413–439. Quoting a letter of 13th Jan 1859, p. 425.

[13] *Ibid.* Quoting a letter of February 1859, pp. 425–426.

[14] Paget J (1850) Letter to Brown-Séquard. GMcCC, Ms 981/15, 30th Apr.

[15] Paget J (1850) Letter to Brown-Séquard. GMcCC, Ms 981/15, 14th Dec.

Furthermore, in the second half of 1857, he won two prizes. The Prize of Medicine and Surgery of the **Académie des sciences**, which amounted to 1,000 francs for his work on artificially induced epilepsy and, for the second time, he won the **Montyon Prize for Experimental Physiology**, this time for his research on the properties of venous and arterial blood. The title of his paper was "Continuing researches on the properties of arterial and those of venous blood."[16]

In February 1858, James Paget wrote to him, suggesting that he should come to London and lecture there. Paget's letter is not available, but this was Brown-Séquard's reply, dated 18th March:

> In your kind letter of February last, you tell me that, if I went to London, I could lecture at the Royal Society, at the Royal Institution and at some Medical Colleges.
>
> I should be most happy to deliver at least one lecture at these two places and a course of six lectures at St Bartholomew.
>
> I do not know what kind of lecture a person, who is not a member of the Royal Society, can deliver there, but I expect it must be a really scientific lecture on some original facts or views?
>
> I know that at the Royal Institution, the audience is not composed of savants, but of ladies and gentlemen who require other things than a mere dry scientific lecture. I have, I hope, a convenient lecture for such hearers: it is on the importance of exercise to develop power.
>
> As to St Bartholomew, I should like to deliver there a course of six lectures on some points of the Physiology and Pathology of the spinal cord, the Medulla oblongata, the Pons Varoli, the Cerebellum, etc., on Epilepsy and Tetanus, and on the transfusion of blood.[17]

Paget replied on March 29, stating that:

> You will be able to lecture at the Royal Society on their conditions: namely that the lecture must be, or must already relate to a paper at the time communicated by you,...[18]

He added that there was no possibility of lecturing at the Royal Institution for the remainder of the season. As to St Bartholomew, no definite arrangements had been made, but he was "quite sure that a lecture will be acceptable at Cambridge,... and the same at Oxford."[19]

So, in May 1858, Brown-Séquard travelled to London to deliver a series of lectures and demonstrations at St Bartholomew's Hospital. James Paget had very close ties with this hospital, occupying quite a number of posts there during his lifetime, including: curator of the pathological museum, lecturer in anatomy and physiology, warden of the students' residential college and, ultimately, a fully fledged surgeon. His reputation is mainly that of a pathologist, who has given his name to half a dozen affections, namely **Paget's disease of the areola and nipple**: an inflammatory skin condition round the nipple of the breast due to an underlying

[16] Egli N (1970) Der "Prix de Physiologie expérimentale" in 19 Jahrhundert. Juris Druck ? Verlag, Zurich, p. 24.

[17] Brown-Séquard CE (1858) Letter to Paget. Wellcome Institute for the History of Medicine. Department of Western Manuscripts N° 50356, 16th March.

[18] Paget J (1858) Letter to Brown-Séquard. GMcCC, Ms 981/76, 29th March.

[19] *Ibid.*

**Fig. 11.1** Portrait of Brown-Sequard aged 40 1857 © Celestin

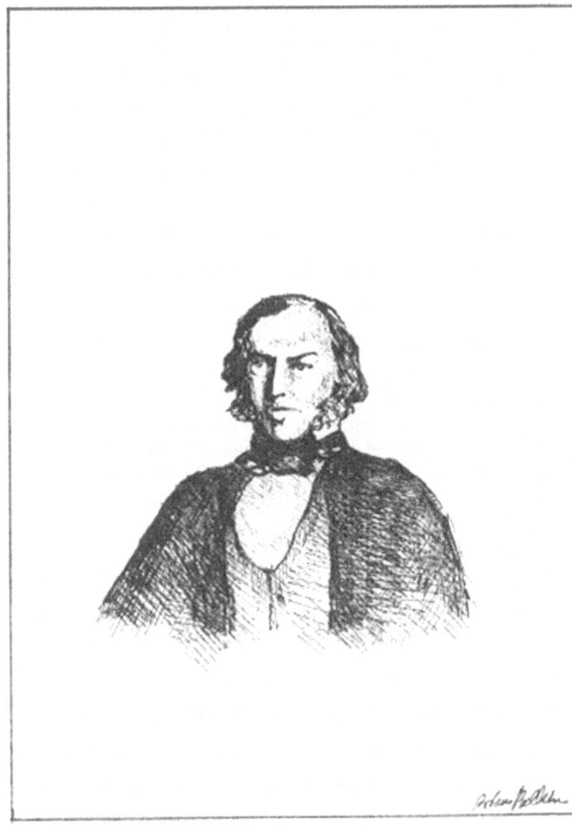

PORTRAIT OF BROWN-SEQUARD AGED 40
1857

carcinoma; a recurrent fibroid: a benign tumour of the uterus; **osteitis deformans** also called Paget's disease of the bone: a chronic disease, particularly of the long bones, the skull and the spine causing them to become thickened and soft and finally the **Paget-von Schroetter syndrome**.

Brown-Séquard's lectures were publicised in the following terms:

> Mr Brown-Séquard, the Marshall Hall of the Continent, has been induced by special invitation to come to London, and is now delivering, perhaps, the most interesting and certainly the most original and beautiful series of clinical demonstrations ever witnessed at St. Bartholomew on the pathology of epilepsy and the general therapeutics adapted to that and other nervous diseases consequent on these novel discoveries of that disease.[20]

Sadly, James Paget had to miss the lectures he had so painstakingly arranged as he was seriously ill with pneumonia. His presence was sorely missed by

---

[20] McCausland C (n.d.) Notebook in her handwriting. GMcCC, Ms 999/6, p. 36.

Brown-Séquard who referred to him as "my only real friend here (among the men of high standing)."[21]

Brown-Séquard's lecture-demonstrations were an outstanding success and considerably boosted his morale. After the first one, he envisaged making a lot of money from lecturing in the United Kingdom, writing to Ellen, he said:

> My lecture was extremely successful. In fact I never had such a success in my life. Most of the men interested in Physiology in London were present yesterday. I am able, I think now to gain money enough by private lectures for our expenses in France.[22]

The attendance at his courses was increasing with every new lecture, and a week later he was able to write:

> I had yesterday, the largest class I have ever had anywhere; nearly 400, almost all old men and, although I have had a bad cold, my lecture is the best I have delivered in England.[23]

While he was lecturing at St Bartholomew's Hospital, he was approached about the possibility of taking a Chair of Physiology at Oxford. He wrote immediately to his wife:

> Would you like to live in Oxford? Some persons are seriously thinking of procuring to me a chair of Physiology at the University. It is a new chair which will give at first £500 (2500 dollars) and in 2 years £800 (20,000 Francs).[24]

Ellen did not share his enthusiasm for living in Oxford and he wrote back:

> Your objections about Oxford are not insurmountable. Now, as to the future, I will certainly have any chair I choose in The United States and we shall go and live at home after three, four or five years passed at Oxford—Oxford is a relay—and an agreeable one which gives the certitude of arriving safe home.[25]

But the financial prospects were not as good as he had been led to believe. The starting salary was not as high as £500 per annum and the creation of the chair was still something like 2 years in the future.[26]

The success of his lectures at St Bartholomew's Hospital whetted his appetite for a life in London, earning money lecturing. He told Ellen:

> I will come here with you and reside in a part of the town which is much more delightful than Bellevue and our expenses will be less than in Paris, and I will be able to earn more than my living.[27]

Six days later, he returned to the subject, speculating about opening a practice in London:

---

[21] Brown-Séquard CE (1858) Letter to his wife, Ellen. GMcCC, Ms 977/12, 11th May.

[22] Brown-Séquard CE (1858) Letter to his wife, Ellen. GMcCC, Ms 977/18, 18th May.

[23] Brown-Séquard CE (1858) Letter to his wife, Ellen. GMcCC, Ms 977/19, 19th May.

[24] Brown-Séquard, *op. cit.*, note 22, above.

[25] Brown-Séquard CE (1858) Letter to his wife, Ellen. GMcCC, Ms 977/17, 17th May.

[26] Brown-Séquard CE (n.d. probably May 1858) Letter to his wife, Ellen. GMcCC, Ms 977/15.

[27] Brown-Séquard, *op. cit.*, note 22, above.

I have the proposal of living in London to give consultations on nervous complaints and especially epilepsy which is the great of lords and myladies… I am told I would easily gain thousands of pounds.[28]

The opportunity of lecturing at the Royal College of Surgeons of England arose unexpectedly for him. On the initiative of Thomas Henry Huxley, the offer was made to him, on the day of his last lecture at St Bartholomew's Hospital and came as a complete surprise, as revealed by the following passage of a letter to Ellen:

I have just received an offer to deliver five lectures at the Royal College of Surgeons, with a fee of £50 (1,250 Francs). This has come to me quite unexpectedly and I must say that I am much disturbed by it.… The offer is the result of the success of my lectures at St Bartholomew. In fact, I know, now, that I am able to earn much money in this country by lecturing and I have no more anxiety for the future.[29]

This five-lecture series began on May 22, 1858, and he enthused:

I have begun my course on Saturday in the presence of the largest audience that has ever been assembled at the College of Surgeons, 350 Physicians and Surgeons and not one student -all men of distinction in London.[30]

He lectured on the anatomy, physiology and pathology of the Central Nervous System and did, indeed, attract a constellation of distinguished medical men. Among the most prominent were Lionel Smith Beale; William Bowman, the anatomist who gave his name to the glomerular capsule of the kidney; William Withy Gull, who was the first to describe myxoedema, a condition resulting from the deficiency of thyroid hormones, as well as anorexia nervosa or slimmer's disease in which avulsion to food is taken to extremes; Thomas Henry Huxley, the biologist and physician and an ardent supporter of Darwinism; John Scott Burdon-Sanderson and Thomas Bentley Todd, both eminent physiologists; William Sharpey, whose pupils included Joseph Lister and Edward Sharpey-Schafer.

Such a large gathering of scientists at the Royal College of Surgeons came to the attention of the lay press and overjoyed Brown-Séquard. He wrote to his wife:

The Queen has been enquiring about me (all the daily papers speaking of me). It is said everywhere that there is no example of such a success as mine, on record. From all quarters, the most flattering compliments.[31]

His successful lecture tour in England was a landmark in his career, establishing him as one of the leading neurologists of his day in English-speaking countries. His lectures were subsequently published in greater details by The Lancet in July 1858.[32] The journal published them for a fee of £50 as well as purchasing the

---

[28] Brown-Séquard, *op. cit.*, note 25.

[29] Brown-Séquard CE (1858) Letter to his wife, Ellen. GMcCC, Ms 977/16, 18th May.

[30] Brown-Séquard, *op. cit.*, note 25, above.

[31] Brown-Séquard CE (n.d. probably end of May 1858) Letter to his wife, Ellen. GMcCC, Ms 977/24.

[32] Brown-Séquard CE (1858) Course of lectures on the physiology and pathology of the central nervous system. Lancet 2: 1–4, 27–31, 53–56, 108–112, 137–140, 165–168, 219–220, 245–247,

printer's block which raised another £30.[33] This is The Lancet's introduction to these lectures:

> When we consider that what are denominated nervous diseases are still the approbia to a class of quacks for plundering the public, we earnestly hope that these lectures will not be read for mere motives of curiosity, but that they will be studied with the degree of attention which their immense importance merits.[34]

Later they were brought in book form in America under the title: **Course of Lectures on the Physiology and Pathology of the Nervous System**.[35]

To launch the book, Brown-Séquard had to appeal to the generosity of two of his friends for financial help and dedicated it to them in these words:

> To Henry J Feltus Esq., of Philadelphia, US, and Jules Chauvin of Port Louis, Mauritius.
> My dear friends,
> Had it not been for the assistance I owe to your extreme kindness, it is probable that the publication of the present edition of these lectures, in book form, would have been much delayed; I, therefore, take, with much pleasure, this opportunity of publicly expressing to you my very best thanks.
> Your devoted friend CE. Brown-Séquard London September 1860[36]

Whether the success of his tour of lectures caused him to delude himself is not clear, but he wrote to Ellen about the prospect of another chair in England:

> I hear the question has been agitated yesterday to create a chair for me here with large emoluments. I do not know where: they have not been willing to tell me.[37]

It was a possibility that did not materialize. However, a proposal of Thomas Wakley, the founding editor of The Lancet, did intrigue him. Wakley talked about a salary of £500, if Brown-Séquard was prepared to render some services to The Lancet. The exact nature of the services, or whether his name was wanted for reasons of prestige, never became clear.[38] He would have considered reviewing books or writing articles, but not editorials.[39] Eventually, the whole project petered out.

On his return to Paris, Brown-Séquard founded his own publication, the **Journal de physiologie de l'homme et des animaux**. Its purpose being to review all the main American and European scientific publications. The journal would appear four times a year and would not be confined to pure physiology but also to

(Footnote 32 continued)
271–274, 295–297, 345–347, 367–369, 391–393, 415–416, 441–443, 467–468, 493–494, 519–520, 545–547, 571–573, 599–601, 625–626, 651–653.

33 Brown-Séquard, *op. cit.*, note 29, above.

34 Lancet (1858) Dr Brown-Séquard's Lectures, 2:25.

35 Published by Lippincott in Philadelphia in 1850.

36 Rouget FA (1930) Brown-Séquard et son oeuvre. Esquisse biographique. General Printing and Stationary Office, Port Louis, Mauritius. p. 23.

37 Brown-Séquard CE (1858) Letter to his wife, Ellen. GMcCC, Ms 977/36, May.

38 Brown-Séquard CE (1858) Letter to his wife, Ellen. GMcCC, Ms 977/27, May or June.

39 Brown-Séquard CE (1858) Letter to his wife, Ellen. GMcCC, Ms 977/43, 15th May.

organic chemistry, hygiene, toxicology, forensic medicine, descriptive and comparative anatomy, tetralogy, histology, and the application of physiology to medical practice.[40] The editorial board was made up of himself, Charles Marie Benjamin Rouget and Désiré Tholozan.

The first volume, due on January 1, 1859, appeared on February 12 and was dedicated to Biot, , Rayer, Flourens and James Paget. To the latter, he wrote:

> I hope you will not blame me to have dedicated my Journal to you, without having previously obtained your consent. I know that I might have met with some objections had I asked your authorization. I think, or at least I hope, there will be no blame from you for my having put your name with those of Messrs. Biot. Rayer and Flourens.[41]

This first volume contained a report from Claude Bernard, two original articles by Charles Robin and not less than 33 from himself, one of which dealt with the importance of the adrenal glands for the survival of animals. By the time that the fourth volume appeared, Martin-Magron and Paul Broca had joined the editorial board. However, the issues were slow to appear and the sixth and last volume came out in 1865, bearing the date of 1863. Broca replaced Tholozan, who had left Paris for Persia (present day Iran). Perhaps the difficulties which Brown-Séquard experienced with the journal's publication were due to Tholozan's departure, for he was the main financial broker.

Joseph Désiré Tholozan was born at Diégo Garcia, the largest island of the Chagos Archipelago, which was then a dependency of Mauritius, lying 2,000 km to its northeast. He was a childhood friend of Brown-Séquard, and both had attended the Singery School in Port Louis. In 1841, he joined the Service de Santé de l'Armée (French Army Medical Corps) and, after studying medicine in Marseilles and Paris, qualified as an army surgeon and a doctor in medicine. In 1849, during the cholera epidemic in Paris, he was attached to the Val-de-Grâce Military Hospital and appointed professor there in 1852. He served in the Crimean War in 1854 and 1855. In 1858, on the request of Persia, the French government appointed him to be the personal physician to the Shah Nasir od-Din of the Qajar dynasty. With the exception of three trips to Europe during the Shah's state visits, he was to spend 38 years in Persia, until his death in 1897. His influence on the state of medicine in that country was very great. There, he carried out a great number of investigations on Asiatic cholera and its spread from India along the trade routes; on plague and its foci of infection; on the various forms of diphtheria and on the epidemiology of influenza. He wrote medical books in Persian. He isolated the soft tick **Ornithodoros tholozani**, as the vector of **Borrelia persica**, the causative agent of a relapsing fever, endemic in the Middle East and Central Asia. In collaboration with Brown-Séquard, he carried out in the 1850s, a series of

---

[40] Printed note giving details of the journal's proposed scope and the names of the members of the editorial panel. GMcCC, Ms 1000/87.

[41] Brown-Séquard CE (1859) Letter to Paget. Wellcome Institute for the History of Medicine. Department of Western Manuscripts N° 51496, 13th Feb.

experiments which led to the first description of a vasomotor reflex. Tholozan was knighted (KCMG) by Queen Victoria.[42]

The impact of Brown-Séquard's lecture tour in London had been so great, that he was invited to lecture in Edinburgh, Glasgow and Dublin at the beginning of 1859. So, early in April of that year, he began a series of 12 lectures at Glasgow and Edinburgh. The attendance was very good and the audiences were enthusiastic. He, however, quickly developed fatigue, writing to Ellen that he felt "like a man condemned to forced work."[43] At the end of the Scottish courses, he was proposed as an Honorary Fellow of the Faculty of Physicians and Surgeons of Glasgow and even offered a chair at the University. He turned it down because he did not like the climate which affected his daily moods and depressed him.

In May 1859, he stayed in Dublin for ten days, where he lectured at the College of Physicians of this town on various affections of the nervous system, including the effects of the stimulation of the auditory nerve. His interests in this nerve led to his becoming the first to describe the symptoms of aural vertigo: dizziness in which everything around the sufferer seems to be revolving and causing inability to keep one's balance.[44] This was before Prosper Ménière, whose name the syndrome bears: **Ménière** disease. It is a disorder of the inner ear which leads to progressive deafness, thought to be caused by excessive amount of fluid in the inner ear and characterised by recurrent attacks of acute vertigo, deafness and tinnitus (Fig. 11.2).

The lectures that Brown-Séquard delivered in Scotland and Ireland were published by The Lancet from April to December 1860.[45] This periodical commenting that

> With regard to a knowledge of the physiology of the nervous system, Dr. Brown-Séquard has attained a position which is altogether unrivalled.

The following year, these lectures were gathered in a condensed book form in America under the title: **Lectures on the Diagnosis and Treatment of the Principal Forms of Paralysis of the Lower Extremities.**[46]

---

[42] The Times (1897) Obituary: Sir Joseph Tholozan. For information detailing Tholozan's career in Persia (present day Iran) consult: (1) Hassenforder (1954) Les Médecins français fondateurs et organisateurs de l'enseignement médical et de la santé publique en Iran. Histoire de la Médecine, 4:57–63. (2) Browne EG (1962) Arabian Medicine. The Fitzpatrick Lecture delivered at the College of Physicians in November 1919 and 1920. Cambridge University press, Cambridge. (3) Caventou (1898) Profil biographique: le Dr Désiré Tholozan, médecine de S.M. le shah de Perse. A Lahore, Paris. (4) Elgood CE (n.d.) Medicine in Persia. A series of primers on the history of medicine. Clio Medica, London. (5) Schneider (1911) La Médecine persane. Les Médecins français en Perse. Leur influence. Société Anonyme des Imprimeries Wellhoff & Rrohe, Paris.

[43] Brown-Séquard CE (1858) Letter to his wife, Ellen. GMcCC, Ms 977/22, 7th April.

[44] Brown-Séquard CE (1861) Note sur la production de symptômes cérébraux à la suite de certaines lésions du nerf auditif. Gaz Hebd Med 8:56–58.

[45] Brown-Séquard CE (1860) Lectures on the diagnosis and treatments of the principal forms of paralysis of the lower extremities. Lancet 1:389–390, 415–417, 437–438, 511–512, 563–564, 613–614.

[46] Published by Collins in Philadelphia in 1861.

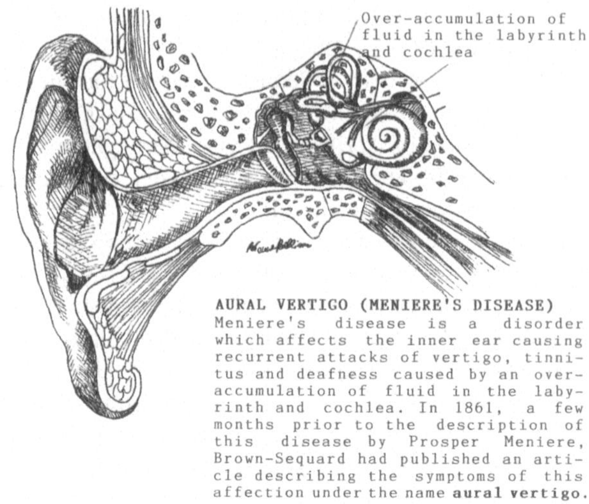


**Fig. 11.2** Aural vertigo (Meniere's disease) © Celestin

On his return to Paris from Dublin, Brown-Séquard became one of the founder-members of the **Société d'Anthropologie**, the brain child of Paul Broca. The aim of the Society was to engage in "the study of the human group, considered in its wholeness, in its details and in its relation with the rest of Nature."[47] The Society's creation had been delayed for years because of laws which suppressed intellectual diversity. But, finally, on May 19, 1859, the first meeting was held, although the Society was only officially recognised in 1864.

One other landmark was completed on December 1859, the change of name of Edouard Charles Brown. The document drafted was what could be called an identity certificate for a scientific nom de plume. It was done by an attested affidavit, in the presence of a notary public, with two witnesses vouching that Edouard Charles Brown and Charles-Edouard Brown-Séquard were one and the same person. The two witnesses were Charles Marie Benjamin Rouget, professor of the Faculty of Medicine in Paris and Aristide Auguste Verneuil, a surgeon and likewise a professor of that Faculty. The reason given for the necessity of an identity certificate was

> That on the occasion of the publication of various scientific works the said Mr. Brown had added to his patronymic that of Séquard which is that of his mother, with the object of avoiding confusion between him and other persons bearing the name of Brown.[48]

At this period of his life, Brown-Séquard's prestige in the United Kingdom was such that there was the possibility that he could secure an appointment there. Very soon, in fact, such an opportunity presented itself.

---

[47] Achard CH (1924) Eloge de Paul Broca. Prononcé à l'Académie de Médecine dans la séance annuelle du 9 décembre 1924. Mason & Cie, Paris.

[48] Affidavit, 17th December 1859. GMcCC, Ms 987/3.

# Chapter 12
# The London Consultant Neurologist: 1860–1864

Early in December 1859, Brown-Séquard learnt of plans for the creation of a hospital in London for the treatment of paralytics and epileptics. He wrote to Neil Arnott, the President of the Royal College of Surgeons of England, seeking his help in securing a physicianship at the proposed hospital. This is his somewhat circumspect letter of December 6, 1859

> My dear Sir,
>
> You treated me with such kindness when I had the honor of seeing you in London, 18 months ago, that I feel authorized to ask you to help me obtain the appointment of Physician to a Hospital for Paralytics and Epileptics soon to be established in your metropolis.
>
> The subjects of the works and of most of the papers I have published and also of the lectures I have delivered to so large classes of medical men, in London, Edinburgh, Glasgow, Dublin and in the principal cities of the United States; - my speciality as a Practitioner, for more than twelve years; - and the kinds of facts and theories for which I have five times received rewards or prizes from the Académie des Sciences of France, might show how much I am prepared to fulfil the duties of a Physician to a Hospital of Paralytics and Epileptics.
>
> Some of my friends think that the Council of the Royal College of Surgeons of England from whom I have already had the honor of being called to deliver a course of lectures, might, as a body, give me a testimonial. However proud I would be to receive such a proof of esteem from the most eminent body of surgeons in the world, and however important and, I might say, decisive for me would such a testimonial be, I would not dare ask for it, not only because it would not become me to make such a demand, but also because it might be in opposition with the rules of the College.[1]

Although Arnott's reply is not available and no testimonial from the body of the Royal College of Surgeons was, ever actually, given, it seems that Arnott acted in Brown-Séquard's interests.

Brown-Séquard also sought help from James Paget. The latter's reply, dated December 9, 1859, reveals that he had been contacted:

> You may be sure that I will promote your interests in every way that I can, and I fully agree with you that the opportunity of being a candidate for the Physicianship to the

[1] Brown-Séquard CE (1860) Letter to Neil Arnott. Wellcome Institute for the History of Medicine. Department of Western Manuscripts N° 72200, 6th Dec.


DOI: 10.1007/978-3-319-03020-3_12, © Springer International Publishing Switzerland 2014

Hospital gives an excellent occasion for your starting to practice in London. Of course I will write a Testimonial for you but, among the Committee for the proposed hospital, the only one whom I know and can apply to is the Lord Mayor. I shall at once write to him, and perhaps, being himself partially hemiplegic, he may have weight with the election…[2]

The following day, Paget wrote to Alderman Wire, the Lord Mayor, who was also the Chairman of a Management Committee which was specifically set to oversee the establishment of the hospital, drawing his attention to Brown-Séquard's unique qualifications for the post of Physician of the proposed hospital:

I can hardly doubt you know well who he is or much of what he had done. Yet, I beg you to let me assure you that I know nothing by which, so much as by the election of Dr. Brown-Séquard, you could promote the best object of the proposed hospital, namely the advancement of the knowledge of the disease for the relief of which it is designed. If the medical profession anywhere could be polled, to return the man best suited for the object, I have no doubt, whatsoever, that Brown-Séquard would be elected by a great majority.[3]

In acknowledgement of Paget's letter, the Lord Mayor assured him that

He fully intended to vote for Dr Brown-Séquard but think it would smooth the matter and make it unanimous if he would write a letter to me making an application.[4]

Another person who wrote to Alderman Wire promoting Brown-Séquard's candidature was the surgeon John Zachariah Laurence. His letter is dated December 12, 1859 and reads:

He is a man of such transcendent abilities, that he will grace any position of an honourable nature. What the Lancet says of him may be safely taken as rather under than over the estimation he is held in by the Faculty, not merely of this country, but of Europe…. It may fairly be asked why, after his long residence in France, he should seek an appointment in this country? His first reason, which should give him additional claim on our sympathies, namely that he is a British subject and as such incapable of an appointment in the Paris hospitals.

I have been accused in advocating Dr Séquard's cause to be opposing other candidates,… I certainly should be very much grieved that our Hospital should be robbed of the great prestige it will acquire amongst the Profession and thus the Public by the rejection of Dr Séquard…. My only desire is to see our Hospital acquire a first-rate position in the Profession: that it can only do by the appointment of the ablest man, irrespective of patronage and influence.[5]

Very soon after, Brown-Séquard took David Wire's advice and forwarded a letter of application which covered two foolscap pages, documenting his career up to that point. Among the achievements that he stated were that he was an Honorary Fellow of the Faculty of Physicians and Surgeons of Glasgow and a member of a string of learned societies: the **Société Philomatique**, the **Société de biologie**, the **American Philosophical Society**, the **Academy of Natural Sciences** of

---

2 Paget J (1859) Letter to Brown-Séquard. GMcCC, Ms 981/78, 9th Dec.

3 Paget J (1859) Letter to David Wire. GMcCC, Ms 988/8, 10th Dec.

4 *Ibid.* Wire's reply was scribbled on the last page of Paget's letter.

5 Laurence JZ (1859) Letter to David Wire. GMcCC, Ms 988/9, 12th Dec.

**Philadelphia** , the **Sengbergische Naturforschende** of Frankfurt, the **Société d'Anthropologie** and the **Society of Arts and Sciences of Mauritius**. He was a Laureate of the Académie des sciences "having five times the honor of receiving prizes from the Académie." He had twice received from the "Royal Society a part of the Grant of the Queen for the advancement of Science." He mentioned the part he played in combating the cholera epidemic in Mauritius and having been awarded a "gold medal by many of the inhabitants of Port Louis;" his professorship at the Medical College of Virginia; the many lectures he had delivered in Great Britain and The United States as well as the lectures at the Royal College of Surgeons of England. He listed the four books that he had published. He mentioned the many original papers which had appeared in the medical press of France, Great Britain and The United States. He ended his application by saying:

> I am a British subject, born in the "Mauritius" a British colony. To my name Brown, I have added my mother's name Séquard, according to a custom followed by many of my countrymen of the Mauritius.[6]

His candidature was supported by joint references from members of medical faculties and by testimonials from individual physicians. The reference from Glasgow was signed by 20 physicians, including six professors and several lecturers.[7] From Edinburgh, a testimonial was signed by professors, lecturers and general practitioners, including Joseph Lister.[8] The testimonial from Dublin was signed by the Regius Professor of Medicine in the University and by the President of the King and Queen's College of Physicians of Ireland.[9] All these recommendations stressed that Brown-Séquard's settlement in Great Britain and his appointment to a London hospital, would contribute to a better knowledge of the physiology and pathology of the nervous system and lead to an improvement in the treatment of nervous disorders.

The individual testimonials were no less auspicious in their praise. Henry Bence Jones, the physician and chemist who isolated albumose or Bence Jones protein in the urine of patients suffering from Kahler's disease or multiple myeloma (also called myelomatosis)—a cancerous disorder characterised by tumours of the bone marrow affecting the skull, the vertebrae, the ribs and the pelvis—wrote to the Management Committee reminding them of the great discoveries that Brown-Séquard had "made respecting nervous action."[10]

---

6 Brown-Séquard CE (1859) Letter of candidacy to the Management Committee of the proposed for Paralytics and Epileptics. GMcCC, Ms 981/1.

7 Physicians of Glasgow (1859) Letter to the Hospital's Management Committee. GMcCC, Ms 988/3, 14th Dec.

8 Physicians of Edinburgh (1859) Letter to the Hospital's Management Committee. GMcCC, Ms 988/4, Dec.

9 Physicians of Dublin (1859) Letter to the Hospital's Management Committee. GMcCC, Ms 988/2, Dec.

10 Bence Jones (1859) Letter to the Hospital's Management Committee. GMcCC, Ms 988/7, Dec.

James Paget, in his letter to the Management Committee wrote:

> Wherever the medical sciences are studied, it if known that Dr Brown-Séquard is second to none in the knowledge of the physiology of the nervous system and in the works by which, of late years, that knowledge has been increased.[11]

George Edward Day, the Professor of Medicine at the University of St Andrews, at that time, commented that

> when it is known that Dr. Brown-Séquard is a candidate, I can hardly think that any Physician will venture to offer himself as a rival competitor.[12]

Some physicians and surgeons wrote directly to Brown-Séquard, offering their best wishes for his candidature. The most interesting of these letters is that of John Struthers—the anatomist and great supporter of Darwin's theory of natural selection—since it associates Brown-Séquard's name with that of two of the most eminent British neurophysiologists. He wrote:

> It seems almost absurd to testify to the fitness of one whose fitness is already well known to the profession not only in all Europe but wherever scientific medicine is cultivated. If you will allow me to say so to yourself, your reputation is already not exceeded by that which Sir Charles Bell or Dr Marshall Hall have left behind them. Like theirs your reputation is not merely as a Physiologist but, likewise, as a practical Physician and, also like theirs, it's especially in connection with the Nervous System. Hence a double fitness in your being physician to such a Hospital.[13]

So, on December 29, 1859, the Management Committee of the proposed hospital appointed Brown-Séquard as one of the physicians,[14] despite the fact that it was still without premises. The same day, a telegram was sent to Brown-Séquard, signed by John Zachariah Laurence, saying: "you are unanimously elected write you have received the message."[15]

Brown-Séquard acknowledged the news of his nomination a fortnight later on January 12, 1860. Writing to the Secretary of the Management Committee, his letter was entered on the minutes of a Committee meeting on January 14, 1860. It reads:

> Owing to the distressing circumstances which have disturbed me for the last ten days, I have neglected to acknowledge, as I should have done, the reception of the letter you wrote to inform me officially of my election for the office of Physician to the National Hospital for the Paralysed and Epileptics.[16]

[11] Paget J (1859) Letter to the Hospital's Management Committee. GMcCC, Ms 988/8, 9th Dec.

[12] Day GE (1859) Letter-testimonial. GMcCC, Ms 988/10, 14th Dec.

[13] Struthers J (1859) Letter to Brown-Séquard. GMcCC, Ms 988/15, 20th Dec.

[14] Gooddy W (1964) Some aspects of the life of Dr. C.E. Brown-Séquard. Proc Roy Soc Med 57: 189–192.

[15] Laurence JZ (1859) Telegram to Brown-Séquard. GMcCC, Ms 988/13, Dec.

[16] Brown-Séquard CE (1859) Letter to the Secretary of the Management Board of the National Hospital. Quoted by Gooddy, *op cit.*, note 14, above.

These "distressing circumstances" were that his wife's health had been a cause for concern[17] and that she was expecting, at any moment, a child. During that month of January, she gave birth to a daughter, Charlotte Ellen who, unfortunately, died after living for seven weeks, on February 29, 1860.[18] Her father, however, had the consolation of embarking on a new phase of his career. He was moving to a hospital which was to have a great influence on British and international neurology.

The original impetus for the founding of such a hospital arose from the experience of two sisters, Johanna and Louise Chandler and their brother Edward who, orphaned at an early age, had been brought up by their maternal grandparents. Their grandmother was crippled by paralysis as a result of a stroke and needed constant care at home. While she was caring for her grandmother, Johanna began to think of the plight of paralysed people who were financially deprived. The prolonged treatment that paralysis requires could not be provided by most hospitals, which meant that the poorer victims were relegated to poor law institutions. Johanna found that "although there were charities in London for the relief of nearly every class of human afflictions, the sufferings of the paralysed have been strongly overlooked."[19] It also came to her attention that the plight of the epileptics, who were consigned to lunatic asylums were no better, if not worse. To raise funds for an organisation which would fulfil this function, the two sisters started to make artificial flowers and bracelets and other trinkets made of sea shells and glass beads, which they sold to friends and neighbours. But, despite all their efforts, after 3 or 4 years work, they had only managed to collect £200.

However, in 1859, Johanna did manage to attract the attention of Alderman Wire, the Lord Mayor of London, who had been left slightly paralysed by a stroke. He called a meeting at Mansion House on November 2, 1859, during which a Management Committee was formed for establishing a hospital to care for sufferers from neurological disorders. The Lord Mayor was appointed Chairman of the Management Committee. The hospital that was proposed was not to be an institution for the chronically sick or incurables. Its aim was the active care, treatment and cure of nervous diseases. The Management Committee was soon replaced by a Management Board chaired by David Wire and comprised of businessmen from prosperous City companies. Their first task was to decide upon the Hospital's name. It was to be: **The National Hospital for the Relief and Care of the Paralysed and Epileptics**.

The Board finally leased a house at 24 Queen Square, Bloomsbury, on January 29, 1860. It could accommodate 8 in-patients and had space for a consultation room, a waiting room for out-patients and a dispensary. 3 months later, the Hospital was opened and started admitting patients. The Lancet wrote:

---

[17] Paget, *op cit.*, note 4, above.

[18] McCausland C (n.d.) Notebook in her handwriting. GMcCC, Ms 999/6.

[19] Holmes C (n.d.) The National Hospital, Queen Square 1860–1948. Livingstone, Edinburgh, p. 8.

> The National Hospital for the Paralysed and Epileptic is opened for the reception of patients. Under the influence of Dr Brown-Séquard, it cannot fail to exercise an important influence on the progress of our knowledge on the pathology of these diseases and to lead to a more scientific treatment.[20]

It was the first hospital exclusively founded for the care and treatment of nervous disorders as well as the first to charge a weekly fee to patients who could afford to pay. Patients who were poor, were admitted free of charge. Over the years, the Hospital's reputation grew rapidly. Within 3 years, the second floor at 24, Queen Square was converted into a ten-bed ward and by 1864, the purchase of an adjoining house increased its bed capacity to 36.[21]

The National Hospital aroused the interest of many physicians. William Ferguson offered his services as a consultant. John Zachariah Laurence competed for and, ultimately, was appointed to the post of active surgeon. He was a general surgeon who had moved into ophthalmology. In 1857, he established the **South London Ophthalmic Hospital**, later to be known as the **Royal Eye Hospital**. Collaborating with Moon, his assistant, he described the **Laurence-Moon syndrome**, a progressive debilitating condition, starting in childhood and marked by mental deficiency and perturbation of night vision, culminating in blindness. The first physician to be appointed, three weeks prior to Brown-Séquard, was Jabez Spencer Ramskill. His appointment might have owed something to nepotism.

Brown-Séquard's attendance at the new hospital began in April 1860, when the first patients had been admitted. His position carried no salary and he soon engaged in private practice. At first, he practised at 82 Wimpole Street, moving later to the more fashionable 25 Cavendish Square, as his clientèle grew. Little is known about the identity of his patients, but it is certain that he saw members of the aristocracy and gentry. One of his known patients was the daughter of George Campbell, the eighth duke of Argyll.

Brown-Séquard arranged to deliver a course of lectures at the National Hospital, at least once a week.[22] The Hospital records of May 17, 1860, show that his lectures were to be "advertised in The Lancet, Medical Journal and Times for a month."[23] They had, however, already come to the attention of the medical press, having been mentioned in The Lancet of May 12, in the following terms:

> We are glad to direct the attention of our readers to the announcement of a Course of Clinical Lectures on Paralysis and Epilepsy, to be delivered at the National Hospital for the Paralysed and Epileptics by Dr Brown-Séquard. By this means, the full pathological and therapeutic value of this institution will acquire its utmost development. The instructions of the distinguished physiologist and physician will be sought with eagerness and profit.[24]

---

[20] Lancet (1860) National Hospital for the Paralysed and Epileptic, 1: 328.

[21] Anonymous (1960) Queen Square and the National Hospital 1860–1960. Edward Arnold Ltd, London, pp. 6–7.

[22] Gooddy, *op. cit.*, note 14, above.

[23] *Ibid.* p. 191.

[24] Lancet (1860) Clinical Lectures on Paralysis and Epilepsy, 1: 475.

Entries in the minutes of the Management Board show that Brown-Séquard attended meetings fairly regularly and that he was concerned with the development of the Hospital and the quality of care for the patients. On April 19, 1860, he requested medical instruments for the physicians and it was agreed that "they procure such as are necessary..."[25] That October, he requested facilities for physical therapy and electro-therapy for rehabilitation purposes.[26]

There is an interesting entry in the minutes of the Management Board's meeting of June 7, 1860, which reveals his stance on a question of medical ethics. He asked that the "names of the Physicians shall not be published nor allusion made to their cure in future advertisements."[27] There had been some highly praiseworthy comments about him in the lay press and in some minor medical periodicals, and even like the following which appeared in The Lancet::

> The great success of this much-needed Hospital for the Paralysed and Epileptic, is mainly owing, under PROVIDENCE, to its chief Physician, Dr Brown-Séquard, of Wimpole Street, who, perhaps, in the peculiar class of cases for the treatment of which the National Hospital is exclusively set apart, has no living rival in Europe or the world.[28]

The Fellowship of the Royal College of Physicians of London was conferred upon Brown-Séquard in May 1860. This College, the oldest of the medical colleges of the United Kingdom, was founded in 1518 by Thomas Linacre, physician to Henry VIII. On June 7 of the same year, Brown-Séquard was elected a Fellow of the Royal Society which is, in fact, the national academy of sciences of Great Britain. The Society was founded in 1610 and its Charter was granted by Charles II in 1663. Brown-Séquard's nomination was supported by Neil Arnott, to whom he had appealed for help when applying for a physicianship at the National Hospital. The other supporters were: William Carpenter, the physiologist and naturalist; James Paget and the surgeon-anatomist, Francis Sibson. Thus, within a year of taking residence in London, Brown-Séquard had received two of the highest scientific distinctions that Great Britain had to offer.

A year after being awarded these two distinctions, he was chosen to deliver both the Gulstonian and the Croonian Lectures. In February 1861, he delivered six **Gulstonian Lectures** at the Royal College of Physicians in Pall Mall East, dealing with **Symptoms of Brain Disease**. They were published from July to December 1861 by **The Lancet** under the title "Lectures on the diagnosis and treatment of the various forms of Paralytic, Convulsive and Mental Affections, considered as effects of morbid alterations of the blood, or of the brain or other organs."[29] The

---

[25] Gooddy, *op. cit.*, note 14, above.

[26] *Ibid.*

[27] *Ibid.*

[28] Lancet (1860) 21st Apr.

[29] The subtitle was: Being a continuation of the Gulstonian Lectures, delivered at the Royal College of Physicians in February 1861 and of the Clinical Lectures at the National Hospital for the Paralysed and Epileptics. 1–2, 29–30, 55–56, 79–80, 153–154, 199–200, 391–392, 415–416, 611–613.

Lectures were a legacy of Theodor Gulston, a sixteenth century physician, who left a sum of money to the Royal College of Physicians for a Lecture to be delivered each year by one of its youngest physicians. It has been read annually since 1639.

On May 16, 1861, Brown-Séquard delivered the Croonian Lecture to the Royal Society. Its subject was **On the Relation between Muscular Irritability, Cadaveric Rigidity and Putrefaction**,[30] in which he sought to establish a law which he had enunciated, namely:

> The greater the degree of muscular irritability at the time of death, the later the cadaveric rigidity sets in and the longer it lasts, and the later also putrefaction appears and the slower it progresses.

This Lecture derives its name from Croone or Croune, a physician of the sixteenth century, who had planned to found two Lectureships: one to be read annually before the Royal Society and the other to be delivered before the Royal College of Physicians at the same time as a sermon was being preached at the Church of St Mary-le-Bow.

In 1862, an assistant-physician was needed at the National Hospital, and John Hughlings Jackson was appointed on Brown-Sequard's recommendations. The Hospital records of May 1862, gives no hint of the role that the latter played in influencing the career of a man, who was later to be known as the **Father of British Modern Neurology**. Jackson was appointed "on the understanding that he should visit the Hospital twice a day and see the out-patients at their homes…"[31]

John Hughlings Jackson was born in Yorkshire, the son of a small landowner. In 1852, he entered the Medical School at York, where the neurologist Thomas Laycock was the most distinguished of its teachers.

The latter had studied physiology and anatomy under Alfred Armand Louis Marie Velpeau and Jacques Lisfranc in Paris. In 1844, he formulated the theory of reflex action of the brain. Jackson graduated from York in 1856 and made his way to London. There, Jonathan Hutchinson, a physician from the same school in York, though several years older than him, had to dissuade him from giving up medicine for philosophy.

How Jackson came to make the acquaintance of Brown-Séquard is not known, but it must have been soon after his removal from York to London. There is no doubt whatsoever of the influence that he had on the future medical orientation of the younger man. This is how Hutchinson sums up his role:

> Although I claim credit for having retained Hughlings Jackson for medicine, I did not specialise him. My friend,… fell under the influence of Dr Brown-Séquard, who told him strongly that it was foolish to waste his efforts in wide observation of disease in general and that if he wished to attain anything, he must keep to the nervous system.[32]

---

[30] Brown-Séquard CE (1860) On the relationship between muscular irritability, cadaveric rigidity and putrefaction. Proc Roy Soc Med 11: 204–214, 1860–1862.

[31] Gooddy, *op. cit.*, note 14, above, p. 192.

[32] Hutchinson J (1911) The late Dr Hughlings Jackson. Recollection of a lifetime friendship. Br Med J 1: 151–154.

Brown-Séquard's advice to Hughlings Jackson, reinforcing that of Thomas Laycock, was his greatest contribution to British neurology. It led to Jackson spending nearly all of his professional life at the National Hospital, where his genius ensured him such an important place in medical history. His name lives on in a form of epilepsy, the Jacksonian type, which was thus named by Charcot,[33] even though it had been described, in 1827, by Louis François Bravais under the name of hemiplegic epilepsy.[34] Jacksonian seizures begin in one part of the body such as a limb and then spread to other parts or even to the whole body.

In 1863, Brown-Séquard resigned his post at the National Hospital and its records of July 15th of that year note: "Dr. Brown-Séquard stated that he intended to give up practice in this country and was reluctantly compelled to withdraw from the Hospital..."[35] Soon after, the Management Board elected him Honorary Physician.

The story goes that he decided to resign his post on an impulse he felt looking through the window of his house in Cavendish Square. He was overawed to see the square full of carriages of his wealthy patients and felt suddenly as though he was wasting his time practising medicine and neglecting his scientific research work. Whether one can rely on these actual details is doubtful, but there is certainly a germ of truth in the suggestion that he left London in order to concentrate on experimental work. Writing long after the event, he said:

> My success was much too great. Charcot, Vulpian and Rouget who saw me in London in 1861 and 62 could tell you that my patients oppressed me and that I had not a minute to spare for science. It was intolerable, however pleasant and useful it was to earn stacks of guineas. I called a halt to the gold digging.[36]

To a colleague, he said that "he was making too much money and did not wish to demoralise his only son by leaving wealth."[37] To others, he said that he had been worried about his health and was totally exhausted by the busy life that he had led. Probably, a more important reason than all these was Ellen's rapidly failing health. Moreover, she wanted to leave Europe and settle in The United States and was anxious to see her only child brought up as an American citizen.[38]

Brown-Séquard's resignation and eventual departure from London brought surprise and disappointment. The Lancet echoed the thoughts of many when it said:

> ... imperfect health, an unconquerable love of purely scientific research, and a desire to revisit the continent to which he is most bound by family ties, have taken Dr Brown-

[33] Jackson JH (1881) Epileptiform convulsions from cerebral disease. Trans Int Med 2: 6–15.

[34] Bravais LF (1827) Recherches sur les symptômes et le traitement de l'épilepsie hémiplégique. Thèse pour le Doctorat en médecine, N° 118, Paris.

[35] Gooddy, *op. cit.*, note 14, above.

[36] Brown-Séquard CE (n.d.) Autobiographical letter. GMcCC, Ms 994/2.

[37] Note in pencil, unidentified handwriting. GMcCC.

[38] Brown-Séquard CE (1858) Letter to his wife, Ellen. GMcCC, Ms 977/17, 17th May.

Séquard from this metropolis, where his success as a practitioner was rapid and lucrative beyond precedent, and where he quickly acquired a large circle of warm friends.[39]

However, if his resignation was a disappointment for his colleagues and a greater one still for his numerous patients, it came as no surprise to his cousin Henry J Feltus. As early as April 1862, Brown-Séquard was complaining to him about his dislike of English weather, of his poor health, of his recurring headaches, of depressive moods on dull days and of his anxiety at earning too much money. In answer to one of his letters, his cousin wrote back, on April 11, 1862:

> The accounts of your health are the cause of great anxiety on the part of all here in our family - to be depressed for the sake of pecuniary advantage would be but a sorry result. It is hoped that with the returning pleasant seasons of the year you may find much improvement.[40]

On the eve of his departure from London, late in 1863, he was very depressed, blaming the arrival of autumn for his alternating buoyant and melancholic moods, for his anxiety, his headaches and his dyspepsia. He wrote to Feltus, receiving the following reply on November 12, 1863:

> I wish your next letter will bring better tidings, though I have some apprehension that such may not be the case, as the climate of England does not seem to agree with you excepting in the summer months. There is also the thought that your mind is overtaxed at the expense of such relaxation as may be necessary for your health. Would that you were prosperous, joyous & happy. But the fortunes and chances of life are coupled with circumstances which are seldom at our option or bidding.[41]

His stay of over three and a half years in London was the longest he had stayed in a post. Only 15 years later, when he was appointed Professor of Medicine at the Collège de France, did he exceed this. He made few friends in England, but strengthened existing ties with many of his colleagues. Through his association with the National Hospital, he kept in touch with Hughlings Jackson,[42] with Edward Henry Sieveking,[43] who joined the Hospital after the expansion of 1864, and with Thomas Buzzard,[44] who was elected a consultant physician to the Hospital in 1896.

Brown-Séquard struck a lasting friendship with Thomas Henry Huxley, the most influential scientist of his time. The former was present at the acrimonious debate of the recently formulated Theory of Evolution, during the meeting of the British Association for the Advancement of Science at Oxford in 1861. In the course of the meeting, Huxley, on replying to Samuel Wilberforce, Bishop of

---

39 Lancet (1864) 2: 719.

40 Feltus HJ (1862) Letter to Brown-Séquard. GMcCC, Ms 981/154, 11th Apr.

41 Feltus HJ (1863) Letter to Brown-Séquard. GMcCC, Ms 981/158, 12th Nov.

42 Jackson JH (1866) Letter to Brown-Séquard. GMcCC, Ms 980/22, 27th Jan.

43 Sieveking EH (1868) Letter to Brown-Séquard. GMcCC, Ms 980/11, 29th May.

44 Brown-Séquard CE (1868) Letter to Thomas Buzzard. Correspondence, Buzzard's file, Letter 5 & 9. Archives of the Library of the Royal College of Physicians of London.

Worcester, and an influential prelate and a ferocious opponent of the **Theory of Evolution**, said:

> If then,... the question is put to me would I rather have a miserable ape for a grandfather or a man endowed by nature and possessed of great means of influence... I would, unhesitatingly, affirm my preference for the ape.[45]

Huxley writing to Darwin said:

> He [Brown-Séquard] is a thoroughly good man, and told me it was worth while to come all the way to Oxford to hear the Bishop pummelled.[46]

Brown-Séquard met Charles Robert Darwin for the first time in 1858. The latter was the grandson of Erasmus Darwin, one of the precursors of **Transformism**, that is the concept of the slow and gradual transformation of animals and plants in the course of geological aeons. In his work **Zoonomia or the Laws of Organic Life**, published in 1794, he advanced an evolutionary theory which stated that the environment has a direct influence on the changes that occur in an organism, a conception of evolution not unlike that of Jean-Baptiste Pierre Antoine Monet, chevalier de Lamarck. Moreover, he was the first, before his grandson, to create the concept of survival of the fittest, when he wrote in his above-mentioned work: "the strongest and most active animal should propagate the species, which should thence become improved."

In November 1859, Charles Darwin, supposedly not inspired by his grandfather's writings, published his famous book: **The Origin of Species by Means of Natural Selection** and found himself very much in need of friends, for his work made enemies among scientists and churchmen. The champions of Immutability or Fixity—that is the theory that since their creation all living organisms have remained unaltered—among them the anatomist and palaeontologist Richard Owen, were bitterly opposed to Darwin's concept of natural selection and, likewise the clergy who maintained that the story of the Creation as expounded in the first chapter of Genesis of the Old Testament, was a divine act and therefore an indisputable one.

Brown-Séquard volunteered to review The Origin of Species in a French periodical. It would be no overstatement to say that Darwin was overcome with joy. He wrote to Brown-Séquard saying:

> I am extremely grateful to hear that you intend noticing my book in some French periodical.... I shall be truly glad to read any criticism from one who stands so very high in one of the highest branches of Science as you stand.[47]

---

[45] Bibby (1972) Scientist extraordinary. The life and scientific work of Thomas Huxley 1825–1895. Pergamon Press, Oxford, p. 141.

[46] Huxley L (1901) Life and letters of Thomas Henry Huxley, vol. 1. Appleton & Co., New York, p. 221.

[47] Darwin C (1861) Letter to Brown-Séquard. GMcCC, Ms 981/96, Jan.

Darwin wrote again to him, four months later, to let him know that a translation of The Origin of Species had been published in French, adding:

> You say in your note "that few men are so near agreeing with you as I am", I cannot tell you how this has pleased me, for I look with profound interest for the judgement of such men as yourself. I have not the least doubt that I have erred most seriously on many points, but now so many (yet few) really good judges concur in the main with me, that I do not fear that some such view will ultimately prevail not withstanding all the abuse and ridicule poured on me.[48]

On Brown-Séquard's resignation from the National Hospital, Hughlings Jackson immediately applied for the post. He was unsuccessful this time and once more in 1864, when two physicians were required. It was not until 1867 that he finally attained the position. Brown-Séquard's successor was Charles Bland Radcliffe of whom it has been written that "he erected no milestone in the progress of medicine, nor indeed added anything to nascent Neurology." He also took over Brown-Séquard's house at Cavendish Square which, much later on, was also occupied by Victor Alexander Haden Horsley. It is interesting to note that, in 1864, another young and promising Mauritian was elected Physician to the National Hospital. This was Pierre Victor Lanougarède Bazire, who occupied this post until his death in 1867.

Although the years that Brown-Séquard spent in London were not really productive for his research work, looking after patients in the National Hospital and at his private practice did make him into an eminent clinician. His lectures contained no new facts, but he did contribute a section entitled **Diseases of the Nerves** to Timothy Holme's four-volume treatise: **A System of Surgery Theoretical and Practical, in Treatises by Various Authors.**[49] A classic of its day whose contributors included some of the most distinguished physicians and surgeons of the time, such as Joseph Lister, who not only introduced carbolic acid as an antiseptic in his operating theatre, but was the first, in 1878, to grow a bacterium in pure culture: **Listeria monocytogenes**. It is present in the environment, producing symptomless lingering infections and is particularly dangerous in pregnant women, causing spontaneous abortion, but also in the unborn child, resulting in stillbirths, premature births or babies born suffering from meningo-encephalitis.

Brown-Séquard left London in November 1862 for Paris. His presence at the Queen Square's Hospital—nowadays known as **The National Hospital for Neurology and Neurosurgery**—contributed to its celebrity.

---

[48] Darwin C (1861) Letter to Brown-Séquard. GMcCC, Ms 981/97, 16th Apr.

[49] Published in London, 1860–1864.

# Chapter 13
# The Harvard Professor: 1864–1867

After leaving London in November 1863, Brown-Séquard spent 6 months in Paris.[1] His intention, however, was to go to The United States to seek an appointment to a professorship. While still working at the National Hospital, he had, the previous May, applied for the Chair of the Institute of Medicine at the University of Pennsylvania. The vacancy had arisen after the resignation of Samuel Jackson, an academic colleague of Professor George Bacon Wood, to whom Paul Broca had written on behalf of Brown-Sequard in 1852. Silas Weir Mitchell was another applicant for the Chair, but it was the third contender, Francis Gurney Smith, an obstetrician, who was appointed.[2]

Brown-Séquard had several reasons for wanting to work in The States. First, there was his wife's desire to live there and to see her son brought up as an American citizen.[3] Then, there was his still precarious financial situation. Despite his success and his monetary gains in London, he was still far from being well off, as he himself wrote:

> Although I had earned a tremendous amount of money in London, I had also enormous expenses, outstanding debts to pay, some of my wife's relatives to assist and other expenses. I had to think of the future and I again left for The United States in March 1864.[4]

But, despite these financial preoccupations, he was not about to compromise his principles. The family stopped in London, in March 1864, en route for Liverpool, where they would take the boat to America. In London, he received a telegram offering him 200 guineas to visit a patient in Liverpool. He replied that he would be in that city the day after tomorrow and he would see the patient for his normal fee of five guineas.[5] A similar situation occurred later in life, when he was Professor of Medicine at the Collège de France. He was asked by Governor Hanford

---

[1] Brown-Séquard CE (n.d.) Autobiographical letter. GMcCC, Ms 994/2.

[2] Corner GW (1965) Two Centuries of Medicine, University of Pennsylvania. J.B. Lippincott, p. 121. Also Konke BA (1997) Standard History of the Medical Profession of Philadelphia, 2nd edn. AMS Press, Philadelphia, p. 243.

[3] Brown-Séquard CE (1858) Letter to his wife, Ellen. GMcCC, Ms 977/17, 17th May.

[4] Brown-Séquard, *op. cit.*, note 1, above.

[5] La République Française (1894) Désintéressement d'un grand savant. Paris, 19th Apr.

L.-C. Celestin, *Charles-Edouard Brown-Séquard*,
DOI: 10.1007/978-3-319-03020-3_13, 

of California[6] to go to Venice to see his son who was sick. He replied that he was not the appropriate specialist for such an affection. Hanford was not satisfied with this answer and offered him £10,000, but he was unmoved, insisting that he could be of no help.[7]

On June 7, 1864, some 10 weeks after arriving in Boston, Brown-Séquard was unanimously elected a member of the Massachusetts General Hospital.[8] The Civil War, also known as the War of Secession was raging between the Union (the North) and the Confederacy (the South) and on June 14th, Brown-Séquard lectured at the Smithsonian Institution to an audience composed mainly of army surgeons. His lecture on **Hospital Practice** dealt with the care of the wounded. Namely, the emergency measures to stop or slow down the loss of blood from haemorrhages due to arterial injuries; the treatment of tetanus: cleansing and disinfecting the wounds with a solution of calcium chloride and administration of potassium bromide to attenuate the painful muscular contractions; the use of prolonged and continuous irrigation of burns with tepid water; the surgical procedures to be adopted in cases of spinal injuries caused by fracture of the spine, such as the removal of bone fragments pressing upon the spinal cord.[9] This was a subject which had been dealt with in his book **Course of Lectures on the Physiology and Pathology of the Nervous System.**[10] It was a theme he referred to, in 1863, in a letter to The Lancet, entitled "Trephining in cases of Fractures of the Spine", in which he said that he had tried

> to prove that in cases of fracture of the spine, trephining and other operations for the removal of pieces of bones pressing upon the spinal cord might be employed with great benefit to many patients. This view is based upon many experiments I have made on animals, and on sixteen or seventeen cases in which the operation has been performed on man.[11]

The Smithsonian Institution, where he delivered his lecture, was founded in early 1864 with a legacy from Jack Smithson, the illegitimate son of the Earl of Northumberland. His whole fortune of half a million dollars was bequeathed to The United States to found "an establishment for the increase of knowledge among men,"[12] in Washington.

Brown-Séquard made it known that he was interested in an academic chair anywhere in The States. On the initiative of Jean Louis Rodolphe Agassiz, the Corporation of Harvard Medical School, voted for the establishment of a **Professorship of the Physiology and Pathology of the Nervous System**. Agassiz

---

[6] McCausland C (n.d.) Notebook in her handwriting. GMcCC, Ms 999/7, p. 91.

[7] *Ibid*, p. 57.

[8] Dexter Mrs (1864) Letter to Brown-Séquard. GMcCC, Ms 984/12, 7th June.

[9] Brown-Séquard CE (1864) Stenographic transcript of lecture delivered at the Smithsonian Institute. GMcCC, Ms 991, 14th June.

[10] pp. 224–260.

[11] Brown-Séquard CE (1863) Trephining in cases of fracture of the spine. Lancet 1: 477.

[12] Leskind MC (1958) The Evolution of medical research in the United States, In: Martin-Ibanez History of American Medicine. A Symposium. M.D. Publishers, New York, p. 123.

strongly recommended Brown-Séquard's candidature[13] who, at the time, he was still not acquainted with.[14] Apparently, it was senator Charles Sumner who, as a member of the same Saturday Club as Agassiz, had drawn the latter's attention to Brown-Séquard's merits.[15]

Agassiz, the eminent geologist, zoologist and palaeontologist, was born in Switzerland. He qualified as Doctor of Philosophy in 1829. He had been the pupil of Frédéric Cuvier at **Le Jardin des Plantes** (later to be known as **Le Muséum national d'histoire naturelle**) in Paris. By the age of thirty, he had achieved a worldwide reputation. In 1846, on the initiative of John Amory Lowell, he was appointed to the Chair of Zoology and Geology at Harvard College. There, he devoted his spare time to raising considerable sums of money for a Museum of Comparative Zoology. His first wife died in 1848 and he remarried in 1850. His second wife was Elizabeth Cabot Cary, who came from an influential Boston family. Popularising Science, through his public lectures and numerous writings, he became a public figure and is held to be the Father of Zoology in The United States.

Brown-Séquard was invited to present his candidature for the new chair. He did so, enclosing with his letter of application for the post, a printed list of all his original papers in chronological order from 1846 to 1863.[16] He was chosen as the titular professor by ballot.[17] He notified the Corporation of Harvard of his acceptance on June 25th, stating that he would "spare no effort to justify the confidence in my usefulness shown by the Corporation."[18] The Boston Medical and Surgical Journal welcomed his "permanent settlement in Cambridge."[19]

The duties of the new professor were "to be such as may be determined from time to time, and the compensation of the Professor to be derived from fees."[20] At that time, professors, in medical schools, had no fixed income, having to support

---

13 Lurie E (n.d.) Louis Agassiz A Life in Science. The University of Chicago Press, Chicago, p. 368.

14 Marcou J (1896) Life, letters and works of Louis Agassiz, vol 2. Macmillan & Co., New York, p. 158.

15 Agassiz EC (1887) Louis Agassiz: Sa Vie et sa correspondence. Traduit de l'anglais par Auguste Meyer. Librairie Fischbacher, Paris, pp. 428–429.

16 Brown-Séquard CE (1864) Notice sur les travaux originaux (spécialement de physiologie) du Dr Brown-Séquard. Mason et Cie, Paris.

17 Corporation of Harvard Medical School (1864) Letter to Brown-Séquard. GMcCC, Ms 984/14, June.

18 Brown-Séquard CE (1864, 15th June). HML/CLC(Harvard Medical Library/Countway Library Collection). Quoted by Tyler HR & Tyler KR. Charles-Edouard Brown-Séquard: Professor of physiology and pathology of the nervous system at Harvard Medical School. Neurology 34: 1231–1236.

19 Quoted by Olmsted JMD (1946) Charles-Edouard Brown-Séquard. A nineteenth century neurologist and endocrinologist. The John Hopkins Press, Baltimore, p. 120.

20 Harrington RF (1905) The Harvard Medical School. A history, narrative and documentary, vol 2. Lewis Publishing CO, New York, p. 543.

themselves by private practice and through lectures which were paid for by the students.

In the 1860s, Physiology at the Harvard Medical School was part of Anatomy and the responsibility of the Parkman Professor, the poet-anatomist, Oliver Wendell Holmes. It was not taught as a science in its own right, but confined to topics such as Respiration and Circulation of the blood. Lectures were combined with practical demonstrations, but there was no laboratory, where the students could carry out their own experiments.

Tragically, within three months of his nomination, Brown-Séquard lost his wife. The exact date of Ellen's death is not known, but judging from a letter of sympathy of Henry J Feltus to her husband,[21] she must have passed away some time during the first half of September 1864. Her exact age, at the time of her death, is not known. She must have been between 32 and 34 years old. She had never enjoyed good health. There have been hints that she suffered from consumption, the wasting disease which, in those days, was due to tuberculosis of the lungs. Moreover, she had a chronic knee effusion which needed removal of the purulent fluid by puncture from time to time.[22] This accumulation of fluid could also have been due to an underlying tuberculous infection. The previous July, she had had a severe bout of rheumatism and had been in great pain. This condition was chronic, having been first mentioned during her stay in Mauritius, in 1854.

There was intermittent correspondence between her and her husband when away from each other between 1853 and 1863. Apart from a few letters that she wrote to her family, in 1854–1856, while staying in Mauritius and Richmond, no other of her letters are available. However, in the period from 1856 to 1859. Brown-Séquard wrote her a total of 41 letters, most of them in reply to hers, from New York, Philadelphia, Charleston, London, Edinburgh, Glasgow and Dublin.[23]

It is possible that the disappearance of her letters was a deliberate, praiseworthy, but regrettable move to protect Brown-Séquard's memory, as their contents would have revealed Ellen's deep unhappiness.

The picture that emerges of the 11 years of married life of the couple is of a wretched existence due to the husband's mental instability. Ellen had to live with a spouse who was always ready to sacrifice a position, a home and the comfort it afforded, as well as the stability of their relationship for the pursuit of an illusion.

Prior to each visit abroad, however short, Brown-Séquard ended the lease of his apartment or house, and stored all his belongings in a furniture depository. From January 1856 to July 1857—an 18-month period—the couple had, three times, moved houses from rue du Dragon to rue Monsieur-le-Prince and from there to Bellevue-sur-Meudon, Seine et Oise. Lacking a permanent abode, they had letter boxes all over Paris: at Broca's home and service at the **Bicêtre** Hospital, at Laverdant's and Tholozan's addresses and even at the **Société de biologie**. Over a

[21] Feltus HJ (1862) Letter to Brown-Séquard. GMcCC, Ms 981/133, 19th Sept.

[22] Brown-Séquard CE (1859) Letter to his wife, Ellen. GMcCC, Ms 977/30 and 977/32, 5th and 6th.

[23] Brown-Séquard CE (1852–1864) Letter to his wife, Ellen. GMcCC, Mss 977/1–43.

period of 12 years from 1853 to 1865, Brown-Séquard's, friends in Mauritius, including his godfather, Emile Gausseran, addressed letters "To Brown-Séquard: care of D. Laverdant."

The lack of money was chronic. The rent often remained unpaid and, to avoid the couple being thrown out on the streets, friends intervened. The lenders were Désiré Laverdant, Charles Marie Benjamin Rouget, Charles Robin, Paul Broca, Joseph Tholozan, the Banking Firm of Donon, Aubray, Gautier and Cie., and even Mason, the well-known Medical Publishing House. In 1858, while on a lecture tour in England, Brown-Séquard, in reply to a letter of Ellen, tells her to go and see Mason père and borrow money from him, to pay the maid's wages! Money was sent by telegraphic transfers from Mauritius by his childhood friend, Jules Chauvin and by his godfather, Emile Gausseran and likewise from America by his cousin, Henry J Feltus. It is said that, during his stay in London, from 1860 to 1863, his earnings exceeded 10,000 guineas, and that three-fifths of that sum was used to clear outstanding debts, some dating as far back as 1848.

In most of his letters to Ellen, Brown-Séquard complains of his headaches, his insomnia, his mood swings, his tiredness and his depression; but when his wife mentions that she is unwell, he shows neither sympathy, nor understanding. In reply to one of Ellen's letters, he admonishes her for suffering from menorrhagia—excessive loss of blood at the monthly period—because she has probably not taken, as she should, some ergot of rye. This parasitic fungus of rye and wheat, **Claviceps purpura**, was used in the nineteenth century as a vasoconstrictor in the management of bleeding from the uterus. Ellen's married life was far from a happy one and the worries and financial difficulties that she experienced on a daily basis, may well have hastened her untimely death.

Her passing affected her husband considerably and triggered a prolonged bout of depression. He complained that his health was not good enough for him to prepare for his forthcoming lectures at the Medical School. So much so, that at a Faculty meeting, at the end of September 1864, it was agreed to release him from any academic duty during the next 2 or 3 months.[24]

But the next 3 months did nothing to improve his health. In November, he informed the Dean of the Medical School, George Cheyne Shattuck, that he intended to resign his professorship, saying that he had given up "altogether the idea of ever being able to deliver a full course of lectures."[25] He complained of constant headaches and of intolerable friction between himself and Ellen's in-laws. He was unhappy about the way they had behaved towards her, during the last days of her life.[26] Hinting that he might be leaving America in the near future,[27] his

[24] Minutes and Records of the Faculty of Medicine, Harvard Medical School 5th September 1864. HML/CLC. Quoted by Tyler & Tyler, *op. cit.*, note 18, above, p. 1233.

[25] Brown-Séquard CE (15th Nov, 1864) Letter to Shattuck. HML/CLC. Quoted by Tyler & Tyler, *op. cit.*, note 18, above, p. 1233.

[26] *Ibid.*

[27] *Ibid.*

resignation was accepted by the Faculty, on November 17. A letter was sent to him, deploring his decision and wishing him a prompt recovery.[28] The Dean reported to the Harvard Overseers, on December 28, 1864, that it was doubtful that Brown-Séguard would "be able to assure the duties of his department."[29]

However, at the beginning of January 1865, he spontaneously offered to deliver a lecture on the physiological effects of a lesion of the lateral half of the spinal cord. His offer was readily accepted, but it is not known whether the lecture was ever given[30] as he had sailed to France by the end of the month. On the way, he stopped in Dublin, where he lectured at the College of Physicians of Ireland, on February 3, 1865. The subject of his lecture was On the **Importance of Physiology to the Practice of Medicine and Surgery**.[31]

He did not return to Harvard for the next 21 months, between January 1865 and September 1866, residing some time in Paris and some time in London. During the whole of his absence from Cambridge, he corresponded with his cousin, Henry J Feltus and with Dean Shattuck. As early as March 1865, he wrote to the latter, telling him of his intention of "returning to America and assuming my duties as professor."[32] This letter was followed by several others of a highly fanciful nature. On March 17, he wrote to Shattuck that he would be returning to The States

> ... to establish a Physiological and Pathological Institute, combining the most important features of Virchow's, Du Bois-Reymond's and Valentine's Institutes with those of Claude Bernard's laboratory. I will return to America quite prepared for the establishment of such an institute on a larger scientific and practical scale than that of any in the Old World, and I will spend all the money necessary to buy the expensive instruments and apparatus. ... Would it be possible to have a building erected at my own expense?[33]

Shattuck wrote back to discourage him with the various difficulties such a scheme would throw up. For example, he wrote that there was a lack of ground space for a building and suggested that the plans be put back for a year.[34] Brown-Séquard replied, on April 28th, that he had no objection to postponing the building of a laboratory,[35] so long as he could be provided with enough space in the College for his own research work. But still, he persisted in detailing his plans for the

[28] Harvard Medical Faculty Committee (18th No, 1864) Letter to Brown-Séquard. Quoted by Tyler & Tyler, *op. cit.*, note 18, above, p. 1233.

[29] Shattuck GD (28th Dec, 1864) Report to the Board of Overseers. Overseers Report, Harvard Archives. Quoted by Tyler & Tyler, *op. cit.*, note 18, above, p. 1233.

[30] Minutes and Records of the Faculty of Medicine (7th Jan, 1865). HML/CLC. Quoted by Tyler & Tyler, *op. cit.*, note 18, above, p. 1233.

[31] Published by John Falconer in Dublin in 1865.

[32] Brown-Séquard CE (17th March, 1865) Letter to Shattuck. HML/CLC. Quoted by Tyler & Tyler, *op. cit.*, note 18, above, p. 1233.

[33] Tyler & Tyler, *op. cit.*, note 18, above, p. 1233.

[34] Shattuck GC (6th Apr, 1865) Letter to Brown-Séquard. HML/CLC. Quoted by Tyler & Tyler, *op. cit.*, note 18, above, p. 1233–1234.

[35] Brown-Séquard CE (28th Apr, 1865) Letter to Shattuck. HML/CLC. Quoted by Tyler & Tyler, *op. cit.*, note 18, above, pp. 1233–1234.

institute and the work that would be undertaken there. This would include: repeating all the experiments previously carried out by other experimental physiologists and pathologists; new experiments to solve the unanswered questions of physiology, medicine and surgery and the study of a score of topics such as the transplantation of organs, epilepsy, diabetes and the consequences of ablation of organs.[36]

By June 1865, his health had deteriorated. He wrote to Shattuck on the 13th, telling him that his headaches had recurred and he would not be able to purchase the apparatuses and instruments for the proposed institute.[37] Likewise, he informed his cousin of his decision not to return to America, to which the latter replied on June 23rd:

> Your decision not to return to America till next year is a disappointment but your reasons are sensible. To undertake such duties as you would have to perform at fixed days and hours would require perfect health and, by attempting it before you were fully recovered, might be the means of a permanent breakdown.[38]

On July 7th, he informed the Dean that he was preparing his course of lectures and would be back in Cambridge by the 20th October.[39] He then wrote to Henry J Feltus that, after a short visit to England, he would be lodging at Asnière, a suburb of Paris.[40] On September 15th, however, he tendered his resignation once again, in a letter to Shattuck which invoked his poor health as a reason.[41] This letter was the last he wrote to the Harvard Medical School in 1865. Late in that year, he delivered a lecture in London on the **Recent Advances of Our Knowledge in the Diagnosis and Treatment of Functional Nervous Affections**, which he enlarged for publication in The Lancet from January to March 1866.[42]

In June 1866, he wrote to his cousin, complaining of his bad health. He was suffering from insomnia, headaches and dyspepsia, and received the following reply:

> Your headaches still continue—and perhaps must continue till you have some fixed plan of enjoying recreations at short intervals and thus be relieved, in some measure, from the constant strain of mind.[43]

[36] *Ibid.*

[37] Brown-Séquard CE (13th June, 1865) Letter to Shattuck. HML/CLC. Quoted by Tyler & Tyler, *op. cit.*, note 18, above, p. 1234.

[38] Feltus HJ (23rd June, 1865) Letter to Brown-Séquard. GMcCC, Ms 981/162.

[39] Brown-Séquard CE (7th July, 1865) Letter to Shattuck. HML/CLC. Quoted by Tyler & Tyler, *op. cit.*, note 18, above, p. 1234.

[40] Feltus HJ (18th Aug, 1865) Letter to Brown-Séquard. GMcCC, Ms 981/164.

[41] Brown-Séquard CE (15th Sept, 1865) Letter to Shattuck. HML/CLC. Quoted by Tyler & Tyler, *op. cit.*, note 18, above, p. 1234.

[42] Lancet (1866) 1: 1–2, 85–87, 139–141, 247–250.

[43] Feltus HJ (12th June, 1866) Letter to Brown-Séquard. GMcCC, Ms 981/163.

His first letter of that year to Shattuck, since the previous one in September 1865, was on July 23, 1866, in which he said: "after reflection, … it would be better for me to deliver my lectures."[44]

This period of his life, following Ellen's death, when he was separated from his son, who was in a boarding school in Boston, was very unsettling for him, as his erratic correspondence with Dean Shattuck reveals. Désiré Laverdant wrote about this period of his life in the Mauritian newspaper, **Le Cernéen**:

> For his only relief from his worries he had his work, and that work extended to 20 h a day. Never did this mind, consumed by thirst for science, allowed him the distraction of a show, a concert, an evening in town, or even a stroll.[45]

In fact, an anecdote from that half year or so he spent in London, illustrates the extremity of his state of mind. He was staying at Victor Bazire's house, who was a Physician to the National Hospital. The story comes from the Mauritian pharmacist, Eugène Curé, who heard it from his father, also a chemist, who had lived at Bazire's house, where he stayed, for the duration of his pharmaceutical studies in London from 1865 to 1867. He often accompanied Brown-Séquard to a shop in Tottenham Court Road, which sold guinea-pigs, helping him to carry them back. So devoted was Brown-Séquard to his experiments on these animals that he could not understand how anyone could spare time for anything but scientific investigations. As Bazire was married to the daughter of the Convent Garden Theatre's orchestra leader, he often invited Curé to accompany him to concerts; but it was necessary to take meticulous precautions so that Brown-Séquard would not know of their escapade. They had the cab stop some way from the house and took inordinate care to enter or leave the house, without Brown-Séquard noticing them. The secrecy could not go on forever though, and he eventually found out and severely admonished the culprits over breakfast.[46]

There were, however, at least some positive developments in these otherwise depressing years. In January 1866, while he was in Paris, Brown-Séquard heard, from Hippolyte Larrey, that he had been elected a Foreign Corresponding Member of the Paris Surgical Society. Larrey had sent a letter to him in New York, to the address he had given to the Secretary of the Société de biologie.[47] A few days later, he was officially informed of his nomination and on January 28th, he was made a Foreign Corresponding Member of the **Académie Impériale de Médecine**[48] as he had given his address in New York. Strangely enough, he remained a

---

[44] Brown-Séquard CE (23rd July, 1866) Letter to Shattuck. HML/CLC. Quoted by Tyler & Tyler, *op. cit.*, note 18, above, p. 1234.

[45] Laverdant D (1st June, 1878) Letter to Le Cernéen. Le Cernéen, Port Louis, Mauritius.

[46] Rouget FA (1930) Brown-Séquard et son oeuvre. Esquisse biographique. General Printing and Stationary Cy, Port Louis, Mauritius. pp. 56–57.

[47] Larrey H (4th Jan, 1866) Letter to Brown-Séquard. GMcCC, Ms 984/13.

[48] Secretary of the Académie Impériale de Médecine (3rd Feb, 1866) Letter to Brown-Séquard. GMcCC, Ms 980/321.

Foreign Corresponding Member until his death, even though he lived in Paris for the last 16 years of his life.

In the spring of 1866, he advised his cousin that he was about to cross the Atlantic. The latter was somewhat surprised by this sudden decision, for he had written in his previous letter that his health was a obstacle to his returning to America in the near future. Feltus wrote back: "I am a little apprehensive about your health and confess to some anxiety in regard to it."[49]

Early in April, Brown-Séquard was in New York, and practised privately there. He chose to stay in that city, so as to avoid any friction with Ellen's relatives. He planned to commute from there to Boston, twice a week, to deliver his lectures at Harvard but, in October, he decided to move to Cambridge.[50]

So, in November 1866, he resumed his professorship. He was invited to give the opening address to the winter course. He greeted the new class of medical students on November 7th with a lecture entitled: **Advice to Students**,[51] which did, indeed, contain a lot of sound advice. He advocated that the students form small study groups as an excellent method of fixing knowledge in the mind,[52] and he emphasized the importance of acute observation in the practical study of physiology by saying:

> How can one have a clear idea of the rhythmical movements of the heart, or the peristaltic movements of the bowels, … if he has not studied these important phenomena with the help of his senses, and especially his sight.[53]

He urged the students "to make good use of these low creatures, endowed with so little sensibility,—the frogs, the fishes and the turtles,"[54] justifying the practice of vivisection by stressing the importance to mankind of experiments on animals, stating that he agreed

> with the worthy motives of the gentlemen composing the English and American societies for the protection of animals, so long as they only want to prevent absolutely useless and wanton cruelty to animals, but I must, and do radically dissent from them in the attempts they have made in Europe and here to check if not to prevent altogether certain modes of scientific research, the great object of which is the good of mankind. I am selfish enough to prefer mankind to frogkind, rabbitkind, etc.[55]

As a scientist who had often carried out experiments upon his own person, he encouraged the students to do likewise:

---

[49] Feltus HJ (7th June, 1866) Letter to Brown-Séquard. GMcCC, Ms 981/164.

[50] Brown-Séquard CE (3rd Oct, 1866) Letter to Shattuck. HML/CLC. Quoted by Tyler & Tyler, *op. cit.*, note 18, above, p. 1234.

[51] Brown-Séquard CE (1867) Advice to Students. Address delivered at the opening of the Medical Lectures of Harvard University. Cambridge Press of John Wilson, Cambridge, Massachusetts.

[52] *Ibid.*, p. 5.

[53] *Ibid.*, p. 7.

[54] *Ibid.*

[55] *Ibid.*, pp. 7–8.

> I will suggest that you should study upon yourselves the effects of the most valuable remedies. I well believe that you will never know fully the action of certain remedies if you have not ascertained, on your own person, what effects they produce on the brain, the eye, the ear, the nerves, the muscles, and the principal viscera.[56]

He warned the students about some of the common pitfalls of scientific research such as "continuing to accept a theory, notwithstanding our recognition that there are positive facts in direct opposition to it;"[57] "neglecting certain circumstances of cases or experiments and drawing consequently erroneous conclusions;"[58] or "denying facts because we cannot explain them."[59] What he said, towards the end of his address, was either a hint of his bitterness at not being given the means of pursuing a career as an experimental physiologist in The States, or a coded appeal to a philanthropist who might be interested in perpetuating his own name. At the same time, however, it was an insensitive, unpalatable and misguided criticism of American progress in medical science:

> But, I am asked, how can we learn to make scientific or practical investigations in physiology or medicine in a country like this, where the teaching of these sciences is yet only rudimentary? I do not deny that there is a great need here of an institute, where the means of prosecuting scientific researches should be taught by competent men. I have no doubt that he who would establish such an institute would be a benefactor of the human race, not only in this Republic but all over the world; while he would also do much, at this time, to place this country on a level with Europe, for things about which the inferiority of America is notorious.[60]

It is worth comparing his diatribe with an account of the state of medical teaching in The United States in the 1860s, as presented by E.C. Atwater:

> By the time of the Civil War there had already been a considerable amount of experimental physiology done in the United States. The idea that answers could be known through conventional scientific methods had gained acceptance; Americans were becoming less believing and more questioning. New teachers trained a generation of experimentalists. Technological innovations provided new methods and there was talk of all students having laboratory experience in physiology as they did in gross anatomy.[61]

The Harvard Medical School catalogue for the academic year 1866–1867 indicates that Brown-Séquard lectured twice a week during the 4 months of the winter term.[62] He was paid from the sale of attendance tickets which were priced

---

[56] *Ibid.*, pp. 8–9.

[57] *Ibid.*, p. 20.

[58] *Ibid.*, p. 21.

[59] *Ibid.*, p. 25.

[60] *Ibid.*, p. 32.

[61] Atwater EC (1978) Squeezing Mother Nature. Bull Hist Med 52: 313–335.

[62] Harrington, *op. cit.*, note 20, above, vol 2, p. 548.

at 10 dollars. He encouraged the students to purchase his books and tried to have them included on the College's recommended list. His lectures were well attended and the following tribute from Henry Pickering Bowditch sums up his teaching ability:

> Those who were privileged to listen to him will not readily forget the enthusiasm which he awakened in his hearers for medicine as an experimental science. It is interesting to note how physiology thus taught was in advance of the then accepted views.[63]

As well as the fees he earned from his lectures, Brown-Séquard also made some money from private practice. He saw patients, twice a week, at his consultation room at Dean Shattuck's city surgery. However, on January 10, 1867, the Boston Medical and Surgical Journal reported that he was giving up the practice of medicine.[64] His decision was due to his patients failing to meet their financial obligations. His cousin, Henry J Feltus, wrote to try to dissuade him from his course, suggesting that he presents his patients with a bill at the end of each consultation.[65] This did not appeal to him and in the end he stopped receiving patients altogether.

He got more involved in the running of the Medical School, and started attending the faculty meetings, grumbling, however, about the meagre payment he received for his lectures.[66] At the faculty meetings of February and March 1867, he expressed his dissatisfaction with his earnings[67] once more and the attendance price was raised from 10 to 12 dollars.[68] That year, 1867, was an unhappy one for him at Harvard. In March, the title of his **Chair of Physiology and Pathology of the Nervous System** was shortened to just Physiology and Pathology.[69] His behaviour started to become irrational. Unhappy with the alteration of the title of his professorship, he was contemplating resigning "both the new and the old appointment."[70] At the end of the month, he wrote to Dean Shattuck asking him for an adjunct professor, who would "deliver a part of the winter course in my place."[71]

Amid all these misunderstandings, he was invited, in May, to take part in an election for a professorship of physiology in the Medical College of the State of North Carolina, which was due to take place in June.[72] It is not known whether he

---

[63] Quoted in the The Harvard Medical School 1782–1906. Boston, p. 89.

[64] Olmsted, *op. cit.*, note 19, above, p. 129.

[65] Feltus HJ (16th Jan, 1867) Letter to Brown-Séquard. GMcCC, Ms 981/14.

[66] Minutes and Records of the Faculty of Medicine, Harvard Medical School (22nd March, 1867). Quoted by Tyler & Tyler, *op. cit.*, note 18, above, p. 1234.

[67] *Ibid.*

[68] *Ibid.*

[69] Harrington, *op. cit.*, note 20, above, vol 2, p. 543.

[70] Brown-Séquard CE (28th March, 1867) Letter to Shattuck. HML/CLC. Quoted by Tyler & Tyler, *op. cit.*, note 18, above, p. 1235.

[71] *Ibid.*

[72] Chisden JJ (28TH May, 1867) Letter to Brown-Séquard. GMcCC, Ms 984/17.

took part in that election, but he was elected a Fellow of the **American Academy of Arts and Sciences** of Boston, in the same month.[73]

In August 1867, an International Congress of Medicine—the first of its kind—was held in Paris, coinciding with the Paris Exhibition. The President of the Congress was Jean-Baptiste Bouillaud. It was an event that brought together delegates from all over Europe and America, who were so distinguished, that Bouillaud ended his inaugural address by quoting the writer Casimir Delavigne: "France it's Paris and Paris it's the World." Brown-Séquard was chosen as delegate of the American Medical Association and was

> The most eagerly awaited of the speakers, ... who was due to discuss the early signs of cerebral disease; but alas for his admirers, the sudden illness and death, ... of his younger former colleague and fellow Mauritian Victor Bazire, ... had called him to London.[74]

In Pierre Victor Lanougarède Bazire, Brown-Séquard lost a very good friend. He had stayed at Bazire's town house in Woburn Square, Bloomsbury, whenever he visited London. Bazire was from a distinguished family of professionals. His brother Eugène was a barrister and his other brother, Emile, a district magistrate. His maternal grandfather, the Commandant Lanougarède had, with a handful of men stopped the advance of the British army on Port Louis in 1810. The courage of this officer won him the admiration of the British commander-in-chief, General John Abercrombie who, at the hour of capitulation of the Isle de France, handed over to him his sword, an honour which was denied to his superior, General Decaen.

In 1853, Bazire commenced his medical studies at University College, London, where it is said of him that "the list of class victories won would suffice for an epic."[75] After being successful at the M.D. examination he was, for a time, the assistant of William Jenner at University College Hospital. At the end of 1858, he attended the Medical School in Paris, graduating M.D., in 1860, with a thesis on diseases of the hip joint.

That same year, he returned to Mauritius, where he was appointed assistant-physician to the **Civil Hospital** in Port Louis. After the death of his wife from cholera in 1862, he returned to London. There, as well as running a consultation room in Harley Street, he held in succession the posts of medical registrar of the Westminster Hospital, Assistant-physician and, finally, Physician to the National Hospital for the Paralytics and Epileptics. He was appointed a member of a commission to investigate the incidence of sexually transmitted diseases in the London area. His clinical observations of lateral lesions of the spinal cord led him to add to the signs of the **Brown-Séquard syndrome**: a diminution of the

---

[73] Certificate of Fellowship of the American Academy of Arts and Sciences. GMcCC, Ms 984/18.

[74] McMenemy WH (1967) International Congress of Medicine and some of the personalities involved. Br Med J 2: 487–489.

[75] Lancet (1867) Obituary: P Victor Bazire, M.D. 2: 213–214.

proprioceptive sensibility on the same side as the motor deficit.[76] He started to translate into English, Armand Trousseau's treatise: **Clinique médicale de l'Hôtel Dieu**. His death, premature at 32, resulted from the rupture of an aneurysm of the basilar artery. In his obituary, the **British Medical Journal** said that "he had barely indicated the rarity and richness of his promise when death stepped in."[77]

On his return to The United States, on November 6, 1867, after attending Bazire's post-mortem examination, Brown-Séquard declared to Dean Shattuck his intention of resigning definitely before the end of the winter term. His letter of resignation stated that he was "in a condition of health that will never allow my fulfilling the duties of the chair."[78] Despite the Dean's attempts at dissuading him, his resignation became effective on December 28, 1867.[79]

His departure from Harvard was very much regretted by his American colleagues, and above all by Silas Weir Mitchell, whose work, in collaboration with William Hammond, on snake venoms and curare, had been reviewed by Brown-Séquard in his **Journal de physiologie de l'homme et des animaux**,[80] in 1859. Mitchell wrote:

> I hear with the utmost regret of your intention to leave us. I for one find so few in this country who sympathize with my studies, that I think every defection from our physiological rank a great loss.[81]

So sincere was Mitchell's admiration for Brown-Séquard's research on the nervous system, that he sent him his articles whenever they were published.[82]

Silas Weir Mitchell, after graduating from Jefferson Medical College in 1850, spent a year in Paris, working with Claude Bernard, . On his return to Philadelphia, he devoted his time to physiological investigations on the nervous system. His combination of physiology and experimental medicine earned him the title of Father of American neurology. He never held an academic post. He was twice rejected as a candidate for professorships in physiology. Competing for the same chair at the University of Pennsylvania, in 1863, he and Brown-Séquard lost to Francis Gurney Smith. Again, in 1868, Mitchell lost to James Atkin Meigs for a

---

76 Bazire P (1865) On a case of partial disease of the left half of the spinal cord, causing anaesthesia on one side, and paralysis of movement on the other, with remarks on the transmission of sensitive impressions in the spinal cord. Lancet 2: 116–118.

77 British Medical Journal (1867) Obituary: P. Victor Bazire, M.D. 2: 141.

78 Brown-Séquard CE (6th Nov, 1867) Letter to Shattuck. HML/CLC. Quoted by Tyler & Tyler, *op. cit.*, note 18, above, p. 1235.

79 Harrington, *op. cit.*, note 20, above, vol 2, p. 548. Also handwritten note, GMcCC, Ms 984/19.

80 Brown-Séquard CE (1859) Appreciation des progrès de la physiologie. J Physiol (Paris) 2: 707–709.

81 Mitchell SW (14th Apr, 1868) Letter to Brown-Séquard. GMcCC, Ms 980/28.

82 Mitchell SW (n.d.) Letter to Brown-Séquard. GMcCC, Ms 980/90.

chair at the Jefferson Medical College. He asked Brown-Séquard for a testimonial to back his candidature to that chair "saying what you can in my favour as a physiologist".[83] This is part of the latter's testimonial:

> I willingly bear witness that in the Old World, as well as here, he is well known as an enthusiastic lover of Science, as a most ingenious experimenter, as a discoverer of very important facts, doctrines and laws in Physiology and in Scientific and Practical Medicine, and a clear, forcible and learned writer, ... few of the competitors could occupy that chair with so much benefit to the students and so much credit to themselves and to the College, as Dr Weir Mitchell.[84]

After his resignation from the Harvard Medical School, Brown-Séquard stayed in The States for the better half of 1868, hesitant to return to Paris. He set up a private practice, taking a passing interest in what was going on at the Medical School. He also received two more honours during this year. He was made an Honorary Member of the Medical Society of the State of New York, and a Fellow of the National Academy of Sciences of Philadelphia.

Of the various acquaintances that Brown-Séquard made in the two and a half years he spent intermittently at Cambridge, he got to know well Edward Hammond Clarke, the Professor of Materia Medica at the Medical School. Other acquaintances included the Wyman brothers, Morill and Jeffries. Morill was the inventor of **pleurocentesis** also known as **thoracocentesis**, that is the withdrawal of fluid from the pleural cavity by means of a hollow needle inserted through the chest wall. Jeffries, who collaborated with the naturalist Louis Agassiz, studied Anatomy at the Paris Medical School and attended courses of Comparative Anatomy and Physiology under Pierre Jean Marie Flourens at the Jardin des Plantes of Paris. Brown-Séquard had quite a close relationship with George Cheyne Shattuck, as demonstrated by his helpful treatment of the former. He had studied in Paris under Pierre Charles Alexandre Louis. His most notable achievement was the differentiation, in America, of typhoid from typhus. Last, but not least, Louis Agassiz who, in 1864, after successfully helping Brown-Séquard to secure the professorship at Harvard, left for a scientific expedition to Brazil. On his return from that country, and especially from 1866 onwards, he struck a lasting friendship with him.

Brown-Séquard's departure for Paris, late in 1868, was not the end of his professional links with America. Throughout the next 10 years, he would return to spend months at a time there. His return to France turned out to be a short interlude in a peripatetic career.

---

[83] Mitchell, *op. cit.*, note 81, above.

[84] Brown-Séquard CE (16th Apr, 1868) Letter to the Board of Trustees of the Jefferson Medical College. Quoted by Fye WB (1983) Weir Mitchell, Philadelphia's "Lost Physiologist". Bull Hist Med 57: 188–203.

# Chapter 14
# The Paris Course Lecturer: 1869–1872

Brown-Séquard departed from The States very much upon the advice of Louis Agassiz, who realised not only that he was unhappy, but also that his investigatory work had stagnated during the whole period of his association with Harvard. To Agassiz, there was no doubt that Brown-Séquard was far more disposed to pursue his researches, when he was in Paris.[1]

Agassiz wrote directly to Napoléon III, asking him to provide an academic chair for Brown-Séquard. It was a request that was to open up a complicated series of ministerial correspondence.

Since 1857, Napoléon III and Agassiz had struck a friendship. The former, convinced that the latter was a French citizen, had tried to lure him to Paris, by offering him the Chair of Palaeontology at the **Muséum national d'histoire naturelle**—previously known as the Jardin des Plantes. The then Minister of Public Education, Gustave Rouland, had written to him that the:

> Chair of paleontology is vacant at the Muséum d'Histoire Naturelle in Paris. You are French, you have enriched your native land with eminent studies and hard work. You are a corresponding member of the Institute. The Emperor would be delighted to bring back to France a distinguished scholar, and a renowned professor. I write to offer you, in his name, the vacant chair, and your motherland will congratulate herself on having back one of her children, most devoted to science.[2]

Agassiz replied:

> Allow me to draw your attention to an error which concerns me personally, I am not French, though French in origin. My family is Swiss and has been for centuries. Despite an absence of ten years from my country, I am still a Swiss national.[3]

For Napoléon, Agassiz was, in Natural Sciences, of the same mould as Claude Bernard in Physiology. A few months after his letter, Rouland again wrote to

---

1 Marcou J (1896) Life, letters and works of Louis Agassiz, vol 2. Macmillan, New York, p. 158.
2 Rouland J (19th Aug, 1857) Letter to Agassiz. Quoted by Agassiz EC (1887) Louis Agassiz. Sa Vie et sa correspondence. Traduit de l'anglais par Auguste Meyer. Librairie Fischbacher, Paris, p. 432.
3 *Ibid.*, p. 433.

L.-C. Celestin, *Charles-Edouard Brown-Séquard*,
DOI: 10.1007/978-3-319-03020-3_14, 

Agassiz,[4] on behalf of the Emperor, with the promise of keeping the chair vacant for one or two years, to give him the time to finish the work he had started in America.[5] The terms of this second offer were extremely generous: a post as overall director of the Muséum national d'histoire naturelle, where he would have been responsible for the financial resources of the institution with the authority to reorganise the whole administrative and research structure of the Muséum; a town house provided by the French government; a lifetime position as senator of France and a professorship at the Collège de France. Agassiz's declination of this auspicious offer earned him **the Légion d'honneur** and the respect of Napoléon III and successive ministers of Public Education, who consulted him on matters of academic considerations.[6]

This is the draft of the letter written to Napoléon, that Agassiz gave to Brown-Séquard. It was dated November 3, 1868:

> To His Imperial Highness Prince Napoléon
>
> My Prince,
>
> You have encouraged me in such a kindly manner to write to you from time to time, that I take advantage of the liberty you have accorded me, in order to recommend a friend to you.
>
> The Chair of Experimental Physiology at the Jardin des Plantes is vacant, and I doubt whether the candidates who have entered the lists are the men most capable of giving a new lustre to that teaching.
>
> There is really, at the moment, only one man in France who is truly equal to this position and my friends write that he does not wish to compete with inferiors, to be, perhaps beaten by them. I do understand the sensitiveness on the part of Dr Brown-Séquard who has received, in the past, the most flattering distinctions from the Académie des Sciences. Crowned over and over again for his work, he has twice received the Monthyon [sic] Prize of Experimental Physiology, but in spite of all that he has not made his way. Too exclusively devoted to his work, he has not applied himself to making a position and today, he should have the right offered, and I do not doubt that it is the sole reason for his abstention. It is this which has prompted me to beg you, in the interests of higher studies and the glory of the Jardin des Plantes, to draw the attention of M. Duruy to the great merits of Dr Brown-Séquard. and if I did not fear to pass in the eyes of the Emperor for an ungrateful person who only cares for my own interest, I would ask you even to tell His Majesty that I am convinced that it would be a real loss for France, should the government let pass the occasion to attach Dr Brown-Séquard to one of the greatest and most illustrious scientific establishments of Paris.
>
> Dr Brown-Séquard is better known abroad than in France and this may be a disadvantage for him at the moment. Yet, the fact is that the Universities of Edinburgh, of Glasgow and several in The United States have disputed the honour of having him to make special courses on his scientific discoveries. Presently, I am having a laboratory set up for him here, but I feel strongly that for him the real centre of action is Paris, and should the steps I am taking deprive me of a devoted friend whom I have always hoped to have in The United States, I would console myself, knowing that I have rendered a service to science in helping to place, in a most advantageous position a man of the highest capability.

---

[4] *Ibid.*

[5] *Ibid.*

[6] *Ibid.*

I would fear to tire your Highness by adding some words concerning me personally etc.
My Prince, please accept my most respectful consideration.
Ls Agassiz[7]

Agassiz was referring to the Chair of Comparative Physiology which was still vacant after the death of Flourens, the previous year. Several candidates had been considered for this chair, namely Achille Dareste, Jean-Baptiste Gris, Jules Emile Planchon, Wilhelm Philipp Schimper and Brown-Séquard. Flourens had succeeded Frédéric Cuvier, who had been Agassiz's teacher. Of all the scientific chairs in Paris, this one was the best, as its laboratory space and facilities were superior to all the others.

The outcome of Agassiz's approach to Napoléon is revealed in the following undated draft of a letter, the Minister of Public Education, Victor Duruy, meant for the Emperor:

Sire,

In order to appoint Brown-Séquard to the Muséum, I would have to make a ministerial coup d'Etat. The Emperor does not want it and, above all, he would not allow it in favour of a man who, even in M. Agassiz's opinion, is not of the first rank.

However, there is an important chair to be awarded, that of Comparative Physiology, I can only suggest to the Emperor understudies like M. Dareste (Achille) or novices like M. Bert, Vaillant, etc. One contrivance would save everything.

The Emperor has established for Claude Bernard a chair of General Physiology which is not in its right place at the Faculty of Sciences for two reasons: first, because the candidates for degrees are never examined in physiology; second, because at the Sorbonne the professor lacks everything necessary for such a course: ample well-aired space, light, tank, paddock, stall, stable for the animals used or to be used for experimentation, amphitheatre for vivisections, etc…

All that is lacking and always will be lacking at the Sorbonne, can be found at the Muséum. Claude Bernard would be at ease, but he does not want to solicit the votes of the professors of that institution who have the right in case of vacancies to present candidates; and he is right, he cannot be a supplicant.

But he is willing to accept if his chair is transferred by decree to the Muséum.

at the Sorbonne[or] at the Collège de France, he has his auditors but he cannot train pupils.

It is pupils we need, however, if the future is to be assured in the same way as discoveries which honour the present. The Emperor sees the sad condition of natural sciences in this country, since I am unable to find anyone, at the present, worthy to occupy M. Flourens' two chairs.

At the Muséum, Claude Bernard will train pupils for us, because he will find there all that he lacks at the Sorbonne and at the Collège de France. …

If the Emperor would approve this solution which, I think, will be applauded by everyone, H[is] M[ajesty] would only have to sign a decree and say a word to the Court Minister.

As for M. Brown-Séquard, whom the professors at the Muséum do not want, I have seen him and told him that I was ready to do everything for him except to violate the law by placing him by brute force at the Muséum. He has asked me to convey his appreciation to the Emperor and has promised me to think about what he could request. I await his answer.

The Emperor's humble and faithful servant, with the deepest respect. V.D.[8]

---

7 Agassiz L (3rd Nov, 1868) Letter to Napoléon III. GMcCC, Ms 981/3.

8 Duruy C (1868) Draft of a letter to Napoléon III. Quoted in full by Schiller J (1966) Claude Bernard and Brown-Séquard. The Chair of Genral Physiology and the experimental method. J Hist Med 21:260–270.

It is clear that there was an exchange of letters between Agassiz and either Napoléon or Duruy. Had Brown-Séquard been considered a real loss to science in France, Napoléon could have issued a decree for his appointment at the Muséum. His nationality would not have been a stumbling block, this much is clear from Napoléon's offer to Agassiz, ten years earlier. It is difficult to accuse Agassiz of duplicity. He had previously been quite embarrassed by Brown-Séquard's mental instability. He had a chair specially created for him at Harvard and, less than three months after his appointment, his protégé was tendering his resignation and went absent from his post for 21 months. Despite his friendship for Brown-Séquard, it was his duty to draw Napoléon's attention to his friend's unpredictable behaviour.

Duruy's letter to Napoléon must have been written late in November or early December 1868, as he had already made arrangements by the 14th December for the transfer of Claude Bernard to the Muséum, the appointment of Paul Bert to succeed the latter at the Sorbonne and for the creation of a new chair for Brown-Séquard at the Paris Medical School. No official announcement had yet been made, but the latter was not fully aware of the situation, for anxious and depressed, he wrote to Napoléon and received the following reply, on December 18th:

> Your worth and your knowledge recommend you above all to the attention of the Minister of Public Education. I have been pleased to back up my friend, M. Agassiz. I believe that M. Duruy is well disposed towards you. I very much look forward to your nomination and there is every hope that it will not be long.[9]

Ironically, his appointment was hampered by his nationality. Enquiries by Broca's secretary revealed that his naturalization could take one year. Disheartened, he wrote to Duruy on December 28, 1868:

> My naturalization cannot be obtained before one year. If it is so, I am compelled, to my great regret to give up the hope of being professor at the Medical Faculty of Paris.[10]

To which, Duruy immediately replied:

> I cannot tell you if it would be absolutely necessary for a waiting period of one year for your naturalization.
>
> It is possible that we shall find, in the terms of the Convention of 1824, a clause which will enable us to eliminate that delay, or some other loophole which will lead to the same thing.
>
> Please send me only the dates and the information which allow me to plead your case, which I long to win.[11]

This setback is due to the fact that to be nominated professor at a medical school, the successful candidate must be a French national.

---

[9] Napoléon III (18th Dec, 1868) Letter to Brown-Séquard. GMcCC, Ms 984/323.

[10] Brown-Séquard CE (25th Dec, 1868) Letter to Duruy. GMcCC, Ms 980/31.

[11] Duruy V (26th Dec, 1868) Letter to Brown-Séquard. GMcCC, Ms 980/32.

Meanwhile, Brown-Séquard's anxiety reached pathological proportions, but he was comforted and kept informed of what was going on in the Ministries by a good friend, the distinguished chemist, Henri Etienne Saint-Claire Deville. On December 31st, he wrote to Brown-Séquard from his laboratory at the Ecole Normale Supérieure:

> I did the right thing in reassuring you, dear friend. I saw du Mesnil yesterday: he will offer the following solution, which I found excellent.
>
> You will be immediately appointed as professor in charge of courses at the Medical School. … During the coming year, your time limit [for naturalization] will run out and on the day of your naturalization, confirmation of it [your appointment] will be given by the Emperor.
>
> Duruy so much wants to help you that he will accept this solution which, in my opinion, is to everyone's satisfaction.[12]

So, finally, on February 6, 1869, Charles-Adolphe Wurtz, the Dean of the Faculty of Medicine, wrote to Brown-Séguard:

> I am pleased to inform you that, by an order of 30th January instant, the Minister has appointed you Chargé de Cours [Course Lecturer] to the Chair of Comparative and Experimental Pathology, and, for this position, you will be paid a fixed salary of 7,000 francs as from February 1st, instant.[13]

By this ministerial order, the Chair of Comparative Medicine, which had been created by Napoléon III for Pierre Rayer, in 1862, and which he vacated, when he resigned as Dean of the Faculty of Medicine in 1864, was now that of Comparative and Experimental Pathology.

At the bottom of this official letter, Wurtz had added a handwritten note, congratulating Brown-Séquard and adding:

> I have asked and obtained from the Minister funds for the construction of a laboratory of experimental medicine. I will submit the plan to you as soon as I have obtained it from the Town [Municipal Council] responsible for the execution of the work.[14]

It is clear from the above-note, that Wurtz envisaged the possibility that Brown-Séquard would, at a future date, enjoy some of the facilities afforded by this laboratory.

Simultaneously to the official confirmation of his appointment, Brown-Séquard was granted an official residence permit. By a decree of Napoléon III, he was "authorised to establish his residence in France and to enjoy civil rights for as long as he continues to be domiciled here."[15] This meant that he had an official work and residence permit. He remained a foreigner. He could hold a Lectureship, but not a Professorship.

---

[12] Sainte-Claire Deville HE (31st Dec, 1868) Letter to Brown-Séquard. GMcCC, Ms 984/2.

[13] Wurtz A (6th Feb, 1869) Letter to Brown-Séquard. GMcCC, Ms 984/24.

[14] *Ibid.*

[15] Decree N°3642 x 2 of the Ministry of Justice and Cults. Authorization for Brown-Séquard to elect domicile in France. GMcCC, Ms 987/7.

As a result of his appointment, he was invited to have dinner, at the Palais Royal , with the Emperor and the Empress, Marie Clotilde, on April 3, 1869.[16]

Soon after his nomination, he was, on April 12, elected a Member of the **Royal Irish Academy** in Dublin, and much later in that year, he was made an Honorary Member of the **St Andrew's Medical Graduate Association.**[17]

During the months of November and December 1868, while he was waiting for a position to be arranged for him, Brown-Séquard devoted his spare time to the launch of another medical periodical. "Scientific journalism had for him a particular attraction, … He loved to write according to his own fancy…"[18] The journal was called **Archives de Physiologie normale et pathologique** and replaced his **Journal de physiologie de l'homme et des animaux**, defunct since 1865.

As editorial collaborators, he chose two of the most prominent specialists of the nervous system: Jean-Martin Charcot and Alfred Vulpian. Since 1862, both had worked at the **Salpêtrière** Hospital, which was a "chaotic welfare institution", where the chronically sick with unclassified and unknown neurological and psychiatric disorders were confined. It was through their association that Charcot became a distinguished neuropathologist, eventually, in 1882, occupying the first Chair of Diseases of the Nervous System. Over a period of ten years at the Salpêtrière, he described the symptoms of many neurological disorders, which he differentiated from each other. It was him, who described the cardinal signs of multiple sclerosis, a disease of the brain and spinal cord, in which there is a loss of the myelin sheath which surrounds the nerve fibres and disrupts their function. With Vulpian, he distinguished this condition from Parkinson's disease. Charcot also described a progressive form of paralysis: Charcot's disease or amyotrophic lateral sclerosis, a form of motor neurone disease. He was the founder of the renowned French School of Neurology, which flourished in the final quarter of the nineteenth century. It has been rightly said that he "entered neurology in its infancy and left it at his coming of age nourished by his own contribution."[19]

Another occurrence, during these two months of inactivity, was the visit to Brown-Séquard of Henry Pickering Bowditch, a student at Harvard Medical School, during the former's professorship there, having just graduated earlier in the year. This was a seemingly minor event for Brown-Séquard, but Bowditch's visit did have a calculable effect on medical history. He travelled to Paris to study there, encouraged by Jeffries Wyman. He was hoping to combine clinical work with physiological investigations under Brown-Séquard's direction. This was impossible as the latter did not have a laboratory; he therefore sent Bowditch to

---

[16] Napoléon III (30th March, 1869) Invitation to Brown-Séquard to dinner. GMcCC, Ms 980/34.

[17] Certificate of the Royal Irish Society and Certificate of St. Andrew's University Ms 984/18.

[18] Berthelot MPE (1898) The Life and Works of Brown-Séquard. From the Smithsonian Report for 1898. Translated from the Revue Scientifique, 4ème série, 1:801–812, Government Printing Office, 1900, p. 687.

[19] Owen ARG (1971) Hysteria, Hypnosis and Healing. The Work of J-M Charcot. Dennis Dobson, London, p. 33.

serve in Broca's service at the Bicêtre Hospital and to courses by Claude Bernard and Louis Ranvier at the Collège de France. Bowditch wrote to Wyman that the conditions in the College's laboratory left much to be desired. It was "dark, poorly provided with apparatus and without proper arrangements for pupils,"[20] and that "the Frenchmen acknowledge… the great advantage that the Germans had over them."[21] This was that their laboratories were better equipped and arranged.

So, Bowditch went to Leipzig, to the laboratory of Karl Friedrich Wilhelms Ludwig. When he returned to The States in 1871, he brought with him German-made laboratory apparatuses and was appointed Assistant Professor of Physiology at the Harvard Medical School. From the modest beginnings of a makeshift laboratory in the attic of one of the old medical buildings there, he organised the first physiological laboratory in America in which students carried out their own experiments. He had succeeded where Brown-Séquard had failed some years earlier.

Bowditch's experience in Paris, namely, the lack of equipment that he found there, was to greatly diminish the influence that France had over the development of the medical sciences in America. It marked the beginning of the trend of young American physicians opting for postgraduate studies in German universities and hospitals.

Returning to Brown-Séquard, he inaugurated his course at the Medical School by the early spring of 1869. His opening lecture was a source of intense joy to him. He felt happy and proud to lecture in an amphitheatre where, as a student, he "had sat amongst the humblest and the poorest."[22] A great number of his friends and colleagues attended his opening lesson, including Claude Bernard, who congratulated him "for the sake of our old friendship and of science that we love so much."[23] From then on, his courses were well attended and the many experiments that he carried out to illustrate the pathology of nervous disorders attracted a large number of students. What appealed mostly to his audience was, that he was not

> A didactic lecturer, nor was he likely to carry his audience by bursts of borrowed eloquence. But he excelled in displaying his own discoveries with a sincerity that was not wanting in finesse.[24]

Sadly for him, his happiness and satisfaction did not last long. Difficulties arose. His immoderate demands for laboratory material, chemicals and animals exceeded the budget that had been allocated to his course. There were not enough rooms to house all his animals at the **Ecole Pratique.** His course was scheduled to continue during the winter term of 1869–1870, but, by the summer of 1869, he had learnt

---

[20] Bowditch HP (14th Jan, 1867) Letter to Wyman. In Fye WB (1982). Why a Physiologist? Henry P Bowditch. Bull Hist Med 56:19–29.

[21] *Ibid.*

[22] Dupuy E (1894) Notice sur M. Le professeur Brown-Séquard, ancient Président de la Société de biologie. Revue Scient 2:737–743.

[23] *Ibid.*

[24] Berthelot MPE (1898) La Vie et les travaux de M. Brown-Séquard. Revue Scient 10:801–812.

that it was going to be curtailed.[25] This was just the kind of setback that would unhinge him and lead to discouragement, depression and despair.

In the summer of 1869, he left Paris for America, where there were two poles of attraction for him: his son, who was in a boarding school in Boston, and his friend Agassiz in Cambridge, who was always good at boosting his morale. Indeed as the latter wrote:

> To dissipate these phantoms which trouble you so often, I have always believed that I was magician enough to help you in this matter and it is a real sorrow for me not to be given the occasion.[26]

But, disastrously, on September 14th of that year Agassiz suffered a stroke which left him completely paralysed and affected his speech. Besides Brown-Séquard, he was attended by two eminent physicians: Oliver Wendell Holmes and Morrill Wyman. Untiringly, Brown-Séquard nursed Agassiz back to health and in due course, the paralysis disappeared. After a long period of convalescence, he was able to resume work. Several letters, over the next four years, express his infinite gratitude to Brown-Séquard, like the following:

> Be assured that every day I remember what I owe you, for I know that it is you who has given to me what remains of my health, and my wish to increase still further this little capital is too much at heart for me not to desire ardently to be nearer you, to receive daily your good advice.[27]

Back in Paris, after attending to Agassiz, the academic year 1869–1870 was a frustrating one for Brown-Séquard. This despite the fact that he was able to admit an American pupil into his own laboratory at the Ecole Pratique. Edward Constant Seguin spent the winter term researching under him.[28] Seguin was born in Paris, the son of Edouard Onésimus Seguin, who had emigrated to The United States after the 1848 Revolution, when he lost his position as the medical director of the **Bicêtre** mental asylum. The young Seguin turned to neurology after working in Paris with Brown-Séquard, Jean-Martin Charcot and Victor Cornil. He is best remembered in America, for the introduction of medical thermometry.

Brown-Séquard was so disappointed with the limits of his budget for his Lectureship that he considered resigning his post in July 1870. This can be seen from the reply letter he received from Augustus Volney Waller, the Paris-trained physician, who had been Professor of Physiology in Birmingham and who, in 1851, described the degeneration of the myelin sheath of a nerve fibre after its

---

[25] Boston Medical & Surgical Journal (1869) Medical Miscellany. 80:444.

[26] Agassiz L (16th Jan, 1870) Letter to Brown-Séquard. GMcCC, Ms 981/9.

[27] *Ibid.*

[28] Denny-Brown D (1975) Centennial Anniversary of the American Medical Association 1875–1975. Springer Publishing, New York pp. 91–92.

severance: **Wallerian** degeneration. He wrote approvingly of Brown-Séquard's intention of taking a break at an English sea resort and advising him that:

> As regards the resignation, my reason agrees with your arguments, but my instinct is opposed to it. If you would only take it quietly, diminish the laboratory expenses or get them allowed by the government like other professors, I would tell you to hold at least another year, before deciding and stepping "out into space again".[29]

In his letter, Waller was concerned about the deterioration in Franco-German relations. Effectively, the day after he wrote, the Franco-Prussian War broke out. A coalition of German States was opposed to France and following the defeat of the French army at Sedan, Paris was besieged from September 1870 to January 1871, when an armistice was signed. Some of the immediate consequences of the conflict were: the fall of the Second Empire of Napoléon III; the loss of the provinces of Alsace and Lorraine and the unification of Germany. Brown-Séquard was away from France for the duration of the war. He learnt, from an English war correspondent that, during the Paris's siege, shells had fallen in the street, where he lived.[30]

In September 1870, on the invitation of Thomas Henry Huxley, the President of the Royal Society, Brown-Séquard lectured in Liverpool at the annual meeting of the **British Association for the Advancement of Science.** One of the two papers he presented was "On the Apparent Transmission of Abnormal Conditions due to Accidental Causes,"[31]in which he stated "that epilepsy induced in the guinea-pig could be transmitted to its offspring."[32] Huxley complimented him on the value and importance of his paper, adding that:

> He was convinced that the observations made by Dr Brown-Séquard would be referred to as having proved an introduction to a great and new path in science. The great theoretical problem that they had now to determine was to know about the effect artificial modifications and external conditions have on living organisms—changes which, by being transmitted hereditarily, become the basis of new races.[33]

Brown-Séquard had been researching the nature of epilepsy since 1850, when he published articles on an epileptic-type of convulsion, experimentally induced in guinea-pigs by the hemisection or transection of the spinal cord.[34] In the days and weeks that followed the operations, the animals exhibited periodic clonic and tonic

---

[29] Waller AV (17th July, 1870) Letter to Brown-Séquard. GMcCC, Ms 980/37.

[30] Unidentified correspondent (10th Jan, 1871) Letter to Brown-Séquard. GMcCC, Ms 980/37.

[31] Lancet (1870) 2:436–439.

[32] *Ibid.*

[33] *Ibid.*

[34] Brown-Séquard CE (1850) D'une affection convulsive qui survient chez les animaux ayant une moitié latérale de la moelle épinière coupée. C R Soc Biol (Paris) 2:195–197. Also (1850) D'une affection convulsive consécutive à la section transversale de la moelle épinière. C R Soc Biol (Paris) 2:169–171.

convulsions.He also noticed that the skin in the facial and cervical regions was particularly excitable and triggered "epileptic fits" when pinched. He called these areas the epileptogenic zones. In 1869, he reported that cutting the sciatic nerve in one hind leg of guinea-pigs resulted in epileptic seizures.[35] In 1892, he was to show that amputating the whole of the hind leg, resulted in an epileptiform condition far more marked than seen in the previous experiment, whereas amputation below the knee joint was much less effective.[36]

It was in 1859, that he first reported the appearance of epilepsy in the offspring of guinea-pigs he had operated upon.[37] He found that not all the young had "inherited" epilepsy and those which had, did not necessarily inherit the same kind of epileptiform condition. He also stated that he had not found a single case of spontaneous epilepsy in guinea-pigs whose progenitors had not had the condition induced. He concluded that the lesion itself was not inherited, but rather a disposition to the epileptic condition. The following year, he made his findings known to the Royal Society of London, in an article which appeared in the Proceedings of the Society.[38]

The notion of heredity of acquired characters was not new. In the 18th century, it had been advocated by Pierre Louis Moreau de Maupertius and it constituted one of the pillars of **Lamarckcism**, the theory devised by Jean-Baptiste Pierre Antoine de Monet, chevalier de Lamarck, which explains the evolution of living organisms to their adaptation to the environment as well as to the inheritance of acquired characteristics.

Brown-Séquard was so engrossed with the heredity of acquired characters that, early in 1870, he presented two guinea-pigs, with defective ear lobes, to the Société de biologie, claiming that the female's defect had been passed on to her by her male partner, via the offspring. This was brought about by the male having lost part of its ear auricle through gangrene, following the section of the sympathetic nerve in the neck.[39] This communication as well as his findings on the transmission of acquired characters in the guinea-pig, were debated at several of the Society's sessions. Paul Bert pointed out that the age-old custom of circumcision had never caused children to be born circumcised!

---

[35] Brown-Séquard CE (1869) Nouvelles recherches sur l'épilepsie due à certaines lésions de la moelle épinière et des nerfs rachidiens. Arch Physiol norm pathol 2:211–220, 422–441, 496–503.

[36] Brown-Séquard CE (1870) Faits nouveaux concernant la physiologie de l'épilepsie. Arch Physiol norm pathol 3:516–522.

[37] Brown-Séquard CE (1859) De la transmission par hérédite chez les mammifères, et particulièrement chez les cochons d'Inde, d'une affection épileptiforme produite chez les parents par des lésions traumatiques de la moelle épinière. C R Soc Biol (Paris) 11:194–196.

[38] Brown-Séquard CE (1860) Hereditary transmission of an epileptiform affection accidentally produced. Proc Roy Soc Lond 7:297–298.

[39] Brown-Séquard CE (1870) Modifications des mères par leurs embryons, d'après des faits observés chez le cobaye. C R Soc Biol (Pairs) 22:5–7.

Undeterred by the storm of criticism, Brown-Séquard made over half a dozen reports on the hereditary transmission of mutilations of the ears and paws of guinea-pigs passed onto the offspring by their progenitors.

He even presented a case which he termed "compensatory heredity". It was a guinea-pig with supernumerary toes, born of parents surgically lacking the normal number of toes.[40] Finally, in 1882, he published his last report on the transmission of acquired characters. It was a complete listing of all the defects that he had observed in the offspring of the guinea-pigs he had operated upon. They included epilepsy, deformities of the ear lobe, drooping of the eyelids, exophthalmia, absence of digits, of phalanges and of nails, corneal opacity and muscular atrophy.[41]

He had published a shorter list of these defects in The Lancet [42] in 1875, which remained a sort of Gospel truth on the hereditary transmission of acquired characters for Anglo-Saxon scientists interested in the study of genetics.

This was, notably, the case for Charles Darwin who, like Lamarck, was a proponent of the heredity of acquired characters. Indeed, his **Theory of Evolution** expounded in his book **The Origin of Species by Means of Natural Selection**, published in 1859, implies that variations selected in a natural way are hereditarily transmitted. This concept, known as Darwinism and commonly referred to as **survival of the fittest** states that the fittest organism chosen by **natural selection** survives to produce more offspring than the less fit one.

Darwin exalted Brown-Séquard's discoveries in three of his books. In **The Variation of Animals and Plants under Domestication**, published in 1868, referring to the latter's article which appeared in the Proceedings of the Royal Society, he states that:

> The most remarkable and trustworthy fact is that given by Dr Brown-Séquard, namely, that many young guinea-pigs inherited an epileptic tendency from parents which had been subjected to a particular operation, inducing in the course of a few weeks a convulsive epilepsy-like disease and it should be especially noted that the eminent physiologist bred a large number of guinea-pigs from animals which had not been operated on, and not one of these manifested the epileptic tendency. On the whole, we can hardly avoid admitting, that injuries and mutilations, especially when followed by disease, or perhaps exclusively when thus followed, are occasionally inherited.[43]

In The Descent of Man and Selection in Relation to Sex, published in 1873, Darwin mentions Brown-Séquard's findings twice. One of these references is as follows:

---

[40] *Ibid.*

[41] Brown-Séquard CE (1882) Faits nouveaux établissant l'extrême fréquence de la transmission par hérédité d'états organiques morbides, produits accidentellement chez des ascendants. C R Acad Sci (Paris) 94:697–698.

[42] Brown-Séquard CE (1875) On the hereditary transmission of effects of certain injuries to the nervous system. Lancet 1:7–8.

[43] Published by John Murray in 1868, vol 2, p. 24.

> We now have evidence that mutilations occasionally produce an inherited effect. ... I allude to Dr Brown-Séquard's observations on the transmitted effect of an operation causing epilepsy in guinea-pigs and, likewise, more recently on the analogous effect of cutting the sympathetic nerve in the neck.[44]

Finally, in the 1875 edition of **On the Origin of Species** by Means of **Natural Selection**, Darwin reminds his readers that, regarding the rejection of inheritance of acquired characters, Brown-Séquard's work on guinea-pigs should "make us cautious in denying this tendency".[45]

Indeed, Brown-Séquard's findings on the inheritance of acquired characters held sway for years to come. Although this theory was challenged by a few scientists towards the end of the nineteenth century, it was accepted by the majority. It was more or less the general consensus then that "hereditary transmission to predisposition to disease, of qualities acquired, of deformities created"[46] was a Gospel truth. In 1896, Wilhelm Ludwig Johanssen, the Danish-born agriculturist, who was the first to show that the nature of an organism is defined by its genes—he created the terms gene and genotype (the inherited characteristics of a species) as opposed to phenotype (the way in which these inherited characters are expressed) - accepted Brown-Séquard's findings.[47] Thomas Hunt Morgan, the eminent Nobel Prize American geneticist, who created a new era of genetics in his study of the giant chromosomes of the salivary glands of the vinegar fly Drosophila melanogaster—writing in 1907, was convinced that Brown-Séquard had proved the inheritance of acquired characters. He stated:

> The experiments [Brown-Séquard's] appear to have been carried out with such care, and the results are given in such detail that it seems that they must be accepted as establishing the inheritance of acquired characters.[48]

However, the appreciation of Brown-Séquard's observations by Darwin, Johanssen, Morgan and other scientists, was made prior to or at the time of the rediscovery, in 1900, of the work of the Moravian monk, Johann Gregor Mendel, by the German botanist Karl Eric Correns, the Dutch plant physiologist, Hugo de Vries and Erich von Tschermak. Mendel, after experimenting by cross-breeding peas, published his findings: **Versuche, Über Pflanzen-Hybriden** in an obscure journal. He noted that there was a disjuncture of hereditable characters as well as an independency of these characters. His findings were, that the hereditable characteristics could be viewed as single, separate entities, thus suggesting that there was a discontinuation in heriditariness. In a way, Mendel, without knowing it, had stumbled on the existence of genes.

---

44 Published by John Murray in London in 1875, pp. 59–60. Another reference is on page 603.

45 1875, p. 101.

46 Lander-Lindsay W (1871) Insanity in the lower animals. Brit For Med Chir Rev 48:172–213.

47 Roll-Hansen (1978) Drosophila Genetics. A Reductionist research program. J Hist Biol 11:159–210; p. 204.

48 Morgan TH (1907) Experimental Zoology. Macmillan New York, p. 54.

Finally, the notion of heredity of acquired characteristics was rejected by the majority of geneticists, beginning with the German biologist, August Weismann who, as early as 1883, in his theory of the continuity of the **germinative plasma**, to be known later on, as **neo-Darwinism**, acknowledges the concept of natural selection but rejects categorically that of the inheritance of acquired characters. This modified form of Darwinism is based upon the sudden and permanent variations of hereditable characters or mutations, which are the basis of new species. These mutations were first observed in the Vegetable Kingdom in the evening primrose plant of the genus **Oenothora** by Hugo de Vries, who published a book entitled **Die Mutations-theorie** in 1901. In the Animal Kingdom, Thomas Hunt Morgan described the many mutations occurring in successive generations of the vinegar fly.

Despite the progress of the science of genetics towards the end of the nineteenth century, Lamarckcism continued to have supporters in the following century, amongst the most well-known, in the 1950s, were the Russian horticulturist, Ivan Vladimirovich Mitchourine and his disciple, the Soviet biologist Trofim Desinovich Lyssenko. The latter backed by Joseph Vissarionovich Stalin, rejected Mendelian inheritance as well as the chromosomal theory of heredity. His theory based entirely on **vernalization**—that is the exposure of seeds during germination to a period of low temperature to accelerate their flowering when planted and especially for winter varieties of cereals—was used as communist propaganda for the elaboration of a **proletarian** science in opposition to the **bourgeois science** of Gregor Mendel and Thomas Hunt Morgan, and seriously hampered Soviet research in the field of genetics.

Ultimately, Brown-Séquard's findings were repudiated. His belief in the inheritance of acquired characters, which misled other researchers for a long time, was based on erroneous observations in animals, and on blind acknowledgements of dubious evidence in humans. In the latter case, the proof was based on stories from parents or grandparents, whose amputated fingers had supposedly been reflected in their offspring. By the 1920s, the inheritance of acquired characters had been totally discredited in the Western world. The geneticist, Emile Guyénot completely rejected Brown-Séquard's observations on guinea-pigs, in these words:

> As to the so-called transmission of anomalies in paws, eyes, ears, etc., it rests simply on the fact, well-known to all those who have raised guinea-pigs, that these animals present spontaneously, and precisely in the proportion stated by Brown-Séquard, diverses anomalies or congenital malformations.[49]

Regarding the rejection of the inheritance of acquired characters, a statement of Thomas Henry Huxley—who at the Liverpool meeting had encouraged Brown-Séquard in his researches—is worth recalling:

---

[49] Guyénot E La Variation et l'Evolution. Quoted by Olmsted JMD (1946) Charles-Edouard Brown-Séquard. A nineteenth century neurologist and endocrinologist. The John Hopkins Press, Baltimore, p. 187.

A theory is a species of thinking, and its right to exist is coextension with its power of resisting extinction by its rivals.[50]

Despite the fiasco of the hereditary transmission of anomalies, Brown-Séquard's study of epilepsy in guinea-pigs, artificially induced by lesions to the spinal cord, was a concrete clinical entity, which came to be known as **Brown-Séquard's spinal epilepsy**, or for short Brown-Séquard's disease. His experiments were repeated and his results confirmed by Vulpian[51] in France, and by Victor Horsley in England. The latter not only provoked seizures by hemisecting the spinal cord, but also by exposing the sciatic nerve, "nipping it, and closing the wound."[52] For Brown-Séquard, this convulsive disorder was akin to epilepsy, if it was not epilepsy per se, it was "at least an epileptiform affection,"[53] drawing an analogy between this artificially induced epilepsy in guinea-pigs and spontaneous epilepsy in humans. This led him to seek a cure for human epilepsy, focussing on the **epileptogenic** zones. In the guinea-pigs, he had noticed that cauterization of these sensitive zones: the face and the neck, with a hot iron, cured the animals of their seizures. This led him to advocate the same treatment for human epilepsy: "the cauterization of the back of the neck by **moxas** or by the red hot iron."[54]

This Liverpool meeting did not just attract scientists, just the opposite in fact. Some supporters of the antivivisectionist movement attended the meeting. Their movement decried the use of animals for scientific research, asserting that their sacrifice did not serve to facilitate scientific discoveries. Experiments on live animals, and especially those carried out in the Veterinary School in Alfort, were attracting the attention of the British press.[55] Reports in the daily papers prompted British veterinary surgeons to sign a mass protest, and to send a delegation from the Royal Society for the Prevention of Cruelty to Animals (RSPCA) to Napoléon III.

Frances Power Cobbe, an Irish woman, who had been present at the Liverpool meeting, campaigned vehemently for animals' rights, targeting some of the best known vivisectionists of the day. Public opinion was eventually mobilised by the protests and especially after the RSPCA, in 1874, proceeded against the French physician, Eugène Magnan. At a congress of the British Medical Association, held in Norwich, in that year, he had operated on dogs in front of his British colleagues to demonstrate the effects that injections of alcohol and absinth had on these

---

50 Huxley TH (1888) Science and Culture. Macmillan London, p. 312.

51 Vulpian A (1869) Epilepsie observée chez un cochon d'Inde qui avait subi la section des nerfs sciatiques. Arch Physiol norm pathol 2:297–299.

52 Horsley V (1886) Epileptic guinea pigs. Lancet 2:975.

53 Brown-Séquard CE (1856) Recherches expérimentales sur la production d'une affection convulsive, épileptiforme à la suite de lésions de la moelle épinière. C R Acad Sci (Paris) 42:86–89, 542–546.

54 Brown-Séquard CE (1858) Course of Lectures on the physiology and pathology of the nervous system. Delivered at the Royal College of Surgeons of England. Lecture XI. On the etiology, nature, and treatment of epilepsy with a few remarks on several other affections of the nervous centre. Lancet 2:571–573.

55 The Times, 8th Aug, 1863.

animals. Cobbe managed to circulate a memorandum, which came to the attention of Queen Victoria, expressing concern over the number of experiments being carried out in Britain and referring specifically to the Magnan affair. Her memorandum collected the signature of 600 influential people. Two years later, Frances Cobbe and George Hoggan founded the first antivivisectionist society which, ultimately became the National Anti-Vivisection Society. Hoggan was a physician, who had once been an assistant to Claude Bernard, the foremost animal experimentalist in France.

At the Liverpool meeting, Cobbe was enraged to hear Huxley extolling Brown-Séquard's experiments on animals. To her, the latter was nothing short of a serial animal killer. His record was to come out much later, during the sessions of the Royal Commission on Vivisection in 1875. He had, over a period of 30 years, carried out some 15–20,000 vivisections. He himself had already stated that:

> My watching over guinea-pigs has been on such a scale (at one time before the Siege of Paris, I had 584 in my laboratory) that I can say that I have had many thousands under observation from 1843 till now, a period of more than 30 years.[56]

For some years after that meeting, Huxley was targeted by the antivivisectionist lobby. He was falsely accused by a segment of the press of recommending the practice of vivisection in front of children. The charge was repeated in the House of Lords, and he was forced to defend himself publicly. The antivivisectionist campaign was so acrimonious that, in 1876, he advised Brown-Séquard not to attend scientific meetings in Great Britain, warning him that:

> A not uninfluential section of the public here is, at present, perfectly mad on the vivisection question & I am afraid that your appearance, would have the effect of a red rag upon a bull, on the fanatics who would be among your audience.[57]

After his lectures in Liverpool, Brown-Séquard travelled to America, where he stayed until the end of the spring 1871. There, he lectured in various cities, sending the proceeds of his lectures back to France, to help care for the wounded soldiers. He did collect quite large sums from his auditors.

In June 1870, he had written to Louis Agassiz from Paris, obviously unhappy about his position, as evidenced from Waller's reply letter of July of that year. Looking at Agassiz's reply, it is clear that he was trying to arrange for another chair at Harvard for Brown-Séquard:

> That which you write to me of your position does not surprise me, and I have had a long talk about it with your friend Dr Clarke; we agree to advise you not to come to The United States, before having received an official invitation to accept a Chair in our School of Medicine. As soon as I am back in Cambridge, I will see those of our friends on whom

---

[56] Brown-Séquard CE. Quoted by Westacott E (1949) A Century of vivisection and anti-vivisection. A study of their effects upon Science, Medicine and Human life during the past hundred years. The C.W. Daniel CO., Ltd, Ashington, Rochford, Essex, England, p. 44.

[57] Huxley TH (1876) Letter to Brown-Séquard. GMcCC, Ms 981/64, 12th March.

> we can count to do what could be done to assure you of an independent position which would allow you to pursue your researches without interruption.[58]

Brown-Séquard resumed his post at the Paris School of Medicine at the end of the academic year 1871–1872. He was still unhappy about the limitations of his budget. Late in February 1872, he left for The United States, before a letter from the Ministry of Public Education reached him, informing him, on April 16, of a grant of 2,000 francs to defray the expenses of his laboratory.[59] His new pole of attraction, in America, was a young woman, whom he had met there, the previous year.

[58] Agassiz L (1870) Letter to Brown-Séquard. GMcCC, Ms 981/21, 25th June.

[59] Ministère de l'Education publique (1872) Letter to Brown-Séquard. GMcCC, Ms 980/39, 16th Apr.

# Chapter 15
# The New York Practitioner: 1872–1874

On leaving Paris, at the end of February 1872, Brown-Séquard travelled to New York where, on March 13, he married Maria Rebecca Carlisle, "the daughter of a wealthy gentleman of Cincinnati, Ohio."[1]

Maria was some 20 years younger than him. As she was passionately attached to her country, unable to contemplate the idea of living abroad, Brown-Séquard decided to settle in The States, and resigned "his provisional chair in Paris, at the moment when measures had been taken to naturalise him, so that it could be permanent."[2] Vulpian was appointed full professor in his place, relinquishing the Chair of Pathological Anatomy, which he had occupied since 1866, when he succeeded Cruveilhier. Jean-Martin Charcot took over the Chair vacated by Vulpian.[3]

Brown-Séquard's marriage and establishment in America did not meet with the approval of his intimate friends, especially Désiré Laverdant, though Charcot did hurry to congratulate him by letter, adding: "Right now, I have a glimpse of very favourable circumstances for Edouard."[4]

Brown-Séquard bought a house in New York, and set up a laboratory there with Eugène Dupuy, a final year medical student, who was preparing his doctoral thesis. Dupuy was 30 years younger than him, and had followed him to New York to be helped in the preparation of his thesis. He intended to stay, for the rest of the year, in America. Their laboratory investigations had to be limited to week-ends, because Brown-Séquard's workload, as a practitioner, kept him busy during the weekdays. He had opened a consultation room in the city, as well as travelling to Boston, once a week, to see patients in the rented hotel room, where he stayed overnight.

---

[1] M.D.C. Editor of the Daily Chronicle (1894) Dr Brown-Séquard. Daily Chronicle, 6th April.

[2] Berthelot MPE (1898) The Life and Work of Brown-Séquard. From the Smithsonian Report for 1898. Translated from the Revue Scientifique 1: 801–812, 1896. Government Printing Office, Washington, 1900, pp. 687–688.

[3] Corlieu A (1896) Centenaire de la Faculté de médecine de Pairs, 1794–1894. Imprimerie Nationale, Paris, p. 378.

[4] Charcot J-M (1873) Letter to Brown-Séquard. GMcCC, Ms 981/100, April.


DOI: 10.1007/978-3-319-03020-3_15, 

He developed a very close relationship with Dupuy, which was to last for the rest of his life. Dupuy was born in Mauritius, in 1847. He studied medicine in Paris, obtaining his doctorate on December 26, 1873, submitting his thesis: Examen de quelques points de la physiologie du cerveau (Examination of some aspects of the physiology of the brain). He dedicated his thesis to Brown-Séquard with the following tribute: "To my illustrious master, to him who gave selflessly the treasures of his heart and mind."[5]

Brown-Séquard had been a good friend of Dupuy's father, as he had been a lodger in the rue Férou town house, in the early 1840s. Twenty-five years later, his son came to Paris and was warmly welcomed by Brown-Séquard, and the two were very soon as intimate as father and son. While a student, at the time of the Franco-Prussian War, Dupuy served in the French Army Medical Corps and, in 1914, though 67 years old, he volunteered to serve as a medical officer in the trenches. He also held an M.D. degree from the University of London and was elected a Fellow of the Royal Society. In 1874, he occupied the Chair of Experimental Medicine at the London School of Medicine for Women. He was closely associated with some of Brown-Séquard's investigations on the physiology of the Central Nervous System. He published quite a large number of original articles. He was married to a French woman, Eléanore Ollivier, and had three children. His son Eugène Louis became an eminent metallurgist. Dupuy died at Versailles in 1924.

The practices that Brown-Séquard opened in New York and Boston attracted a never ending flow of patients. Writing to a friend in April 1872, he said:

> I arrived from Boston today (April 20). I have never seen anything like the scenes that occurred yesterday. From 7 o'clock in the morning to 8 o'clock in the evening, when I refused to see any more sick, there was an uninterrupted flow of very patient patients. The last of whom I saw had been waiting for their turn for five or six hours.[6]

Writing to his wife, Maria, a year later, he said:

> I am now gaining more money than I ever did except in that exceptional period of April 2nd to April twentieth last year, when masses of patients had been waiting for me a long time. Up to last night, I have gained this month (11 days) $1,275, and there is a great possibility of my continuing to gain nearly at that rate the rest of the month.[7]

His practice in Boston was no less successful. On April 7, 1873, he wrote: "I do not know how I will manage today. I expect more than 20 patients.[8] Of the same day, he later wrote: "I gained $650 in Boston and received at once $470. A trip of that kind once a month would pay my rent."[9]

---

[5] Rouget FA (1930) Brown-Séquard et son oeuvre. Esquisse biographique. General Printing and Stationary Cy, Port Louis, Mauritius pp. 83–85.

[6] Berthelot MPE (1898) Notice sur la vie et les travaux de M. Brown-Séquard. Typographie Firmin-Didot et Cie. Paris, pp. 24–25.

[7] Brown-Séquard CE (1858) Letter to his wife, Maria. GMcCC, Ms 978/12, 12th Apr.

[8] Brown-Séquard CE (1858) Letter to his wife, Maria. GMcCC, Ms 978/7, 7th Apr.

[9] Brown-Séquard CE (1858) Letter to his wife, Maria. GMcCC, Ms 978/8, 8th Apr.

Busy as his practices were, he still managed to find time for other pursuits. In January 1873, he brought out his third medical journal, the English language **Archives of Scientific and Practical Medicine**, while still maintaining his editorship of his Paris-based Archives de **Physiologie normale et pathologique**. His co-editor was Edouard Constant Seguin, who had worked in his laboratory at the Paris Medical School during the winter term of 1869–1870.

The journal was aimed at practitioners and sought to publish medical and scientific papers of clinical relevance. Although there was an annual subscription of only 4 dollars,[10] the journal lasted for five monthly issues, the last one of these appearing in June 1873. Apparently the publishing cost proved too much and Brown-Séquard was somehow put off by the attitude of the publishers, Lippincott. He vented his feelings in a letter to Maria, written in April of that year:

> Will they [Lippincott] try to show that they have the right to keep the Journal in their hands till January 1874? If they do. I will have either to give up the Journal or to sue them. Anyhow, I see nothing but great causes of anxiety & trouble about this Journal. I expect that the best thing is to give it up at once (i.e. after one more number has appeared) if Lippincott is not willing to part with it. If it were not for that Journal, I would perhaps be able to bear many unpleasant things.[11]

Sometime after this letter to his wife, he wrote to Lippincott:

> My mind is now made up, I will publish one more N°. and then stop the publication altogether.
>
> My only object in publishing a Journal was to compel myself to give to the public a good many papers.... I did not undertake that task for the sake of my gaining money. I knew full well that I would lose money during the first year. I did not think that the expenses would be as great as they are.[12]

However, short-lived this periodical was, it still proved to be significant as it contains his first paper on **inhibition** and **dynamogenesis** in affections of the brain, in an article entitled: "On the mechanism of production of symptoms of diseases of the brain." The terms **inhibition** and **dynamogenesis** refer to a property of the nervous system whereby a restraining or an enhancing effect respectively is transmitted from one part of the brain to another. He wrote:

> All parts of the brain are able,... to act on any other of its parts, modifying their activity, so as to destroy or diminish, or to increase and to morbidly alter it.[13]

His first studies on inhibition of the nervous system had been undertaken in 1850. He repeated then, the 1845s experiment of the Weber brothers: the application of an electric current to the vagus nerve causes it to slow down the heart and even to stop it beating.[14] Although the honour of the discovery of the inhibitory

---

[10] Prospectus of Archives of Scientific and Practical Medicine. GMcCC, Ms 999/7.

[11] Brown-Séquard, *op. cit.*, note 8, above.

[12] Brown-Séquard CE (1873) Letter to Lippincott. GMcCC, Ms 989/7.

[13] Archives of Scientific and Practical Medicine (NY) (1873) 1: 251–256.

[14] Brown-Séquard CE (1853) Nouveau fait relatif à l'arrêt du coeur par la galvanisation du nerf vague. C R Soc Biol (Paris) 5: 153–154.

action of a nerve belongs to these brothers, Brown-Séquard was the first to draw attention to the inhibitory role of the Central Nervous System. In 1863, Ivan Mikhailovitch Sechenov had mentioned **inhibition** and **facilitation** of nervous origin. Facilitation being the reaction which follows repeated electrical stimulations of a nerve, whereas stimulations of the same intensity, fired individually, have no effect.

Brown-Séquard was eventually awarded the **Prix Lallemand** , in 1884, for this work by the **Académie des sciences**, but he received little recognition from his contemporary physiologists. His concept that these two mechanisms were responsible for regulating the activity of the nervous system in health and disease, was ignored or swept aside by many. Nevertheless, his work attracted the attention of one of the most distinguished neurophysiologists of the next generation: the Nobel Laureate, Charles Scott Sherrington, who wrote in 1893:

> It is interesting for the study of the functions of the cerebral cortex to note that experimentally it has not only an excitatory but also an inhibitory action on muscular contraction and on muscular tone.
>
> Mr. Brown-Séquard has for a long time emphasized this dual action, and in his writings, he refers to dynamogenic and also inhibitory activities of the cortex. Some experiments which I have carried out this winter on the monkey (Macacus rhesus) confirms this view-point.[15]

In 1932, Sherrington shared the Nobel Prize of Physiology with Edgar Adrian. In his Nobel Lecture entitled **Inhibition as a coordinative factor**, which he delivered on December 12 of that year, he reviewed the role of inhibition in the Central Nervous System "since the very first suggestions of Descartes to the most recent researches;"[16] but did neither mention the name nor the studies of Brown-Séquard. He spoke about inhibition in the following terms:

> The role of inhibition in the working of the central nervous system has proved to be more and more extensive and more and more fundamental as experiment has advanced in examining it. Reflex inhibition can no longer be regarded merely as a factor specially developed for dealing with the antagonism of opponent muscles acting at variable hinge-points. Its role as a coordinative factor comprises that, and goes beyond that. In the working of the central nervous machinery, inhibition seems ubiquitous and as frequent as excitation itself. The whole quantitative grading of the operations of the spinal cord and brain appears to rest upon mutual interaction between the two control processes 'excitation' and 'inhibition', the one no less important than the other.[17]

For Brown-Séquard, these two opposing mechanisms: **dynamogenesis** (excitation) and **inhibition** (restraint) led him to incorporate them in his own conception of the **localization of functions of the brain**, which is dealt with later on.

---

[15] Sherrington CS (1893) Sur une action inhibitrice de l'écorce cérébrale. Rev Neurol (Paris) 2: 318–319.

[16] Eccles JC, Gibson WW (1979) Sherrington. His Life and Thought. Springer International, New York, p. 71.

[17] Sherrington CS (1932) Nobel Prize Lecture, 12th Dec. Quoted by Eccles and Gibson, *op. cit.*, note 16, above.

Despite his financial success as a general practitioner and the free week-ends he had for research, Brown-Séquard was profoundly unhappy. One of the main reasons for this, was the failure of his second marriage. In a letter, dated February 13, 1873, to Eugène Dupuy, who had returned to Paris, the previous December, he is explicit about his unhappiness:

> You are young and you have a numerous family. You have, as compensation for your exile, the constant assurance of sincere affection. But I, who am growing old with frightful rapidity, have near me only people destitute of any tender feeling. Alas! what will become of me?... Your departure is the greatest misfortune that has happened to me for a long time. Not only were you a consolation to me by your sincere attachment, you were also a living reminder of the Société de Biologie and of my Parisian friends. I cannot endure the idea of living here for the rest of my life. I am very unhappy.[18]

Sensing the unhappiness that was gnawing at him, Agassiz planned to help him secure a future devoted entirely to research, by the creation of a private chair of experimental physiology.

In March 1873, John Anderson, a wealthy New York merchant and landowner, gave Agassiz Penikese Island in Buzzard's Bay, on the southern coast of Massachusetts, where he could set up a summer school for the teaching of natural history.[19] To this gift, which included the residential home and a barn which stood on the island, Anderson added a 50,000 dollars' donation. Agassiz started building a dormitory to house 50 students, and converting the barn into a conference hall and laboratories. **The Anderson Natural History School** was opened on July 8, 1873 and courses started soon after.

Agassiz planned to establish a physiological laboratory on the island for Brown-Séguard, as evidenced by the following letter of the latter to his wife, on April 6th:

> He [Agassiz] received yesterday a letter from Mr. Anderson telling him that he can employ at once the $50,000 to organise laboratories. He will go to work at once, building not only a natural history museum but also a Physiological Laboratory.[20]

The next day, he added that "Agassiz is ready to pay me a very large sum if I will teach Physiology in his school (at Penikese) every summer."[21] To a friend, he reveals the extent of Agassiz's generosity:

> Agassiz has asked me directly the question: "How much per year do you want in order to accept the chair of experimental physiology that I propose to found? Include all your expenses, for I wish you to give up the practice of medicine."[22]

---

[18] Berthelot, *op. cit.*, note 2, above.

[19] Agassiz EC (1887) Louis Agassiz: Sa Vie et sa correspondence. Traduit de l'anglais par Auguste Meyer. Librairie Fischbacher, Paris, p. 577.

[20] Brown-Séquard CE (1858) Letter to his wife, Maria. GMcCC, Ms 978/6, 6th Apr.

[21] Brown-Séquard, *op. cit.*, note 9, above.

[22] Berthelot, *op. cit.*, note 6, above, p. 25.

Such an offer was a dream come true for him, who enthused:

> Agassiz is going soon to have thousands of rabbits, guinea-pigs, birds, cats, dogs and living cold-blooded animals, all of which he will put at the disposal of experimenters. Why am I not again 30 years old![23]

Despite the prospects of working on Penikese Island, Brown-Séquard was extremely depressed during this month of April 1873. An offer from Agassiz for the delivery of a course of lectures at the Lowell Institute, embarrassed him and was a source of pathological anxiety. He wrote to Maria on April 10:

> A letter from Agassiz this morning, urging me to deliver this month, either 2 or 4 lectures at the Lowell Institute ($125 a lecture and $500 for 4 lectures). I am very anxious to earn this money as I need it very imperatively (although now & for the first time since I left Boston in 1871, I have more than $1,000 ($1,370) in the Bank), – but it is difficult to do what Prof & Mrs Lowell urge me to do. I know, I will gain a good deal more from patients during my stay in Boston.
>
> That, of course, is an additional reason to accept, but, on the other hand, when will I find a moment to prepare my lectures? I will anyhow make the effort even if I break down from it.[24]

His anxiety and depression increased during the next few days and he wrote: "If I do not prepare my lectures to day, I do not see also when I will have time to do that."[25] By the 15th April, his anxiety had turned into a panic attack:

> I am very unwell and certainly hardly in a condition to deliver a very difficult lecture in the presence of an audience entirely unknown or new to me.[26]

It can only be assumed, however, that he gave the lectures after all, as there was no further mention of them in his correspondence.

At that time, all sorts of pressures were building up in his life. He deeply regretted having sacrificed all "the joys of my French homeland" for "a bitter exile in New York". It was becoming increasingly difficult for him to relax and he was being dragged slowly into deep depression. Maria had left him for a stay of undetermined length in Cincinnati. He felt abandoned and wrote to her:

> Are you to stay 5 weeks away or still longer? On the 25th April there will be 5 weeks you have left me. Please let me know at once.[27]

Though the company of Agassiz did seem to liven him up, the following letter to Maria only highlights his underlying unhappiness:

> Yesterday was the first day of real enjoyment, if not happiness, I have had for a long time.... I got away from the hotel at about 1.P.M. and went to Cambridge, where I passed the whole afternoon and evening till 9, with my dear and most charming friend Prof.

---

[23] *Ibid.*

[24] Brown-Séquard CE (1873) Letter to his wife, Maria. GMcCC, Ms 978/11, 10th Apr.

[25] Brown-Séquard , *op. cit.*, note 7, above.

[26] Brown-Séquard CE (1873) Letter to his wife, Maria. GMcCC, Ms 978/15, 15th Apr.

[27] Brown-Séquard , *op. cit.*, note 9, above.

Agassiz and his hardly less charming wife. My headache disappeared and I felt another man as if the burdens had suddenly been taken away from my shoulders.[28]

During the months of May and June 1873, his health deteriorated. Physically exhausted and suffering from constant and violent headaches, he sought refuge, with his wife, in Brighton, in July of that year. He was deeply concerned about the prospects of his marital life, and especially about "Maria's chronic illness." This was the reason why he had chosen to take her to an English seaside resort. From there, he wrote to a friends: "I am in the depth of despair, life is odious to me. It is possible that I will never return to America."[29]

On top of all these problems was the continuing worry of his son's studies. Edouard was now 17 years old and did not seem to be living up to his father's expectations. He had mentioned his apprehension to Maria in a letter, written prior to their trip to Brighton:

I found Edouard much less hopeful than his letters had shown him to be and his tutors (2 brothers) seem to think that he cannot succeed. I am almost sure from their statements that Edouard will fail [his admission to Harvard]. What to do for him if it is so, I have not decided yet.[30]

However, in August, while the couple were in Brighton, Agassiz wrote with a much more encouraging view:

I had much pleasure in seeing Edward (or Edouard). He appeared very well, very desirous to prepare himself well for Harvard and I hope that he will be admitted as I am sure that once in the fold he will make his way.[31]

By October, the couple was back in New York. The stay in Brighton had not improved the health of either of them. Brown-Séquard was afflicted with hypochondria, imagining that he was terminally ill: "I have a constant headache. I think I am fatally affected."[32] He worked out that his patients owed him nearly 4,700 dollars and that he "would be bankrupt if an illness should keep me for a month without making anything."[33] His domestic circumstances were even more disturbing for him than his financial worries. He wrote to Dupuy: "Despair and uncertainty: these are my lot."[34] The latter, in replying, played down the seriousness of his condition, and he wrote back:

How I wish to have you near me! I have so much need of your sympathy and assistance. I can rely no longer on my own health. I fear that I may die suddenly, or fall sick, good for nothing - I am afraid that I have a serious cerebral affection. If you have more confidence than I in my health, come to me as soon as possible. As soon as I have no

28 Brown-Séquard CE (1873) Letter to his wife, Maria. GMcCC, Ms 978/17, 16th Apr.

29 Berthelot, *op. cit.*, note 6, above, p. 26.

30 Brown-Séquard CE (1873) Letter to his wife, Maria. GMcCC, Ms 978/9, Apr.

31 Agassiz L (1873) Letter to Brown-Séquard . GMcCC, Ms 910/10, 24th Aug.

32 Berthelot, *op. cit.*, note 6, above.

33 *Ibid.*

34 *Ibid.*

longer any depressing influence near me everything becomes easy. My wife is always sick; as for myself, I am exhausted.[35]

Quite used to the older man's depressive moods, Dupuy replied with an emotional attempt to fortify his resolve:

> You must look after yourself and not let yourself go, for, apart from the interests of humanity.... you have to think of Edouard, whom you would leave at a time when he needs support which he would not receive from most of your friends, full as they are of tenderness and concern in your regard. Those who could do something for him are very few indeed, therefore it is vital that you have the will to carry on. I know that nothing is impossible to you when you wish it.[36]

The end of that year though, was marked by a shattering blow for him. On December 6th, Agassiz suffered another stroke. When he heard about it, he left New York immediately for Cambridge. He stayed at Agassiz's house until the latter's death on December 14th. As soon as he reached Agassiz, the latter who always spoke and wrote to him in French, reverted to speaking only this language. At the final moments of his life, he sat up in bed, exclaiming: "Le jeu est fini!"[37] The game was over too for Brown-Séquard. His dream of a private chair and a laboratory of experimental physiology had vanished. The Anderson School of Natural History did not survive its founder. The following February, as a tribute to his departed friend, Brown-Séquard delivered a course of six Lectures on the **Nerves**[38] at the Lowell Institute.

Louis Agassiz was not the only member of his family whom Brown-Séquard cared for. He also treated Agassiz's son Alexander and Quincy Adam Shaw, the husband of Pauline Agassiz, Louis's youngest daughter, a wealthy man, with considerable interests in the mining industry. His son, Louis Agassiz-Shaw, in 1927, with Philip Drinker invented the ventilator, nicknamed the Iron Lung to maintain the breathing of patients paralysed by poliomyelitis.

Although Brown-Séquard's prospects in The United States were bleak after Agassiz's death, he carried on practising and lecturing. Thus, on April 2, 1874, he delivered the Toner Lecture at the Smithsonian Institution. His Lecture was on the **Dual Character of the Brain**.[39] This was a subject that had interested him for quite a while. He referred to it in one of his lectures at the meeting of the British Association for the Advancement of Science, in Liverpool, in 1870.[40] It was also the

---

35 *Ibid.*

36 Dupuy E (1873) Letter to Brown-Séquard . GMcCC, Ms 981/94, 22nd Oct.

37 Marcou J (1896) Life, letters and works of Louis Agassiz, vol 2. Macmillan, New York, pp. 213–215.

38 Brown-Séquard CE (1874) Lectures on the nerves. Delivered at the Lowell Institute, Boston. February–March. Extracts from the New York Daily Tribune. Lecture and Letters extras. N°15, pp. 12–35, 9th April. GMcCC, Ms 999/43.

39 Smithsonian Miscellaneous Collection 15: 1–21, 1878.

40 British Association for the Advancement of Science. Meeting of Liverpool, 14th–21st September 1870. Lancet 2: 436–439, p. 346.

subject of an article entitled "The brain power of man. Has he two brains or has he only one?" which appeared in the Cincinnati Lancet and Observer.[41] In 1878, he was to mention it in his inaugural lecture at the Collège de France[42] and, In 1890, he published an article in Forum entitled: "Have we two brains or one?"[43]

The concept of a dual brain, however, was not new. It originated in the findings and statements of such eminent physicians as Philippe Pinel, Pierre Honoré Bérard and Jean-Baptiste Bouillaud. Further more, Arthur Ladbroke Wigan had published a book in England, in 1844, called The Duality of the Mind, in which he stated:

> The two hemispheres of the brain are really and in fact two distinct and entire organs, and each respectively as complete (indeed more complete), and as fully perfect in all its parts, for the purpose it is intended to perform.[44]

Brown-Séquard's concept of the dual character of the brain was not far from that of Wigan's. For him:

> Each hemisphere is a complete brain endowed with all the powers that we know belong to the whole cerebrum. ...that, in the same manner that we have two eyes, two ears, etc., we also have two great nerve centres, each of which is capable of performing in its full extent, every physical cerebral function.[45]

The prevailing doctrine then was, that each hemisphere controls voluntary movements and sensitivity in the opposite side of the body. That is to say, that from combined sensory and motor centres, in each of the hemispheres, the nervous pathways going to each side of the body cross somewhere along the cerebro-spinal axis. Brown-Séquard categorically rejected the existence of such centres. He attributed any motor or sensory malfunction, in one lateral half of the body, following a cerebral lesion of the opposite side of the brain, to an "inhibitory influence acting on other regions of the cerebro-spinal centre."[46] He claimed that "all the voluntary movements of the two sides of the body can be performed by either of the two halves of the brain."[47] And that only

> one cerebral hemisphere might be sufficient for the perception of all the impressions coming from the various parts of the two sides of the body.[48]

---

[41] 17: 330–333, 1874.

[42] Brown-Séquard CE (1878) Doctrines relatives aux principales actions du centre nerveux. Leçon d'ouverture du cours de médecine au Collège de France fait le 2 décembre 1878. G. Mason, Paris.

[43] 9: 627–643, 1890.

[44] Wigan AL (1985) A new view of insanity. The duality of the mind proved by the structure, functions and diseases of the brain and by the phenomena of mental derangement and shown to be essential to moral responsibility. Reprint by Joseph Simon, USA, 1985.

[45] Brown-Séquard, *op. cit.*, note 43, above, p. 627.

[46] Brown-Séquard CE (1887) Dualité du cerveau et de la moelle épinière, d'après des faits montrant que l'anesthésie, l'hyperesthésie, la paralysie et des états variés d'hypothermie et d'hyperthermie, dus à des lésions organiques du centre cérébro-spinal, peuvent être transférés d'un côté à l'autre du corps. C R Acad Sci (Paris) 105: 642–652.

[47] Brown-Séquard, *op. cit.*, note 43, above, p. 636.

[48] *Ibid.*

He maintained that the dual function was proven by the existence of both crossed-over and direct nervous pathways:

> The crossing-over [of nervous pathways] in the cerebro-spinal axis, as revealed to us by [the study of] anatomy are composed, at least in part, of nervous fibres serving the voluntary movements and the sensitive and sensorial impressions. These crossing-overs are no doubt useful to facilitate communication between the two halves of the encephalon and the body, but they are not essential, because each of these halves are related to both sides of the body by direct conductors as well as by crossed-over conductors.[49]

He supported his theoretical arguments with examples from clinical cases, stating that in man facts abound showing that destruction of every individual part of one hemisphere can take place without the disappearance of the voluntary motor functions.[50]

He strongly objected to the general opinion that each half of the brain serves only the opposite side of the body.[51]

Regarding the functional specialization of each of the cerebral hemispheres, he believed that the left one was the major one, serving

> the mental functions, either in speech, or in intelligence, or in gesture, or in writing. That organ, therefore, is the important organ in our system adapted to the life of communication between ourselves and our brethren in a mental way.[52]

He explained the leading role of the left hemisphere on the control it exerts on the movements of the right limbs, which are the limbs preferred by most individuals since a very early age. By the end of the nineteenth century, the concept of left cerebral dominance which he had advanced, was an universally recognised fact.

As for the right cerebral hemisphere, he considered it as a minor one "more important for organic life than the left,"[53] serving "the emotional manifestations, hysterical manifestations included"[54] and concerned with "the needs of nutrition of the body in various parts."[55] He held the view that this hemisphere was responsible for bedsores, which were then attributed to a nutritional malfunction accompanying lesions of that hemisphere.[56] He suggested that given proper education

> the right side of the brain, in some individuals,... can be educated to become as good a leader in mental faculties as the left side of the brain.[57]

---

49 Brown-Séquard, *op. cit.*, note 42, above, pp. 6–7.

50 Brown-Séquard, *op. cit.*, note 43, above, p. 636.

51 Brown-Séquard, *op. cit.*, note 39, above.

52 *Ibid.*

53 Brown-Séquard, *op. cit.*, note 43, above, p. 636.

54 Brown-Séquard, *op. cit.*, note 39, above, pp. 14 and 18.

55 *Ibid.*

56 Brown-Séquard CE (1871) Symptômes variables suivant le côté de l'encéphale qui est le siège des lésions. C R Soc Biol (Paris) 23: 96–98.

57 Brown-Séquard, *op. cit.*, note 39, above, p. 10.

His concept of the functional difference between the two cerebral hemispheres, in which he attributes the organic life to the right side of the brain, and the intellectual life to the left side, highlights the influence on his thinking of Marie François Xavier Bichat's assertions. This physician—one of the precursors of Histology—was a **vitalist**: a believer in the philosophical doctrine that each individual possesses a **vital principle** distinct from both matter and mind and which, therefore cannot be explained in pragmatic terms. Bichat in his book **Recherches Physiologiques sur la Vie et la Mort** (Physiological Researches on Life and Death), defines life as an "ensemble of functions that offers resistance to death." He conceives of the existence of two lives: an **organic life** common to plants and animals, which presides over the major functions of nutrition, digestion and respiration and an **animal life or life of relations** which is concerned with the relationship of the organism to the external world through intelligence and motion.

In the 1960s and 1970s, nearly a 100 years after Brown-Séquard's concept of the duality of the brain, this question received a new impetus, which confirmed some of his utterances, following the studies of the American neurophysiologist, Roger Walcott Sperry, the 1981 Nobel Laureate, and that of his collaborators. These scientists unearthed major facts regarding the functional specialization of each cerebral hemisphere.[58] In **split-brain** individuals, that is patients who had undergone surgical section of the corpus callosum for intractable epilepsy,—that is whose cerebral hemispheres had been unlinked—these researchers studied the specialized functions of each cerebral hemisphere. They found that the right one of these patients had the ability for some verbal capacity[59] and for expression by writing[60] and that this hemisphere was the starting point for emotive reactions more impulsive and violent than those originating from the left hemisphere.[61] They confirmed, in right-handed individuals, the lateralisation of language in the left hemisphere.

The final part of Brown-Séquard's **Toner Lecture** touched on the subject of **aphasia**, which is not just the loss of speech, but the impossibility of understanding the various spoken or written signs which, for an individual, facilitate the means of communication between him and his fellow human beings. This disorder affects the region of the brain that governs the activities involved in language skills. It is located in the dominant cerebral hemisphere—the left one for almost all right-handed persons and for many left-handed ones—Two clearly defined areas in

---

[58] Gazzaniga MS, Bogen JE, Sperry RW (1965) Observations on visual perception after disconnection of the cerebral hemispheres in Man. Brain 88: 221–226.

[59] Sperry RW, Gazzaniga MS (1967) Language following surgical disconnection of the hemispheres. In: Milikan CA, Darloey FL Mechanism underlying speech and language. Grune-Stratton, pp. 108–115.

[60] Levy J, Treverthan C, Sperry RW (1970) Perception of bilateral chimeric figure following hemisphere disconnexion. Brain 95: 61–78.

[61] Gazzaniga MS (1970) The Bissected Brain. Appleton, New York, p. 573.

that hemisphere, as well, as the nervous pathways connecting them, constitute what is commonly referred to as the **speech centre**. Aphasia resulting from a lesion of this centre can be sensory or motor, for it is divided into an afferent or sensory area and an efferent or motor one. The afferent or sensory area of Wernicke lies in the upper part of the temporal lobe and is responsible for the comprehension of the spoken and written language. The efferent or motor area of Broca is located in the lower part of the frontal lobe and is responsible for the **expression** of language. A lesion affecting Wernicke's area produces word deafness, in which the words cannot be understood although hearing is intact and word blindness or alexia in which written words cannot be read, although vision is intact. A lesion affecting Broca's area produces motor aphasia, when the attempt to speak produces unintelligible noises and **agraphia** in which writing is impossible, although the hand is functionally normal. However, injuries to and diseases of the brain often affect a mixed area of the speech centre, resulting in a varied symptomatology.

The discovery, in 1861, of a speech centre by Paul Broca, at the foot of the third frontal convolution in the left cerebral hemisphere, had considerably strengthened the position of those who argued that the brain was a dual organ. This led Brown-Séquard to state that

> The very fact that the loss of speech depends on a disease in the left side is itself an evidence that the left side of the brain is quite distinct in itself as regards that particular function of the organ we call a brain.[62]

Anticipating the work of Pierre Marie in the early part of the twentieth century, he declared that though speech was a mechanical act, aphasia was the translation of a mental malfunction: a speech dementia-like affection. In 1865, he had, in the course of a lecture in Dublin, defined aphasia in the following terms:

> The deprivation of speech... usually unaccompanied by any loss of movement in the tongue; the patient being unable to give expression to his thought; and this inability extends not merely to speech, he is equally powerless to express ideas either by signs or by writing. The paralysis, in fact, is a "paralysis of the organ of expression of ideas."[63]

He also attributed the deprivation of speech, in part, to a loss of memory and, in 1864, he drew attention to the persistence of speech in songs, dreams and delirium in aphasic patients.[64] This alteration to the memory process was not an entirely new idea. The great clinician, Armand Trousseau, had said that "the aphasic is, in fact, an amnesic who has lost the memory of the means by which thought may be expressed in speech, writing and gesture."

---

[62] Brown-Séquard , *op. cit.*, note 39, above, p. 14.

[63] Brown-Séquard CE (1865) On the importance of the application of physiology to the practice of medicine and surgery. Falconer, Dublin.

[64] Brown-Séquard CE (1884) Persistence de la parole dans le chant, dans les rêves et dans le délire chez des aphasiques. C R Soc Biol (Paris) 1: 256–257.

In the last days of May 1874, Brown-Séquard suffered another tragic blow. Maria died a week after giving birth to a daughter, Charlotte. She was the victim of what was then called childbed fever and nowadays puerperal fever: a septicaemia caused by an infection of the uterus after childbirth. In 1843, the contagious nature of childbed fever had been recognised by Oliver Wendell Holmes in America and, in 1846, the Hungarian obstetrician Ignaz Semmelweis had shown that, in labour wards, the fever was spread by students' hands, which carried the contamination from the dissecting rooms, and that the washing of hands reduced the spread of the disease. However, it was left to Joseph Lister to realise that a lack of cleanliness accounted for the fact that infections were common in surgical wounds. In 1865, he introduced carbolic acid as an antiseptic in his operating theatre.

Practically nothing is known of Maria. Judging by a reference in one of her husband's letter, there is a possibility that she was a musician: "when is your musical festival to take place? I saw, last night, in a paper, that a rehearsal is to be had on 2nd May."[65] Maria suffered from some sort of neurosis, labelled "Maria's chronic illness" by her husband. It has been reported that "her state of mind was a source of perpetual torment" to her husband (l'état moral était pour lui une source de tourments perpétuels").[66] For the sake of Maria's good name, it should be pointed out that the above-quoted passage in French was mistranslated as "her conduct had been a source of perpetual torment for him (Brown-Séquard)" in Berthelot's biographical notice **The Life and Works of Brown-Séquard** , in the Smithsonian Report for the year 1898.[67] The French état moral means mental well-being and not moral conduct.

Although Maria and her husband were in regular correspondence, when away from each other, during their 26 months of married life—Brown-Séquard wrote her 23 letters from Boston, New York and Paris between October 1872 and July 1873—none of her letters are available. In the foremost collection of Brown-Séquard's private and personal papers: the **Gooddy-McCausland Collection** in the Archives of the Library of the Royal College of Physicians of London, apart from her husband's letters addressed to her, only two documents bear witness to her existence: a large multi-coloured and ornamental copy on imitation vellum of her marriage certificate[68] and a letter of sympathy, written by her sister-in-law, Mrs John Carlisle, addressed to Brown-Séquard, on May 29, 1874.[69]

The unavailability of Maria's letters is bewildering. When the 26 months of married life of the couple is assessed, one is struck by the sadness, the regrets and the despair evident in Brown-Séquard's letters to his intimate friend, Eugène Dupuy. Maria was the daughter of a wealthy man and used to a life of comfort and

---

[65] Brown-Séquard, *op. cit.*, note 28, above.

[66] Berthelot, *op. cit.*, note 6, above.

[67] Berthelot, *op. cit.*, note 2, above.

[68] Marriage certificate of Brown-Séquard and Maria Rebecca Carlisle, 13th March 1872. GMcCC, MS 999/76.

[69] Carlisle Mrs John. (1874) Letter to Brown-Séquard. GMcCC, Ms 980/42, 29th March.

leisure. In marrying, at around the age of 35, a 55-year old widower, an eminent man of science of worldwide reputation, she expected, above all, an affluent lifestyle. Hard-pressed to provide for this, Brown-Séquard acquired a permanent address by purchasing a house in New York and chased after money by assiduously practising medicine from morning to evening in two cities. It is possible that, like the unavailability of his first wife's letters, the absence of Maria's was the result of an intentional act to safeguard her memory or that of her husband, or of both.

# Chapter 16
# The Indigent Physician: 1874–1877

During the eighteen months which followed Maria's death, Brown-Séquard was haunted by illness, depression and indecision. He moved from New York to Boston, and from there, to Dublin, London and Glasgow, commenting that "to choose is very perplexing; there are difficulties everywhere."[1] In the midst of all this uncertainty, he gave lectures on both sides of the Atlantic, on a variety of neurological topics. In New York, he lectured on amaurosis caused by disease of the brain and the optic nerve; in Boston, on localization of the functions of the cerebral cortex; in Dublin on aphasia and anaesthesia caused by damage to sensory nerves, the spinal cord and the brain. In London, he delivered a course of three lectures to demonstrate that the same lesion of the cerebral cortex can produce different symptoms in different parts of the body, and that there is no direct relation between cause and effect of a cerebral lesion and a concomitant paralysis. On a visit to Glasgow, he turned down the offer of a chair at the University.

In the spring of 1875, with the permission of Agassiz's family, he experimented in the private laboratory, which was attached to their summer cottage by the sea, on the Nahant river, 25 km from Cambridge. There, he attempted to graft whole or parts of guinea-pigs' testicles on to old dogs.

In the autumn of that year, he left The United States for Paris, accompanied by his baby daughter, Charlotte. The previous year, his son, Edouard, who had failed the entrance examination to Harvard, had moved to Paris to study medicine.

In Paris, Brown-Séquard regularly attended the sessions of the Société de biologie. In the course of the session of December 4, 1875, he clashed with Charcot on the localization of functions of the cerebral cortex. This debate between these two scientists was echoed in all medical circles of the time, and was widely reported by the medical press. The prevailing doctrine then was that in the anterior region of the cerebral cortex of each hemisphere were centres presiding over the voluntary movements and the sensitivity of the opposite side of the body.

---

[1] Berthelot MPE (1898) The Life and Work of Brown-Séquard. From the Smithsonian Report for 1898. Translated from the Revue Scientifique 1: 802–812, 1896. Government Printing Office, Washington, 1899, p. 690.

L.-C. Celestin, *Charles-Edouard Brown-Séquard*,
DOI: 10.1007/978-3-319-03020-3_16, 

This localization theory had just been worked out. The first half of the nineteenth century had seen the confrontation between Josef Gall and Pierre Flourens. The latter viewed the encephalon as an homogenous organ, in which all the parts were functionally equivalent. It was generally accepted that the disturbances caused by damage to the brain were proportional to the amount of brain substance destroyed; although Philippe Pinel, Achille Louis de Foville and Jean-Baptiste Bouillaud had suggested that certain regions of the cerebral cortex had different functions. On the other hand, Gall, a phrenologist, asserted that the cerebral cortex was made up of several functional and independent organs. In 1861, Paul Broca reported the case of an aphasic patient, whose brain, at autopsy, was found to have a lesion in the inferior area of the third left frontal convolution.[2] Despite the significance of this discovery, Flourens's concept of the homogeneity of the brain prevailed until 1870.

In that year, Gustav Theodor Fritsch and Eduard Hitzig in Germany, showed that the electrical stimulation of the anterior cortical region of each cerebral hemisphere, in the dog, caused muscular contractions of the limbs and of the face on the opposite side of the body.[3] They had thus shown that, on the one hand, the cerebral cortex was excitable, thus disproving Flourens and confirming the results of the studies carried out by L. N. Simonoff[4]; and on the other hand that motor function is located in a restricted area of the cortex. The findings of these two German researchers were confirmed, in 1873, by David Ferrier in England, who carried out his experiments on monkeys.[5] The following year, similar results were obtained on a human being. A woman of Cincinnati, in The United States, authorized her physician, Robert Bartholomew, to implant, through the granular tissue of a cerebral abscess, electrodes in the dura mater, covering the left posterior convolutions. The passing of an electric current caused contractions of the right limbs.[6]

From 1875 onwards, the majority of neurophysiologists shared the view that several distinct and separate motor and sensory centres were located in the anterior region of the cerebral cortex. One of those who held a different view was Brown-Séquard, who rejected the existence of such centres. His concept was that

> The nerve cells of the encephalon which form centres endowed with a special function, … far from forming a group or an agglomeration in a distinct and well delimited area are, on the contrary, disseminated in such a way that each function has elements for its

[2] Broca PP (1861) Remarques sur le siège de la faculté du langage articulé; suivies d'une observation d'aphémie (perte de la parole). Bulletin de la Société anatomique (Paris) 6: 350–357, 397–407.

[3] Fritsch G, Hitzig E (1870) Uber die elektrische Errbarkeit des Grosshirns. Arch f Anat Physiol und wiss Med 37: 300–332.

[4] Simonoff LN (1866) Die Hennmungmechanismen der Saugethriere experimentell bewiesen. Arch Anat Physiol (Leipzig) 33: 545–546.

[5] Ferrier D (1876) The Functions of the Mind. Smith, Elder & Co, London.

[6] Bartholomew R (1874) Experimental investigations into the functions of the human mind. Am J Med Sci 67: 305–313.

> exercise, in various parts of the encephalon. The localization of functions does exist, but in cells disseminated and not forming, as it is believed, distinct clusters.[7]

His concept of networks of connected cells within the cortical substance, subserving the same functions and linked to each other by nervous fibres, enabled him to explain that lesions occupying different areas of the brain produced the same symptoms and that certain functions were not suppressed in cases of extensive lesions of the encephalon.

He therefore, categorically, rejected the existence of a speech centre. Thus, in 1877, in the course of a lecture in Dublin on aphasia, he produced evidence to show that lesions, outside the foot of the third frontal convolution (Broca's area) could affect speech, and he stated:

> If we follow the mode of proceeding of the localizers, these facts would lead us to say that, in certain individuals, the centre of speech is in the posterior lobe - that in certain other individuals, it is in the very front part of the anterior lobe - that in other individuals, ... it is in the top part of the middle lobe, very near the longitudinal sinus - that in other individuals it exists in the corpus callosum on the left side - ... that it also exists in the optic thalamus, and in the pons Varoli.

Furthermore, he added:

> Concluding that, because aphasia comes from an irritation of these organs, they are the centres of the faculty of speech, is doing just the same thing as we would if we concluded that the soles of the feet are the centre for the emotional power of laughter, because we laugh when the soles of the feet are tickled.[8]

He also asserted that a lesion acting by irritation, exercised an action à distance, producing the inhibition of one or several functions. According to him, the phenomena observed in various brain diseases "are phenomena of irritation, actions of restraint exerted on distant regions by regions in the neighbourhood of a focus of irritation."[9] As to Charcot, he had reached the conclusion that

> the brain is not an homogenous, unitary organ, but indeed an association, ... a federation composed by a certain number of different organs. To each of these organs are linked physiologically distinct properties, functions and faculties. Once the physiological properties of each of these parts is known, it should be possible to deduce the conditions of the pathological state, since this would only be an alteration, more or less marked of the normal state.[10]

---

[7] Brown-Séquard CE (1878) Doctrines relatives aux principales actions du centre nerveux. Leçon d'ouverture du cours de médecine au Collège de France, faite le 2 décembre 1878. G. Mason, Paris.

[8] Brown-Séquard CE (1877) Aphasia as an effect of brain disease. Dublin J Med Sci 63: 209–225.

[9] Brown-Séquard CE (1875) Sur les localisations cérébrales. C R Soc Biol (Paris) 24: 400–401.

[10] Charcot JM. Quoted by Gassner JL (1988) JM Charcot et la découverte des localisations motrices chez l'homme. Gesnarus 45: 501–520.

Charcot was thus the first to show that a lesion in a given cortical area always produces the same symptoms, though different from those of a lesion in a another cortical area. For him, there exists on the surface of the cerebral hemispheres:

> A certain number of regions which, when diseased, express themselves, for sure, by motor symptoms: paralysis, contractures, partial convulsions, according to the nature and extent of the lesion. These symptoms do not show up, at least as direct phenomena, following a lesion of any other region at the surface of the hemispheres, however extensive this lesion might be.[11]

At the session of the **Société de biologie** of December 4, 1875, Brown-Séguard offered the Society, the text of his Boston lecture of last June, on **Localization of Functions of the Brain.**[12] in which he held on to his own concept of localization, stating that:

> The character of symptoms in brain diseases is not in the least dependent on the seat of the lesion, so that a lesion of the same point may produce a great variety of symptoms, while, on the other hand, the same symptoms may be due to the most various causes, various not only as regard the kind, but also the seat of the organic alteration.[13]

Charcot opened the debate by commenting on a report of bedsores concomitant with lesions of the occipital region, saying: "There certainly exist in the brain, regions whose lesions inevitably leads to the appearance of the same symptoms."[14] Brown-Séquard intervened, saying: "I regret to be in complete disagreement with M. Charcot. I cannot accept the theory of localization as it is presently expounded."[15] For him, the problem was not to determine that a lesion in a given cerebral area always exhibited the same symptoms, but to ascertain whether or not "destruction of certain regions of the encephalon resulted in the abolition of some of the functions."[16] He quoted cases from the medical literature, such as the absence of hemiplegia in lesions of the internal capsule, and findings in experimentation on animals. These latter examples were rejected by Charcot on the grounds that the brains of animals are not identical to those of human beings. Finally, Brown-Séquard confronted Charcot with the following question:

> I would like to know now, from M. Charcot what are, according to him, the regions of the encephalon whose alteration is necessarily followed by a suppression of functions, not of properties.[17]

Putting an end to the debate, Charcot replied:

---

11 *Ibid.*, p. 513.

12 Boston Medical & Surgical Journal (1875) 93: 119–125.

13 *Ibid.*

14 Débat entre Charcot et Brown-Séquard sur les localisations cérébrales (1875). C R Soc Biol (Paris) 24: 400–404.

15 *Ibid.*

16 *Ibid.*

17 *Ibid.*

> I do not have to occupy myself with functions and properties. I am empirical and I will stay empirical. The destruction of the anterior wall of the internal capsule always causes hemiplegia on the opposite side.[18]

For Brown-Séquard, localization of symptoms was not the equivalent of localization of functions. His view would be in agreement with that which prevailed at the beginning of the twentieth century, as expressed by Morton Prince, in 1910:

> … anatomical localization is in no way denied or abridged. It is only the mechanisms of functions and of symptoms that is concerned. The conventional cortical centres, as at present conceived, are symptoms producing centres and not centres of function as conventionally ascribed to them.[19]

So convinced was he that symptoms of brain disorders were not dependent at all on the seat of the lesion that, in 1877, he wrote a long letter to the editor of The Lancet, protesting against the proposed surgical intervention in certain diseases of the brain. The following is one of the passages from that letter:

> Anyone who would be led to apply the trephine to the cranium simply by a supposition that there is a pressure upon certain convolutions, or group of convolutions, because certain symptoms appear, would commit a dangerous blunder.[20]

Brown-Séquard's localization theory, his concept of action à distance, and his belief in a network of inter-connected cortical cells, have been often adversely criticized. However, in the course of the twentieth century, theories which were formulated and experiments which were carried out, have granted him the status of a scholar who had lived long before his time. The first three decades of that century saw a group of scientists who totally or partially rejected the classical and rigid concept of cerebral localization of functions formulated by Broca, Ferrier, Fritsch and Hitzig. These scholars were: Kurt Goldstein in Germany, Henry Head in England, Shepperd Ivory Franz and Karl Lashley in America, Pierre Marie in France and Constantin von Monakow in Switzerland. They interpreted cerebral functions in holistic and dynamic terms, taking into consideration the ontogenetic and phylogenetic development of the brain. As early as the 1880s, when the theory of cerebral localization of functions was an accepted fact, Camillo Golgi who, for his work on the structure of the nervous system, was awarded with Ramón y Cajal, the Nobel Prize for Physiology in 1906, had been opposed to that concept of well-defined cortical centres, arguing for an holistic approach, taking into consideration the way in which the whole of the brain functions.[21]

---

18 *Ibid.*

19 Prince M (1910) Cerebral localisation from the point of view of function and symptoms. Journal of Nervous and Mental Disease 37: 337–354.

20 Brown-Séquard CE (1877) The localisation of functions of the brain applied to the use of the trephine. Lancet 2: 107–108.

21 Golgi C (1883) Continuation of the study of the minute anatomy of the central organs of the nervous system. Alienist & Neurologist 4: 383–416.

In 1906, Pierre Marie rejected the existence of a speech centre in the Broca's area,[22] as well as the existence of a variety of aphasias, which were said to be located in separate cortical centres, presiding over the various components of language. Through his studies, he concluded that aphasia was a unique and unitary affection characterised by an impairment of intelligence, a sort of dementia compromising that part of the thinking process dependent upon language.[23] Marie's work dealt a severe blow to the traditional theory of the cortical localization of functions.[24] Nowadays, the concept is that there are two main cortical areas concerned with speech: **Broca's area** and **Wernicke's,** The latter located behind Broca's in the postero-superior temporal convolution. Lesions of Broca's area causes difficulties in articulating words but the ability to recognise them, whereas lesions of the Wernicke's area results in a lack of comprehension, with the ability to speak, but the words uttered are unintelligible.

Shortly after the publication of Marie's work, it was the turn of Constantin von Monakow to formulate his **diachisis** theory of cerebral malfunctions, akin to Brown-Séquard's concept of action à distance, namely that the disturbances that occur, following a localized cerebral lesion, are not the consequences of that lesion itself, but of an inhibitory action triggered by distant regions of the brain.[25] In the 1980s, M. Mesulam in the United States brought back to life Brown-Séquard's concept of networks of interconnected cortical cells.[26]

Today, on the threshold of the twenty first century, it is widely accepted that some functions or components of functions are controlled from specific cortical areas and that, for example, a cortical motor centre might be the output area of several different motor sub-centres. Moreover, the idea that several different cortical regions, interconnected by a network of nervous fibres, preside over various cerebral functions, has not been ruled out, vindicating, in part or wholly, Brown-Séquard's concept of the localization of cerebral functions.

After his clash with Charcot at the Société de biologie, Brown-Séquard set about looking for a house or apartment, from where he could practice medicine. At the beginning of 1876, he considered a luxury flat on the corner of rue de Rivoli and rue de Castiglione,[27] not far from Eugène Dupuy town house at 176 rue de Rivoli; but he was put off by the high rent. His search for accommodation,

---

[22] Marie P (1906) Révision de la question de l'aphasie. La troisième circonvolution frontale gauche ne joue aucun rôle spécial dans la fonction du langage. Semaine médicale 241–247.

[23] Marie P (1906) Révision de la question de l'aphasie: que faut-il penser des aphasies sous-courticales (aphasies pures) Semaine médicale 493–500. Also: Maire P (1906) Révision de la question de l'aphasie de 1861 à 1866; essai critique historique sur la genèse de la doctrine de Broca. Semaine médicale 565–571.

[24] Prince, *op. cit,* note 19, above, p. 339.

[25] Monakow C von (1911) Lokalisation der Hirufunktionen. Jornal fur Psychologie und Neurologie 1&: 185–200.

[26] Mesulam MM (1985) Pattern in Behavioural Neurology. F.A. Davis, Philadelphia, pp. 1–70.

[27] Brown-Séquard CE (1873) Letter to Emma Doherty. GMcCC, Ms 979/109, Oct.

followed a letter from Désiré Laverdant urging him to settle down permanently in Paris. The latter wrote:

> You have very few needs, therefore, you do not need wealth. A moderate comfort is enough for you to raise your children and leave them the essential. But ... but ... but for that, it is absolutely necessary for you to settle down in a stable position. You tell me: my health is broken down. You have always been sick, always coming back to life again. It is not changing residence which will help you to recover. On the contrary ... there is here a vicious circle.[28]

But he continued to be restless and undecided. He applied for chairs abroad or canvassed his colleagues on helping him to secure an academic post in Paris. In March 1876, he was appointed Professor of Physiology at the University of Geneva but, even before filling the post, he tendered his resignation on 21st March.[29] The Public Education Department of the Republic and Township of Geneva confirmed his resignation on the following day.[30]

During the month of May, he paid regular social visits to Alfred Vulpian at the Medical School. The latter had, the previous year, been appointed Dean of the Medical Faculty, replacing Charles Adolphe Wurtz. At the end of May, Vulpian stood as a candidate for a seat at the **Académie des sciences,** and Brown-Séquard wrote to several members of that Academy, including Edmond Isidore Louis Bertrand, asking them to back Vulpian's candidature. Elected on May 28, 1876, the latter wrote to Brown-Séquard:

> I thank you very much for your letter of congratulations. It is one of those which has pleased me most. I know how much interest you have taken in my being a candidate.
>
> M. Bertrand told me that you wrote him a long letter on this matter, but he was too much pro-Bernard ['s candidate] to change course.[31]

In June, happy at having tried to help in securing Vulpian's election to the Academy, Brown-Séquard approached the latter, on several occasions, asking him to apply for a Chair that was then vacant, so that he himself could recuperate the Chair of Comparative and Experimental Pathology that he had given up in 1872—and now occupied by Vulpian himself—or failing that of promoting his giving a course of lectures at the Medical School. Vulpian wrote to him on June 23rd:

> I have not written to you for I had hoped to see you again in Paris, a few days after our last meeting. I was so busy that I had little time to think about the subject of our conversation. However, presently it does not seem possible to change position.
>
> A change round of chairs will imply new efforts on my part and an enormous amount of work, well above my capabilities.

[28] Laverdant D (n.d. probably Feb or March) Letter to Brown-Séquard. GMcCC, Ms 981/72.

[29] Brown-Séquard CE (1876) Letter of resignation to the University of Geneva. GMcCC, Ms 984/35, 20th March.

[30] Republique et Canton de Genève (1876) Acknowledgement of letter of resignation of Brown-Séquard. Extract from the Register of the State Council. GMcCC, Ms 984/36, 21st March.

[31] Vulpian A (1876) Letter to Brown-Séquard. GMcCC, Ms 980/44, 28th May.

Regarding your wishing to be permitted to give a course of lectures at the Medical School next winter, I would be very happy to bring about its realization, but there will be great difficulties to overcome, given the present organization of Education.

As long as we cannot win round the titular teaching professors who, up to now, do not help each other, it would be difficult to ask the Authorities to grand permissions for courses by individuals who are not linked to the Faculty by an official title. (I refer of course to lectures at the Medical School itself and not to those that are given at the Practical School.)

We recently had an exchange of heated arguments regarding M. Dareste who, by an error of wording in a ministerial document, was appointed course lecturer at the Practical School. Think what it would have been for a course at the Medical School.

I have already told you of such difficulties and there are other impassable obstacles.[32]

Brown-Séquard was greatly disappointed and upset by Vulpian's letter and complained to Laverdant that Vulpian lacked gratitude. Instead of commiserating with him, Laverdant rebuked him:

The Dean's answer, you had anticipated it yourself. Your friend does not tell you all the reasons which stand in the way. I happen to know that the Faculty has not yet digested your resignation and your departure, although it had paid a very deserved homage to you in creating a Chair especially for you.

Institutes and Academies are not individual and sentimental persons. These gentlemen did not take into account what you owed your wife. They only took into account the rapidity of your resignation and they remember it.[33]

The reason that made Brown-Séquard give up, overnight, the chair at the University of Geneva and seek either a professorship or a lectureship in Paris, was his starting up a close friendship with Elizabeth Emma Doherty, née Dakin, the 39-year old widow of the newspaper illustrator, Thomas Doherty, who had an apartment at 82 Boulevard Saint-Germain. Brown-Séquard was by no means a stranger to Emma, having known her and her husband for some while. He had dinner with Thomas Doherty, a man of his age, during his lecture tour of London, in 1858. And, he had been in attendance on the night of December 9/10, 1875, when Doherty lay dying in the Paris apartment, as the result of a cerebro-vascular accident.[34]

Brown-Séquard's relationship with Emma started when she was looking after the 20-month old Charlotte, for whom she had developed a liking. In the summer of 1876, she took this baby girl away with her for a stay in Britain, feeling that she owed a debt of gratitude for what Brown-Séquard had done for her late husband. He followed them both and spent the month of June with them in Brighton. There, he prepared a lecture on the **Physiological Pathology of the Brain**, which he delivered in July, at the Royal College of Physicians of London, on the invitation of its President, James Risdin Bennett.

---

32 Vulpian A (1876) Letter to Brown-Séquard. GMcCC, Ms 980/45, 23rd June.

33 Laverdant D (n.d., probably June 1876) Letter to Brown-Séquard. GMcCC, Ms 981/73.

34 Brown-Séquard CE (1876) Letter to Emma Doherty. GMcCC, Ms 979/10, 8th Dec.

After his London conference, he travelled to Brussels, where the Emperor of Brazil, Dom Pedro II, consulted him about the Empress's health, following a pre-arranged appointment with both him and Charcot.[35] This was not the Emperor's first visit to Europe. In 1871–1872, he had spent a couple of months in Paris, where he visited Pasteur at his laboratory at the **Ecole Normale Supérieure**, as well as going to see Brown-Séquard in his laboratory at the Medical School. The consultation took place on July 25th.[36]

From Brussels, Brown-Séquard travelled to Sheffield where, in early August, he delivered a lecture in front of an audience of 500.[37] From there, he returned to Paris, although Emma and Charlotte were still staying in Brighton. He was particularly worried about the progress of an article he was writing for The Lancet. It was an enlarged version of his July's lecture at the Royal College of Physicians.[38] He wrote to Emma:

> I have not my Library at my command. So that I am often stopped in my work and annoyed at being unable to make use of powerful arguments which I consider as well nigh essential, and which, however, I am compelled to leave.[39]

The fact was, that his 'Library' was in 44 cases, waiting at a warehouse in Le Havre, where it had arrived from New York.[40] It was still there, because he had no place to store it in Paris.

He decided after all, to go to Brighton and join Emma and Charlotte and there write the article, where he felt he would be better organised and where he would appreciate the tranquillity. It was an article which caused him quite a lot of concern:

> So much is at stake about it! Think of it: any fault in the argumentation, however slight, it would be and however little: it would really affect the rest, would at once be seized by all those whose opinions I offend or shock and they would make use - and above - of it to prove that everything I advance is wrong. I do not care about myself, but that I know science progresses so slowly that if I had to be put down now, all these new and important truths (as I believe them to be) which I try to establish, would be left aside, perhaps for half a century. I am fighting, therefore, for a very great object, and I cannot but dread to be defeated by committing some slight mistake or error, and I am, therefore, in a painful "quivive" all the time.[41]

The article was one that The Lancet intended to publish with full details of "not only what Dr. Brown-Séquard delivered at the College of Physicians, but a

---

[35] Pedro II (1876) Letter to Brown-Séquard. GMcCC, Ms 981/21, 24th Feb.

[36] Brown-Séquard CE (1876) Letter to Emma Doherty. GMcCC, Ms 979/6, 25th July.

[37] Brown-Séquard CE (1876) Letter to Emma Doherty. GMcCC, Ms 979/9, 3rd Aug.

[38] Brown-Séquard CE (1877) Lectures on the Physiological Pathology of the Brain. Lancet: 39–40, 77–79, 117–119, 155–157, 265–267, 339–340, 485–486, 599–601, 709–712, 827–829.

[39] Brown-Séquard CE (1876) Letter to Emma Doherty. GMcCC, Ms 979/11.

[40] McCausland C (n.d.) Notebook in her handwriting. GMcCC, Ms 999/7.

[41] Brown-Séquard, *op. cit.*, note 39, above.

number of facts which, for want of time, he was unable to narrate on the occasion."[42]

Brown-Séquard returned to Paris on the 1st September. Emma and Charlotte remained in Brighton until the end of the month, then spent part of October in Malvern, a spa in Worcestershire, in the Malvern Hills, eventually coming back to the apartment in Boulevard Saint-Germain. Thinking of renting a place, both to live and to practice medicine, Brown-Séquard sought again the advice of Désiré Laverdant and had dinner with him, during which he told the latter of his intention of marrying Emma.[43] But, despite, his conversation with Laverdant, he continued to be restless and undecided and spent time at the Practical School of Medicine setting up experiments[44] or long hours at the Library of the Faculty of Medicine. His restlessness brought him a letter from Laverdant, telling him:

> You need to practise a little to earn the money you need and the freedom to pursue your scientific researches. To attain this goal, it is absolutely, unquestionably necessary that you settle down, here or there or over there ... without a fixed abode, you are bound to see the clientèle diminish day by day.[45]

Accordingly, he decided to open a practice in London, in November. He wanted to publicise his intention in **The Lancet**, but this was judged unethical by Radcliffe, the physician who had succeeded him at the National Hospital[46] in 1863, although it turned out that there were no grounds for the latter's action.[47]

The practice was not successful. The public knew little of him and was unaware or had forgotten that, 15 years previously, he had been an eminent neurologist at the Queen's Square Hospital.[48] He considered opening a joint practice with John Hughlings Jackson, but was too embarrassed to proceed.[49] So, as time passed, his financial difficulties deepened.

In London, most of the days, receiving no patient or anticipating none, he called upon his colleagues, John William Ogle and William Dakin Waterhouse. He visited Cambridge, Oxford and even Dublin. While staying in the latter city, late in November, he gave a lecture on aphasia.[50] Many patients consulted him there, but he soon returned to London, only for his practice to fare no better in December. By now, he was acutely short of money which, henceforth, was the constant theme of his letters to Emma Doherty. On November 8th, prior to his visit to Dublin, he had written to her:

---

42 Lancet (1876) Dr Brown-Séquard's Lectures. 2: 203.

43 Brown-Séquard CE (1876) Letter to Emma Doherty. GMcCC, Ms 979/15, 1st Sept.

44 Brown-Séquard CE (1876) Letter to Emma Doherty. GMcCC, Ms 979/11, 5th Sept.

45 Laverdant D (n.d. probably Sept 1976) Letter to Brown-Séquard. GMcCC, Ms 981/73.

46 Brown-Séquard CE (1876) Letter to Emma Doherty. GMcCC, Ms 978/48, 3rd Nov.

47 Brown-Séquard CE (n.d. probably Nov 1876) Letter to Emma Doherty. GMcCC, Ms 979/197.

48 Brown-Séquard CE (1876) Letter to Emma Doherty. GMcCC, Ms 979/57, 8th Nov.

49 Brown-Séquard CE (1876) Letter to Emma Doherty. GMcCC, Ms 979/60, 9th Nov.

50 Brown-Séquard, *op. cit.*, note 8, above.

I am not willing to drop down to the condition of a beggar. Laverdant has offered to help me and I have refused his assistance. I know that I have only to ask and that ten persons here will at once give me what I need. I cannot do that.[51]

Emma wrote back that he should have swallowed his pride long ago, to which he replied:

Do not accuse me to be proud. Don't think of blaming me for not having written a month, two months ago to Agassiz [Alexander. Louis's son] to send me 2, 3, 4 and 5 hundred pounds or more. I know - I have no doubt - that he would have sent me anything I had asked. He would have been glad of it but, indeed I cannot ask, I cannot.

Nearer me there are friends who would be quite willing, but I must say that the difficulties for me to beg of them for help would be even greater than to ask Agassiz. Once, last spring, Agassiz was asked by my Attorney, in New York, to send £200 - the next day the cheque for that amount was provided. I heard of it and gave order immediately to return the money and that was done.

When I was sinking last spring, ... I wrote to Mr Shaw [Pauline Agassiz's husband] asking him to lend me £200, ... he sent me more than double the amount, he sent me £500, and insisted of never troubling myself to return that to him. I know that Agassiz would act in the same way. In fact, they both think they are my debtors. But, ... I pray you don't blame me to be unwilling to ask. It is too humiliating.[52]

A week later, his state of mind had taken a turn for the worse, and he wrote to Emma:

I cannot conceal from you that I am again falling into a frightful despondency. I cannot face my poverty quietly. I am indeed at present feeling just as miserable as I did before I went to Paris. I see no possible way of getting out of this horrible poverty. I have lost all hope of gaining enough here [London] to be able to organise myself in a decent way.[53]

Four days after, he was talking of destitution:

I have suffered & felt humiliated all night at the thought of my not having a home and having this constant plague of moving about, packing, unpacking & repacking. Oh! if I could be in a quiet place.[54]

Financial difficulties, despondency, lack of patients and lack of a home were not his only concern at this period of his life. He was greatly worried about his son's inability to settle down to a normal student's routine. After Edouard had failed the entrance examination to Harvard in the autumn of 1873, his father had toyed with the idea of sending him immediately to Paris, but had changed his mind. It was late, in the summer of 1874, when Edouard finally left The United States for Paris. A letter of Eugène Dupuy, dated June 30, 1874, is revealing, for it shows that Brown-Séquard's off-key attitude towards his 18 year old son was not propitious to the maintenance of a close relationship between father and son. Dupuy wrote:

---

[51] Brown-Séquard, *op. cit.*, note 48, above.

[52] Brown-Séquard CE (1876) Letter to Emma Doherty. GMcCC, Ms 979/61, 9th Nov.

[53] Brown-Séquard CE (1876) Letter to Emma Doherty. GMcCC, Ms 979/65, 16th Nov.

[54] Brown-Séquard CE (1876) Letter to Emma Doherty. GMcCC, Ms 979/73, 20th Nov.

> I regret that you have given up the idea of sending Edouard here [Paris], but after all you are perhaps the better judge in this matter. Should you keep him with you, I beg you most sincerely, please talk to him as a young man and not as to a little child. By constantly telling someone that he is a fool, he believes it and once he has believed, he behaves like one.[55]

In October 1874, Edouard registered as a medical student at the Faculty of Medicine of Paris, but his father's restlessness and bohemian life-style appear to have had a negative influence on his. Time and again, Laverdant, like Dupuy, had warned Brown-Séquard that he was tampering with his son's mental well-being. This is one of such letters of Laverdant:

> How can you hope to provide a comfortable life for your children by moving around without cease and without rest.
>
> The intellectual upbringing of Edouard has thus continuously suffered. And the charming Baby will in turn suffer too.[56]

It had been Ellen Brown-Séquard's wish that her son be brought up in America. So, from the time of her death in 1864, when Edouard was 8 years old, he was brought up in a boarding school in the Boston area, not knowing when his father would visit him and aware that the latter had no permanent residence anywhere, safe for a short period in 1873–1874 in New York. He must have felt deprived not only of affection, but also of a place which he could look upon as a home. Now that he was in Paris, his father was making no effort to settle down. This situation had not escaped Laverdant's attention. He wrote to Brown-Séquard:

> I beg you in the name of your adorable Charlotte, as in the name of your admirable glory, do make up your mind and settle down permanently.[57]

By November 1875, the relationship between father and son was taking a turn for the worse. Emma Doherty became the father's confident in matters relating to his son. Brown-Séquard wrote to her: "I am full of anxiety … you do not realise to what extent I suffer and dread the future about that poor boy."[58] This note brought back the following answer the very next day:

> About this poor boy, I wish something could be done; some place thought of which might keep him near a person who could insist on work. I am not certain that he might not be better with a stranger than yourself. In this on account of restraint as he is restive to your correction.[59]

Three weeks after he had written the above note to Emma, Brown-Séquard was very depressed and when questioned by her on the cause of his depression, he answered:

---

55 Dupuy E (1874) Letter to Brown-Séquard. GMcCC, Ms 981/83, 30th June.

56 Laverdant D (n.d. probably June 1876) Letter to Brown-Séquard. GMcCC, Ms 981/72.

57 Laverdant D (n.d. probably June 1876) Letter to Brown-Séquard. GMcCC, Ms 981/73.

58 Brown-Séquard CE (1876) Letter to Emma Doherty. GMcCC, Ms 979/10, 22nd Apr.

59 Doherty E (1976) Letter to Brown-Séquard. GMcCC, Ms 979/12, 23rd Aug.

... my depressed spirits have a very natural cause. In the first place, Edouard's bad health, his laziness, his gross carelessness about everything, his impoliteness towards all but a few people.[60]

In the same letter, he advanced the opinion that Edouard could be an epileptic, because of his biting his tongue at night, of his recurrent headaches and of his staying late in bed in the morning.

Moreover, he resented the fact that the young man did not address him by such endearing name as 'Papa'. He felt that by thus abstaining, his son was depriving him of affection which he was entitled to. At the end of November 1876, while in Dublin he wrote to Emma:

When I see Dr. R. McDonnell treating his father with much respect and tenderness, I could not help feeling how sad it was for me to be deprived of such treatment. Dr. R. McDonnell (who is 42 years old) calls his father "Papa", the word which Edouard considers good only in the mouth of an infant. Dr. Stoke's son - who is 45 - calls his father, as I found out yesterday "Papa" - but Edouard most likely thinks that a man loses his dignity if he is the son of another man.[61]

This craving for his son's affection, takes us back to the time when Edouard was an infant and his father was moving about lecturing in The United Kingdom. He was very resentful that his baby son—not seeing him—did not appear to be concerned by his absence. His letters of May and June 1858 to his first wife, Ellen, at a time when Edouard was only 2 years old, are somehow pathetic. It appears that the child referred to him as 'grandpapa' and, on learning this, he wrote back to Ellen, an ironic note:

I am happy of what you say of the feeling of my dear child concerning Grandpapa. You should show him my likeness and speak of me to him, as frequently as you can.[62]

In another letter, he was quite upset that "Monsieur Edouard did not mind more than he seems to the absence of his father."[63] Often, his affection for the child was subject to the latter behaving at his best: "Kiss him for me if he wishes to be better and promises to do his best to be good."[64]

On the other hand, Edouard was not making any effort to genuinely study medicine, though he was quite good at practical work. At the beginning of the autumn term of the Medical School, in 1876, Brown-Séquard wrote to Emma.

I am sorry that Edouard persists in asking to study medicine. He will not study. All he will do will be, at great expense, go to a dissecting room almost everyday during the winter and lay bare muscles and nerves and vessels but he will not know more about them at the end of the winter than any one does who has never studied their relations, size, plan of passage and insertions, etc. He dissects very well but does not study at all. What then is

[60] Brown-Séquard CE (1876) Letter to Emma Doherty. GMcCC, Ms 979/27, 7th Sept.

[61] Brown-Séquard CE (1876) Letter to Emma Doherty. GMcCC, Ms 978/86, 27th Nov.

[62] Brown-Séquard CE (1858) Letter to his first wife, Ellen. GMcCC, Ms 977/25, 29th May.

[63] Brown-Séquard CE (1858) Letter to his first wife, Ellen. GMcCC, Ms 977/30, 15th June.

[64] Brown-Séquard CE (1858) Letter to his first wife, Ellen. GMcCC, Ms 977/40, 30th June.

the use of spending time and money in that way? Since October 1874 he has been a so called "Student of Medicine" and he has not learned the least thing.[65]

The father concluded that his son's insistence on studying medicine was a ploy to draw money out of him:

At present, he knows I cannot give him much money; ... As regard the future, he hopes that I will be successful and that I will then yield to his entreaty & give him money & pay his debts. Here lies the secret of his wishing to "study medicine."[66]

Four days prior to writing thus to Emma, he had served Edouard with an ultimatum, and was somewhat surprised that the young man had not made known his decision: "He should have written, because I asked him to let me know what he would do, whether to study medicine or something else."[67] He believed that Edouard was keeping bad company and that he had "fallen in with gambling, races' book-makers and that he will himself engage into that shameful race-gambling.[68]"

However, while he was still in Dublin, Emma wrote that Edouard was behaving very well and he wrote back

I am glad that Edouard behaves better. If he studies a little this winter, I will send him to Brooklyn next March to follow a full course there. The Medical School of that city has its session in the spring and beginning of summer.[69]

Edouard's conduct seemed to have improved for, in July 1879, Brown-Séquard who was, at that time, on a short visit to England, wrote to Emma:

I saw Dr. Redier and I am very much pleased with him. He thinks well of Edouard and has great hopes of his success. He knows and finds that Edouard is lazy, but he thinks he will gradually change for the better.[70]

After that date, there is no more mention of Edouard in Brown-Séquard's private papers. It is not known whether he completed or not his medical studies. However, he is known to have gone and settled in The United States. An entry on a mutilated page of one of Brown-Séquard's diaries reads, under the date of February 7, 1893: "Edouard that I can't give him money nor help him as regards the organic fluid."[71] On March 23 of the same year, another entry in Brown-Séquard's diary reads: "To Edouard, a few stamps."[72] The latter seems to have inherited his mother's weak constitution. He died aged 40, 2 years after his

---

[65] Brown-Séquard CE (1876) Letter to Emma Doherty. GMcCC, Ms 979/50, 5th Nov.

[66] *Ibid.*

[67] *Ibid.*

[68] Brown-Séquard (1876) Letter to Emma Doherty. GMcCC, Ms 979/60, 9th Nov.

[69] Brown-Séquard CE (1876) Letter to Emma Doherty. GMcCC, Ms 978/89, Nov.

[70] Brown-Séquard CE (1879) Letter to his third wife, Emma. GMcCC, Ms 979/123, July.

[71] Brown-Séquard CE. Pages from one of his diaries. GMcCC, Ms 999/3.

[72] *Ibid.*

father's death.[73] He had married in The States and left behind a daughter, Ellen Grace.

The existence of this child is known because her name appears in her grandfather's will and in the correspondence of Charlotte McCausland, Brown-Séquard's daughter. In 1898, on relinquishing the ownership of her father's **Archives de physiologic normale et pathologique**, she instructed Mason, the Publishers, to send some of the proceeds of the sale to her niece in America.[74]

On a more joyful note, on March 7, 1877, Brown-Séquard and Emma Doherty were joined in matrimony at the British Embassy in Paris, in the course of a religious ceremony, officiated by the Reverend Robert A Mansell.[75] Emma was the daughter of the late William Dakin, a wholesale tea merchant from Fairfield in Derbyshire, who normally lived in Dulwich. A relative of hers' was William Dakin Waterhouse, a London physician, who was acquainted with Brown-Séquard. Emma was a woman of independent means with freehold property in Derbyshire, stocks and shares and ground rent for premises in Great Carter Street in London. After the wedding, the couple went to live in Emma's apartment at 82 Boulevard Saint-Germain.

[73] Kelly Ha, Burrage WL (1920) Charles Edouard Brown-Séquard. In: American Medical Biographies. The Norman Remington Co., Baltmore, pp. 155–157.

[74] McCausland C (n.d.) Notebook in her handwriting. GMcCC, Ms 989/10.

[75] Cutting from an unidentified newspaper. GMcCC, Ms 999/7, p. 53.

# Chapter 17
# The College De France Professor: 1878–1894

Two months after his wedding, Brown-Séquard went to the United States, accompanied by Emma and Charlotte. He practised in New York and Boston, while his wife and daughter lived in the latter town. Their stay in America was short-lived however, barely a year, because in February 1878, they received news of Claude Bernard's death. Brown-Séquard immediately returned to Paris, to apply for the now vacant Chair of Medicine of the Collège de France.

The main obstacle to Brown-Séquard's appointment to this Chair was his nationality. It was mandatory to be a French citizen to apply for a professorship of the Collège de France or be elected a Member of the Académie des sciences. Brown-Séquard had taken advantage of his dual British and American nationality several times in the past but, nevertheless, he had always felt French at heart and consequently found the need to apply for French nationality rather humiliating. In private, he confided that he had never approved Britain's annexation of the Isle de France and felt that he had spent his childhood and adolescence under the heel of a foreign power. He used to say:

> I have learnt to love France with all the passion of French people who have been through war and conquest under the yoke of a foreigner.[1]

Nevertheless there was nothing for it but to apply for naturalisation. Therefore, on May 21, 1878, Marshall Edme Patrice Maurice Mac-Mahon, the President of France decreted that:

> Brown (Edouard Charles), Doctor in medicine, born on April 8, 1817 in Port Louis (Mauritius) resident in Paris. Is permitted to enjoy the rights of a French citizen.[2]

It appears that the alacrity with which the whole process was completed, within weeks, was due to decisions taken at inter-ministerial level:

> To facilitate this election (to the Chair of Medicine of the Collège de France), the French government granted (Brown-Séquard) the highest degree naturalization. …

---

[1] Brown-Séquard (n.d) Autobiographical letter. GMcCC, Ms 999/7, p. 43.

[2] Presidential decree, 21st May 1878. GMcCC, Ms 987/6002E.


DOI: 10.1007/978-3-319-03020-3_17, © Springer International Publishing Switzerland 2014

M. Bardoux, Minister of Public Education, wrote on the spot to the Minister of Justice to recommend the prompt execution of the resolve.[3]

Despite such conclusive evidence of the change, Brown-Séquard's nationality had been the subject of much confusion and speculation. It was only, in 1930, that his daughter, Charlotte McCausland, clarified the situation, in a letter to Dr Rouget of Mauritius. Up to that year, it was generally believed that Brown-Séquard had not renounced his British nationality. The Mauritian poet and journalist, Léoville L'Homme, editor of a local newspaper, Le Journal de Maurice, wrote in 1894, at the time of Brown-Séquard's death that:

> He laid down as condition that he would not be naturalized French. The French government made some objections, but in the end put aside the regulations, and Brown-Séquard was appointed to the Collège de France.[4]

The 1910 edition of the Encyclopaedia Britannica refers to him as a

> British physiologist and neurologist. ... His father was an American and his mother a Frenchwoman, but he himself always desired to be looked upon as a British subject.[5]

The Minister of Public Education, Agénor Bardoux was aware that Brown-Séquard's claim to the Chair was unrivalled. Paul Bert and Marcelin Berthelot, who were often consulted by the Ministry,[6] had canvassed the opinions of the professors of the Collège de France, and made sure that there would be no repeat of the incident of 1868, when Brown-Séquard first applied for naturalization, only to be told that it would take a year to come through. This time, his naturalization became effective five days prior to his election to Claude Bernard's vacant Chair. The professors of the Collège de France were to assemble on May 26, to choose two candidates for recommendation to the Ministry of Education.

Brown-Séquard's appointment may have seemed a foregone conclusion, but he did not neglect the necessary steps to support his candidature. He presented a catalogue, listing all his original papers to that date, entitled Notice sur les travaux scientifiques de M. C.E. Brown-Séquard (Bibliographical Information on the Scientific Works of C.E. Brown-Séquard).[7] This catalogue lists more than 300 titles, two-thirds of which deal with the physiology and pathology of the nervous system.

So, at the Professors' Assembly of the Collège de France, on May 26, 1878, the President and Administrator of the College, the legal expert, Edmond Réne Lefevbre de Laboulaye, announced the candidatures of Camille Dareste, Elie de Cyon and Brown-Séquard for the Chair of Medicine, presenting also a copy of the latter's naturalization certificate. After an exposition of each of the candidates'

---

[3] Laverdant D (1878) Letter to Le Cernéen. Le Cernéen, Port Louis, Mauritius, 1st June.

[4] Le Journal de Maurice (1894). Port Louis, Mauritius, 5th Apr.

[5] The Encyclopaedia Britannica (1910), vol 4. Cambridge University Press, Cambridge, p. 674.

[6] Delhoume L (1939) De Claude Bernard à d'Arsonval. Baillière, Paris, p. 251.

[7] Published by Mason in 1878.

scientific achievements by Edouard Balbiani, Louis Antoine Ranvier and Etienne Marey respectively, 30 professors voted for the two candidates they would recommend to the Ministry of Public Education. In the first ballot, for the choice of the first candidate, Brown-Sequard received 25 votes, Dareste 4 and there was one blank vote. The second ballot, for the choice of the second candidate, gave Dareste 25 votes with 5 blank ones.[8] It therefore, came as no surprise when, on August 3, 1878, Brown-Séquard was informed that

> The President of the Republic has appointed you to the Chair of Medicine of the Collège de France, in succession to M. Claude Bernard deceased.[9]

During the 19th century, the Collège de France was the research centre for the most eminent scholars. It is a unique institution, with no attachment whatsoever to formal education in France. Situated in the Latin Quarter, not far from the Sorbonne, the seat of the Paris University, it was founded in 1530 by King François 1er on the recommendation of the humanist, Guillaume Budé. Known as the Collège du Roy, its first two chairs were of Hebrew and Greek, whose occupants were known as the Lecteurs du Roy. As the centuries passed, new Chairs were created and, by the 19th century, the scientific courses were prominent. Right from the beginning, the College has retained its own essential educational characteristics, which are: its independence from the teaching of the Paris University; the personal element in the professors' teaching, who express their own views and opinions, and the freedom for each scholar to carry out his own research. It is this total liberalization of its activities and teaching that has placed this institution in the forefront of French scientific research.

Finally, at the age of 61, Brown-Séquard was saying goodbye to the days of ceaseless wandering, of self-inflicted poverty and chronic financial difficulties. It has been calculated that, up to then, he had spent 6 years at sea, had crossed the Atlantic 66 times and had sailed 60,000 km across the oceans.

After the death of Claude Bernard, and while waiting for the appointment of the next Professor of Medicine, his préparateur (assistant), Arsène d'Arsonval took charge of the medical research laboratory at the Collège de France. Brown-Séquard, as soon as he was back from America, anticipating his nomination, asked d'Arsonval to be his future préparateur.

Jacques Arsène d'Arsonval came from a family of the old French nobility, from the region of Limoges, whose family seat was the Château de la Borie at St Germain-les-Belles. The men of his family had been country doctors for four generations. D'Arsonval had studied medicine, but he was persuaded to pursue physiological research as a career by Claude Bernard, for whom he worked as a préparateur from 1873 until Bernard's death. He was a brilliant physicist with an acutely inventive mind. He unravelled the physical and electrical properties of

---

[8] Minutes of the meeting of the Assembly of the Professors of the Collège de France, 26th May 1878. Document provided to the author by M. Yves Laporte, Professor of Neurophysiology and Administrator of the Collège de France.

[9] Presidential decree, 3rd August 1878. Archives, Collège de France, Paris Ms c-xii-1A.

striated muscles. He constructed various appliances to study body temperature and animal heat. He devised improvements for the telephone and microphone. He was the first to store liquids in a bottle surrounded by a vacuum jacket, an invention which was later improved by James Dewar, who used a vacuum jacket with reflecting walls to keep a liquid hot or cold. From 1882, although in charge of the medical lectures at the Collège de France, in place of Brown-Séquard, during the winter months, he was appointed Director of the Laboratory of Biological Physics of the rue Saint-Jacques, attached to the Chair of Medicine at the College. In 1894, the Académie des sciences honoured him with a seat. On the death of Brown-Séquard in that same year, he was chosen to be his successor at the Collège de France.

From the winter months of 1878 until those of 1882, Brown-Séquard lectured all the year round at the College. In November 1878, with the help of d'Arsonval, he prepared the course which started on December 2nd of that year, with his inaugural lecture on Doctrines relatives aux principales actions du Centre Nerveux[10] (Doctrines relating to the principal actions of the Nervous Centre). His first series of lectures was devoted entirely to the nervous system.

In late June 1879, he and d'Arsonval were preparing a series of lectures on the circulatory system when a misunderstanding, between these two men, arose. In the speech that d'Arsonval delivered at the Collège de France, to commemorate the Centenary of the birth of Claude Bernard, on December 30, 1913, he relates how this misunderstanding came about:

> In the course of experiments on circulation, I said to my new master: "Claude Bernard did not work like this, Claude Bernard thought otherwise." These remarks were meant to be laudatory, but their utterance in a loud voice was, I admit, out of place. Brown-Séquard in the end, visibly annoyed, criticized sharply my attitude. I answered back impertinently; but the strangest thing was what followed: the laboratory washer-up took my side and without conniving with me, we both left the amphitheatre. The washer-up, who had been there since Magendie's time, was known to us as le père Lesage.[11]

When both left the amphitheatre, they took refuge, for a few weeks, in the laboratory of Etienne Jules Marey, which was separated from Brown-Séquard's by a small courtyard.

The painter Léon L'Hermite has immortalised 'le père Lesage' in his famous painting of Le Laboratoire de Claude Bernard. In this painting, old Lesage is seen standing in the company of d'Arsonval, Paul Bert, Louis Ferdinand Nestor Gréhant, the physiologist Albert Dastre and the histophysiologist Louis Charles Malassez.

Happily, d'Arsonval and Brown-Séquard were soon reconciled. On August 2, 1879, the latter wrote to his wife, who was in England:

---

[10] Published by Mason, Paris 1878, 24 pages. Also: Gaz Med 13: 805–818, 1878.

[11] Chauvois L (1937) D'Arsonval. Soixante-cinq ans à travers la Science. Editions J. Oliven, Paris, p. 116.

Il y a du nouveau, d'Arsonval is to be again my Préparateur. He went to Rouget yesterday and implored Rouget to urge me to take him again. He said (and Marey said to Rouget) that he was extremely poor and had no chance of earning anything. So that if he lost this place he would have to give up science and go to the country to practice Medicine. I have consented to have him again. He came today, was very humble and helped Hénocque and me in some experiments.[12]

Lesage was also reinstated and in his old age, Brown-Séquard managed to get him appointed as concierge to the College and even gave him a monthly allowance from his own pocket.[13] Hénocque, who is mentioned in Brown-Séquard's letter was his other Préparateur, for the first year, he spent at the College. He also helped him, using his influence, to obtain him a post of Assistant-Administrator to the Laboratoire des Hautes Etudes.[14]

On July 14, 1880, the Order of Chevalier de la Légion d'honneur was conferred upon Brown-Séquard by the President of the Republic on the recommendation of the Ministry of Public Education and Fine Arts, "in reward for your eminent work on physiology and the services rendered to Public Education."[15]

The preceding May, Brown-Séquard had been notified by the Vice-Chancellor of Corpus Christi College of the University of Cambridge, that he had been selected for the award of the LL.D degree, which is "the highest Honorary Degree which is in the power of the University to confer,"[16] as the Vice-Chancellor described it to him, in a letter dated May 4, 1880. The official ceremony for the conferring of the degree, took place on August 11th. At the same time as Brown-Séquard, four eminent British scientists were honoured: William Bowman, William Gull, William Jenner and Joseph Lister.[17]

During the 1880s, Brown-Séquard was showered with awards, honours and honorary memberships of learned societies. In 1881, the Académie des sciences awarded him the Prix Lacaze, which was worth 10,000 francs. It was awarded every two years to the most significant contributor to Physiology. It was Alfred Vulpian who chaired the awarding committee and who outlined what the Academy considered to be Brown-Séquard's outstanding achievements.[18] They were; the decussation of the sensory pathways in the spinal cord; the irrigation of dying tissues; the artificial production of epilepsy in guinea-pigs and its transmission by heredity; the response of vasomotor nerves to electrical stimulation and finally, the demonstration of inhibition as a property of the Central Nervous System. This Academy award is named after Louis La Caze, a physician who was a great art collector. He donated 275 pictures to the Louvre, which included works by

[12] Brown-Séquard CE (1879) Letter to his third wife, Emma. GMcCC, Ms 979/125, 2nd Aug.

[13] Role A (1977) La Vie étrange d'un grand savant: le professeur Brown-Séquard. Plon, Paris, 1977, p. 167.

[14] Brown-Séquard, *op. cit.*, note 12, above.

[15] Presidential decree, 4th May 1880. GMcCC Ms, 984.

[16] Vice-Chancellor of Corpus Christi (May 1880) Letter to Brown-Séquard. GMcCC MS, 984.

[17] Lancet (1880) The Honorary Degree. 2: 304–305.

[18] Vulpian A (1892) Prix Lacaze. C R Acad Sci (Paris) 94: 321–323.

Rembrandt, Franz Hals, Jean Antoine Watteau. He left legacies for prizes to be awarded by the Institut de France and the Paris Medical School. In February of that same year, Brown-Séquard was made a Foreign Honorary Member of the American Academy of Arts and Sciences.[19]

From the 2nd to the 9th August 1881, the Seventh International Congress of Medicine was held in London. "The greatest and most historical congress ever held."[20] Charcot, Brown-Séquard and Pasteur were invited to take part. The latter was France's official representative. Under the patronage of Queen Victoria, the Congress was officially opened at St James's Hall by the Prince of Wales, who would later become Edward VII.

One of the first things that the Congress decided upon was to elect James Paget as its President and Pasteur, Charcot and Brown-Séquard among its Honorary Vice-Presidents. An honour which can be seen in its true perspective only when we consider the galaxy of eminent scientists that the Congress had attracted from around the world, amongst 200 French, 300 Germans and an equal number of British participants. To name but a few, from Europe: Jules Frank Dastre, Emile François Frank, Raphaël Lépine, Frederick von Esmarch, Robert Koch, Rudolph Virchow and Richard von Volkman. From England came William Bowman, William Gull, Thomas Henry Huxley, John Hughlings Jackson, Joseph Lister and Thomas Spencer Wells. From North America: John Shaw Billings, Austin Flint, Robert Palmer Howard and William Osier. There were a total of 3,000 participants in the whole event. The official languages were English, French and German. The British Medical Journal commented that:

> The number of medical men who have poured into the city from all parts of the world has no precedent in medical history, nor are they undistinguished persons, but from every country may be recognised names which can be counted as among the most highly representative.[21]

The Congress was divided into 15 sections, each representing a particular field of medicine. It organised many well-attended discussions in the Section of Physiology, but these had to be restricted to invitations only, because of fears that antivivisectionists would disrupt the proceedings. Pasteur, Brown-Séquard, Ferrier and Virchow were then the targets of a virulent antivivisectionist press. This danger was especially acute at meetings where animal experiments were actually going to be carried out.[22]

In the Physiology Section, one of the most important discussions was on the Localization of the Functions of the Cerebral Convolutions.[23] A subject on which

[19] Certificate of Foreign Honorary Member of the American Academy of Arts and Science, 9th Feb 1881. GMcCC Ms, 984/42.

[20] Sakula A (1992) Baroness Burdet-Coutt's Garden Party. Medical History 26: 183–190.

[21] British Medical Journal (1881) The International Medical Congress, 1: 234.

[22] Reidman SR (1973) Masters of the Scalpel. The Story of Surgery. Bailey and Swinfen Ltd, Folkestone, England, p. 229.

[23] Lancet (1881) The International Medical Congress. Section II. Physiology. 2: 326–328, p 326.

Brown-Séquard was in complete disagreement with most neurophysiologists and neurologists of his generation. Leopold Goltz and David Ferrier presented contradicting views in the debate, but Brown-Séquard chose not to take part. He did take part, however, in a debate on the Mechanism Regulating and Maintaining the Heartbeat,[24] which was opened by Charles Emile François Frank. Here reference was made to Brown-Séquard's first observation of the rhythmical contraction of involuntary muscles, in 1849. Finally, he participated in the last debate on the Vaso-Dilatator Nerves,[25] along with Leopold Goltz, Raphaël Lépine and Albert Jules Franck Dastre.

In the Pathology Section, Brown-Séquard took part with Thomas Buzzard and Jonathan Hutchinson in the discussion on The Influence of Injuries and Morbid Conditions of the Nervous System on Nutrition.[26] The debate centred on some disorders which were supposed to be due to the influence of the nervous system on the nutrition of tissues, namely on bedsores which interfere with the blood supply to areas such as the sacrum, the heels, the shoulders and the elbows and cause necrosis of the tissues. The influence of the vasomotor nerves was thought to be important in the normal and pathological 'nutrition' of the skin and underlying tissues. Brown-Séquard did not contest this influence, but stated that "there were other influences of the nervous system on nutrition than the mere contraction and dilatation of blood-vessels."[27] He cited gangrene as an effect of a nervous influence, since a cessation of circulation could not account for its appearance one or two days after injuries to the spinal cord.

Besides the sessions of the Congress, a busy social calendar was arranged for the participants. The Lord Mayor of London gave a banquet at Mansion House for a select number of delegates. Brown-Séquard was seated at the head table opposite Louis Pasteur and at the same table as William Bowman, John Scott Burdon-Sanderson, Jean-Martin Charcot, Leopold Goltz, James Paget and Rudolph Karl Virchow.[28] There was a great reception at the Guildhall for all the participants to the Congress. Many eminent British physicians and surgeons, as well as some aristocrats, gave private receptions and garden parties in their homes. Naturally, Brown-Séquard was entertained by several colleagues. Paget even invited him to lunch with the Prince of Wales. On the last evening of the Congress, there was an informal dinner at Crystal Palace, followed by a firework display.

For the last time in 1881, Brown-Séquard gave lectures at the College de France, during the winter months. In the spring of each year, he was always very busy. In 1879, writing to his friend and colleague, John William Ogle of London,

---

[24] *Ibid.*

[25] *Ibid.*, p. 328.

[26] British Medical Journal (1880) The International Medical Congress. SectionG. Pathology. 2: 384.

[27] Brown-Séquard CE (1880) Remarks on some of the physiological and pathological influence of the nervous system on nutrition.Br.Med.J. 2:915–916

[28] Plan of tables and programme of music, Banquet to the President and Members of the International Medical Congress, 4th Aug 1881. GMcCC Ms, 999/80.

he said: "My lecturing and some patients take all my time."[29] Indeed, he had at that time, a fairly large clientèle. Apart from relatives and friends of acquaintances, and those patients sent to him by his colleagues and his cousins, Alexandre Séquard, senior and junior,[30] he was physician to many foreigners especially Americans as well as to wealthy members of the French aristocracy. Among them, Leland Stanford , the owner of Central and Southern Pacific Railroads,[31] who suffered from locomotor ataxia and Baroness Rothschild,[32] the widow of Baron James of Paris. From 1889 onwards, he treated, with a liquid extract of testicular tissues, a great number of colleagues, scientists, politicians and writers, the like of Pasteur, Alphonse Daudet and Emile Zola.

In 1882, following a visit he had paid to the Middlesex Lunatic Asylum during the Seventh International Medical Congress, he had conferred on him the title of Honorary Member of the **Medico-Psychological Society**.[33] Later in that year, he was made an Honorary Member of the **Société Royale des Sciences Médicales et Naturelles de Belgique**.[34] The following year, he was awarded the Baly Gold Medal of the Royal College of Physicians of London. This Medal is awarded to "the person who shall be deemed to have most distinguished himself in the science of physiology, especially during the two years immediately preceding the award." The previous continental recipients of this Medal had been Claude Bernard and Karl Ludwig, to be joined at later dates by Rudolph Peter Heinrich Heidenhain and Moritz Schiff. This Medal commemorates the late William Baly, a lecturer in forensic medicine at St Bartholomew's Hospital, who had been elected a Fellow of the Royal College of Physicians in 1846 and a Fellow of the Royal Society in 1847. He was killed in 1861, in a railway accident.

For the most part and for many years, Brown-Séquard lectured to attentive audiences at the **Collège de France**. There was, however, one lecture, in 1883, that was markedly different from the rest. While he was performing an experiment on a monkey to demonstrate the analgesic effect of carbonic acid, the animal screamed, and a woman rushed forward and hit him with a parasol. He suffered a minor facial scratch, but was visibly shaken by the disruption.[35] This incident was widely reported by the Parisian press and "in a matter of hours, it earned Brown-Séquard

---

[29] Brown-Séquard CE. Letter to JW Ogle. Quoted by Olmsted JMD, (1946) Charles-Edouard Brown-Séquard. A nineteenth century neurologist and endocrinologist. The John Hopkins Press, Baltimore, p. 166.

[30] Brown-Séquard CE (1881) Letter to a lady, née Blaize. Wellcome Institute for the History of Medicine. Department of Western Manuscripts, 7th Dec.

[31] Stanford L (1883) Letter to Brown-Séquard. GMcCC, Ms 980/50, 31st Aug.

[32] Baroness Rothschild (1883) Letter to Brown-Séquard. GMcCC, Ms 980/82.

[33] Certificate of Honorary Member of the Medico-Psychological Society, 30th Jan 1883. GMcCC, Ms 984/44.

[34] Certificate of Membre Honoraire de la Société Royale des Sciences médicales et naturelles de Belgique, 12th Aug 1882. GMcCC, Ms 984/48.

[35] Le Matin (1855) Le fait du jour. M. Brown-Séquard. Paris, 30th June.

**Fig. 17.1** Portrait of Brown-Séquard aged 65, 1882

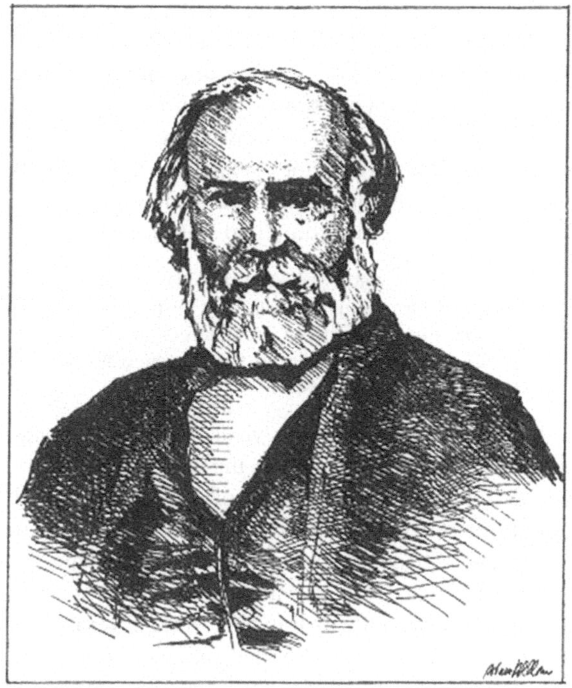

PORTRAIT OF BROWN-SEQUARD AGED 65
1882

more fame than his discoveries."[36] The objector was an English woman by the name of Anna Kingsford. She described the incident in a letter dated May 1883, saying that "the monkey screamed terribly when its throat was treated with carbonic acid in the course of the investigator's search for an anaesthetic" (Fig. 17.1).[37]

Anna Kingsford had studied medicine, but qualified without ever using an animal in an experiment. She founded the **Société Française contre la Vivisection**, early in 1883, inviting the great poet and novelist, Victor Hugo to become its first president, who readily accepted the offer. She spent her time in Paris, visiting laboratories such as those of the **Pasteur Institute** or the **Collège de France**, where vivisections were commonly carried out. She said of the Practical School of Medicine that it was "horrible to see and hear what goes on daily in those infamous dens."[38] A firm believer in the occult, she claimed that she had "been

[36] *Ibid.*

[37] Westacott E (1949) A Century of vivisection and anti-vivisection, A study of their effect upon Science, Medicine and Human life during the past hundred years. The CW Daniel Co., Ashington, Rochford, Essex, England, p. 173.

[38] *Ibid.*, p. 179.

divinely used as an instrument for the destruction of Claude Bernard."[39] She was summoning supernatural powers to kill the "devil Louis Pasteur and the physiologists Charles Richet and Brown-Sequard."[40] She used disruptive techniques in her fight against vivisections, instigating her young female followers to disturb the laboratories where animals were used.

Brown-Séquard did not escape the antivivisectionists' attention and was targeted. The comments of a London newspaper at the time of his death in 1894, reveal that their endeavours had not passed unnoticed:

> No doubt, he was a great physiologist, but he had earned the infamous name of being the greatest torturer of animals next to Pasteur himself. His discoveries were made by intolerable tortures inflicted on hundreds of dumb creatures ... Brown-Séquard has not lived in vain. He has shown to what extent a bottomless abyss of selfishness vivisectors and their patrons may descend.[41]

In 1884, in reward of his work on inhibition and dynamogenesis in the normal and pathological working of the Central Nervous System, Brown-Séquard was awarded the Prix Lallemand of the Académie des sciences. The awardening committee was made up of Paul Bert, Charcot, Athenese Lèon Gosselin, Charles Richet and Alfred Vulpian.[42] The Prize's name is derived from Claude François Lallemand, who was the author of a classic treatise Sur l'Encéphale (On the Encephalon), which was translated into several languages. He left 50,000 francs to the Institut de France to honour and encourage research on the nervous system. In that same year, Brown-Séquard was made an Honorary Member of the Medico-Chirurgical Society of Edinburgh.[43]

The following year, he was awarded a yet bigger prize, the Prix Biennal of 20,000 francs, which is awarded every two years by the five constituent Academies of the Institut de France. It honours any outstanding discovery or research work of the preceding 10 years. Every second year, one of the 5 Academies takes it in turn to select a candidate who has to be approved by the other 4. The year 1885, being the turn of the Académie des sciences to choose a candidate, Brown-Séquard was chosen by the Section of Medicine and Surgery, while the Section of Geography and Navigation chose Pierre Brazza de Savorgnan, a naturalized French citizen, who was originally Italian. He was the explorer who established French presence in the Congo. Brown-Séquard was elected by ballot and the Institut ratified the choice by a majority of 67 votes out of a total of 74 cast.[44]

In 1886, Brown-Séquard was elected to occupy a seat at the Institut de France, as a Member of the Académie des sciences. Thus, on June 21st, the Permanent

---

[39] *Ibid.*, p. 172.

[40] *Ibid.*, p. 179.

[41] The Echo (1894) Dr Brown-Séquard. London 3rd Apr.

[42] Bert P (1885) Prix Lallemand. C R Acad Sci (Paris) 100: 535–537.

[43] Certificate of Honorary Memeber of the Medico-Chirurgical Society of Edinburgh, May 1884. GMcCC, Ms 984/46.

[44] Lancet (1885) The Prize awarded to Dr Brown-Séquard. 2: 168.

Secretaries of the Academy, Edmond Isidore Louis Bertrand and Alfred Vulpian wrote to him:

> We have the honour to inform you that the Académie des Sciences, today, in the course of its session, has appointed you to occupy the seat in the Section of Medicine and Surgery left vacant by the appointment of M. Vulpian as Permanent Secretary.
> As soon as the Academy has received the certified copy of the Decree approving of your election, we will be eager to invite you to take part in our works.[45]

It was not the first time that Brown-Séquard had tried to be elected a Member of the Academy. In the election of April 1882, in replacement of the late Jean-Baptiste Bouillaud, only one vote was cast in his favour, while Paul Bert received 30, ahead of Casimir Joseph Davaine, who was second with 26 votes.[46] In 1883, Brown-Séquard was again a candidate for the seat left vacant by the death of Jules Germain Cloquet. He had then backed up his candidature with the fourth catalogue of his original papers, bearing the same title as his 1878s one for his candidature to the Chair of Medicine of the Collège de France: Notice sur les travaux scientifiques de M. C.E. Brown-Séquard (Bibliographical Information on the Scientific Works of Mr. C.E. Brown-Séquard),[47] but Charcot was elected.

The news of his nomination to the Institut de France was received enthusiastically in his native Mauritius, and a delegation of his countrymen, who were resident in Paris, presented him with the congratulations of all the corporate bodies of his native island.[48] On August 4th, the Medical Society of Mauritius elected him their Honorary President,[49] an honour which he greatly appreciated as his reply to Dr Edwards's letter, the President of the Society, reveals. The then governor of Mauritius, Sir John Pope-Hennesy, "recommended to the British Government that the Cross of St Michael and St George (CMG) be conferred upon the illustrious Mauritian."[50] This request was, apparently, turned down, due to his notoriety as an unrepentant vivisectionist in the United Kingdom. This could have hardly been a great blow for him as awards were coming in from all over the world. Even Sioux City, Iowa, honoured him by electing him an Honorary Member of the North-western Literary and Historical Society.[51]

---

[45] Permanent Secretaries of the Académie des sciences (1886) Letter to Brown-Séquard. GMcCC, Ms 984, 21st June.

[46] Lupovici C, Chapius M, Chapius J (1979) Paul Bert 1833–1886. Centenaire de "La pression barométrique." Académie de médecine, Paris, 12 décembre au 23 janvier 1970, p. 12, note 27. Also C R Acad Sci (Pairs) 94: 925, 1882.

[47] Published by Mason, Paris, 1883.

[48] Rouget FA (1930) Brown-Séquard et son oeuvre. Esquisse biographique. General Printing and Stationary Cy, Port Louis, Mauritius. p. 35.

[49] Dr. Edwards (1886) Letter to Brown-Séquard. Société médicale de l'île Maurice. GMcCC, Ms 984/59, 28th Sept.

[50] Revue Historique et Littéraire de l'île Maurice (1894), p. 13.

[51] Certificate of Honorary Member of the North-Western Literary and Historical Society, 16th June 1886. GMcCC, Ms 984/57.

The Institut de France holds a position of great prestige in France. Created in 1795, it comprises 5 Academies which represent the various branches of Art, Science and Literature, which rank according to the date of their foundation. Thus, the most illustrious is the Académie Française founded in 1635 by Cardinal Richelieu, the chief minister of Louis XIII. This Academy has only 40 members. The other Academies are the Académie des Inscriptions et Belles-Lettres; the Académie des sciences, the Académie des Beaux-Arts and the Académie des Sciences Morales et Politiques. As expounded in Harper's New Monthly Magazine:

> The title of Member of the Institute is the highest distinction to which a Frenchman of culture can aspire. It is the crowning honour of his career, the canonization which makes him a rounded whole; the supreme glorification of the savant, of the sowers and propagators of ideas, of the soldiers of thought, who are esteemed to be as true representatives of the French race and genius as the peasant in the field and the soldier at the frontier.[52]

At the age of 70, the exacting demands of his post, compelled Brown-Séquard to have d'Arsonval appointed substitute professor. The latter had, as Director of the rue Saint-Jacques Laboratory of Biological Physics expounded his own discoveries in the course of lectures on animal heat, electrophysiology and electrotherapy. Brown-Séquard had no intention of retiring. The law on pension's age, postponed for five years for Members of the Institut de France, did not apply to professors of the Collège de France who could occupy a chair for life. By having d'Arsonval appointed substitute professor, Brown-Séquard was indicating that he had no intention of retiring, and that death only would deprive him of a laboratory, where he was free to engage in research work. He reckoned continuing "so long as I have a breath of power left of mind and body."[53]

The best gift for his seventieth birthday was that of being appointed President of the Société de biologie. The position became vacant as a result of Paul Bert's death, a victim of amoebic dysentery in French Indochina (presently made up of Vietnam and Cambodia), where he had been appointed governor-general of the provinces of Annam and Tonkin. So, in 1887, Brown-Sequard competed for the position with Jean-Baptiste Chauveau, a physician, physiologist and veterinary surgeon and was elected to the presidency. On his first day as President, he addressed the members with tears in his eyes:

> My debt of gratitude to the Society dates of old. In the very year of its foundation, in 1848, it honoured me by placing me amongst its first four secretaries and, twice, it has elected me vice-president. But I owe it much more than that, for it was the encouragements, it was the examples that I found here, that have led me to reach the position that I occupy today.[54]

---

[52] Child T (1889) The Institute of France. Harper's New Monthly Magazine 78: 501–520.

[53] Brown-Séquard, *op. cit.*, note 29, above.

[54] Dupuy E (1894) Notice sur M. Le professeur Brown-Séquard, ancient Président de la Société de biologie. Revue Scient 2:742–743.

The honours that he received in 1888 and 1889 were still quite significant. In February 1888, he was made a Corresponding Member of the Neurological Society of London,[55] a society which had been founded in 1876, mainly by botanists and biologists. Among the founding members were Edwin Ray Lankaster, Professor of Zoology at University College, London; Thomas Henry Huxley, Michael Foster and John Scott Burdon-Sanderson, the last two being the leading physiologists of their age in Britain. In October, he was made an Honorary Member of the Société Française d'Hygiène,[56] and in January 1889, a Honorary Member of the Société d'Anthropologie of Paris[57] which had been founded by Paul Broca in 1859.

From 1879, when Charcot started using hypnotism to treat some of his patients, he agreed that Brown-Séquard use his patients, hospitalised at La Salpëtrière, for experimental therapy.[58] The latter attributed the hypnotic state to an inhibition of the Central Nervous System. His interest in this condition led him to attend the International Congress of Experimental Hypnotism, held under the presidency of Victor Alphonse Amédé Dumont-Palier where, together with Charcot and Brouardel, he was chosen as one of the presidents of honour of the Congress. His views on hypnosis influenced the elaboration of several theories to explain this artificially induced state of passivity as a total or partial cerebral inhibition. Thus, Ralph Harry Vincent, in England, in his book Hypnotism, explains it on the basis of Brown-Séquard's concept of inhibition and dynamogenesis as "an inhibition of one set of functions—with an increased capacity of action in the others."[59] A somewhat similar explanation is to be found in Psychology of Suggestion, the work of the American Boris Sidis . A theory attributed to Eduard Rückardt, which was upheld by Camillo Golgi and Santiago Ramón y Cajal, considers the hypnotic state as influencing the histological structure of brain tissue, namely as "an inhibition of the amoeboid movements in the pseudopodic, protoplasmic prolongations of the neurospongium."[60]

Inhibition in the normal and pathological functioning of various systems of the organism was one of the many studies, which Brown-Séquard undertook from 1878 to 1893. The 16 years that he spent at the Collège de France were marked by a spate of experimental activity as great, if not greater, than during the previous 32 years of his research carrier, as attested by his many publications, over 250 papers. Apart from continuing his experiments on artificially induced epilepsy in

---

[55] Certificate of Corresponding Member of the Neurological Society of London, 7th February, 1888. GMcCC, Ms 984/61.

[56] Certificate of Membre Honoraire de la Société française d'hygiène, 10th Oct, 1888. GMcCC, Ms 984/62.

[57] Certificate of Membre Honoraire de la Société d'Anthropologie, 21st Jan, 1889. GMcCC, Ms 984/63.

[58] Delhoume, *op. cit.*, note 6, above, pp. 472 and 475.

[59] Bramwell JM (1921) Hypnotism. Its History, Practise and Theory. William Rider & Son, London, p. 304.

[60] *Ibid.*, p. 305.

guinea-pigs and its hereditary transmission, he devoted his labour to the aetiology of primary shock, to the analgesic action of several chemical substances, to the noxious effect of vitiated air and, from 1889 until 1893, to the therapeutic effects of extracts of endocrine glands and of various organs.

The influence of the nervous system in modifying the metabolic exchanges between blood and the tissues, in conditions of severe injury and morbid states, was the subject of several of his reports to the Académie des sciences and the Société de biologie between 1880 and 1882.[61] In the course of morbid states, he had noticed that the red colour of venous blood indicated the presence of oxygen; that there was a reduction in the blood content of carbon dioxide and that the blood vessels were contracted. These signs were accompanied by a fall in body temperature and by marked respiratory and circulatory malfunctions. In the laboratory, he had been able to replicate this clinical picture, not only by inflicting injuries to animals, but by the cutaneous application of various chemical substances. In clinical practice, he drew attention to a similar picture in cases of peritonitis, angina pectoris, drowning, strangulation and diaphragmatic wounds. The symptoms and circumstances of the appearance of this 'syndrome' led him to conclude that, in certain morbid conditions and severe injuries, the nervous system prevented the exchange of nutrients between the tissues and the blood. What he was describing was, in fact, the signs of primary shock which is mainly nervous.

He had noticed signs of shock after the cutaneous application of chloroform. He undertook a series of experiments on dogs, cats and guinea-pigs and reported:

> If chloroform is dropped on the skin of one of these animals, a reflex contraction of the subcutaneous muscles is immediately produced. The respiration, as a rule, rapidly lessens, the temperature falls, the animal becomes lethargic and sinks upon its flank or back, without any attempt to resume the normal posture. … Later, especially in guinea-pigs, tremor occurs in all four limbs. After a quarter of an hour, or sometimes 3–4 h, the animal wakes up, begins to move, and gradually returns to the normal condition.[62]

He pointed out that

> Another curious effect was the arrest of exchange of material between the tissues and the blood, shown by a rapid fall in temperature, and the pallor of the venous blood.[63]

He insisted that this morbid picture was not the consequence of inhalation of chloroform, having taken precautions to avoid this, by having the animals "to breathe by means of a tube fixed to the trachea, air coming from a distant part of the laboratory."[64] He explained this reaction as the result of an irritation of the nervous centres by the cutaneous nerves in the area where the chloroform was

---

[61] Brown-Séquard CE (1881) Sur l'inhibition (arrêt) des échanges entre le sang et les tissus. C R Soc Biol (Paris) 32: 238–240. Also: Recherches sur une influence spéciale du système nerveux. C R Acad Sci (Paris) 94: 491–494, 1882. Likewise: Researches on some of the physiological influence of the nervous system on nutrition. Br Med J 2: 915, 1881 and 1: 313, 1882.

[62] Lancet (1881) 1: 183.

[63] Lancet (1881) 1: 715 and 1036–1037.

[64] *Ibid.*

applied. Its application to mucous membranes brought about a more rapid and energetic reaction than when applied to the skin.[65] The application of chloral hydrate or prussic acid gave similar results.[66]

He had experimented with the gas carbon dioxide in the 1850s. During his first visit to America in 1852, he was convinced that this gas was active in the maintenance of the heartbeat, and that it had an excitatory role, while oxygen was a tissue nutrient. His views had been rejected by Claude Bernard who had shown that oxygen was an excitant, when placed in contact with some specific histological elements.[67] Brown-Séquard was now experimenting on the analgesic properties of carbon dioxide. In a letter to the editor of The Lancet in 1883, he summarised the results of the action of carbonic acid on the mucous membrane of the larynx:

> My experiments, some already published, others quite new, show than an irritation of the laryngeal mucous membrane (and also, but in a slighter degree, of the lining of the upper part of the trachea) can, through the superior laryngeal nerves, or even through one of them only, ... act on the nervous centres in such a way as to produce a more or less complete inhibition of either the power of perceiving impressions able to give rise to pain, or the power of transmitting these impressions. Every kind of irritation (mechanical, thermic, chemical or galvanic) of the terminal ramifications of the superior laryngeal nerves can produce that effect; but none in the same degree and with so great persistence (in monkeys the analgesia lasts more than 24 h) as the excitation due to carbonic acid.[68]

He undertook similar experiments on his own person,[69] but the results were not as good as in the monkey. He had obtained similar results using chloroform to irritate the laryngeal mucous membrane.

In collaboration with d'Arsonval, he studied the noxious effects of carbon dioxide breathed out of the lungs. They came to the conclusion that, in a confined space, it was toxic. Following a series of experiments on various animals, they attributed the toxicity of expired air in a confined space, not to the accumulation of carbon dioxide, but to the presence of an "organic alkaloid akin to the ptomaines."[70] Ptomaines are nitrogenous organic compounds produced by the putrefaction of animal matter under the action of bacteria. In fact, both these researchers were wrong, the adverse effects of expired air, in a confined space, are caused by the gradual diminution of the amount of oxygen in the air.

---

65 Bernard C (1960) Cahier de Notes 1850–1860. Edition intégrale du "Cahier Rouge". Presentée et commentée par Mirko Grmek. Gallimard, Paris, p. 234, note 117.

66 Brown-Séquard CE (1883) Letter to the Editor of the Lancet, September 1883. Analgesia by the proposed method. Lancet 2: 598. Also: Production d'anesthésie générale sous l'influence de l'irritation de la muqueuse laryngée par l'acide carbonique ou le chloroforme. C R Soc Biol (Paris) 34: 799–801, 1882.

67 Lancet (1885) 2: 30.

68 Lancet (1880) 2: 900–902.

69 *Ibid.*

70 Brown-Séquard CE, d'Arsonval A (1888) Ressemblance entre l'action toxique de certaines ptomaïnes et celles du poison pulmonaire. C R Soc Biol (Paris) 48: 108–110.

Their confining of laboratory animals to a restricted space, with a limited supply of air, reminds one of the experiments undertaken in the preceding century by Joseph Priestley who discovered oxygen and above all, those of Antoine Laurent Lavoisier, who came to the conclusion that in the course of breathing, oxygen is drawn from the surrounding air and carbon dioxide breathed out. He showed that a sparrow confined to a small, fully enclosed cage containing a small volume of air, dies in less than 1 h and that the "air" breathed out, when passed through lime-water, causes it to go milky, thus indicating the presence of carbon dioxide.

In 1869, Brown-Séquard had studied the effect of confined air on the development of tuberculosis in the guinea-pig. The animals inoculated with tuberculous matter, placed in the most favourable conditions: living in an open shed in a garden, with regular changes of bedding, manifested no signs of tuberculosis; whereas, animals inoculated in a similar way, confined to a restricted area in the laboratory, with a limited supply of fresh air, nearly all died of phthisis.[71] He concluded that phthisical patients would benefit if they lived in the open air. In 1887, with the help of d'Arsonval, he conceived and built an apparatus to extract air breathed out by phthisical patients in a hospital ward, and expel it outside.[72]

This interest in the pure air treatment of phthisical patients led him to attend the First Congress for Tuberculosis, held in Paris from July 23–31, 1888. There, he was pilloried by several participants to the Congress on account of the undefined poisonous substance that he had isolated from the air breathed out of the lungs.[73] For many researchers, among them Albert Jules Franck Dastre, had failed to find such a poison, supposedly related to the ptomaines. Though, many believed that pure air could have no direct influence on the bacillus, Mycobacterium tuberculosis, many agreed that pure air, as recommended by Brown-Séquard, could improve both the well-being and the appetite of patients suffering from tuberculosis of the lung. His interest in the management of this disease had a happy outcome: the setting-up of sanatoriums in pure air mountainous regions. In 1882, Carlo Forlanini invented the artificial pneumothorax for the treatment of pulmonary tuberculosis. This procedure, also known as collapsotherapy, is the introduction of air or nitrogen in the pleural cavity by means of a hollow needle introduced through the chest wall to collapse the lung and so rest it and prevent the spread of infection. This operation, and sometimes partial or unilateral total lobectomy, together with rest and long sojourns in remote mountainous regions, was practically the only palliative treatment of tuberculosis of the lung, until the advent of potent tuberculostatic drugs in the 1950s.

---

[71] Lancet (1887) Confined air and development of phtisis. Lancet 2: 1195.

[72] Brown-Séquard CE, d'Arsonval A (1888) Sur quelques points importants relatifs à la durée de survie des lapins après injection du liquide contenant le poison de l'air expiré. C R Soc Biol (Paris) 40: 151–152.

[73] Brown-Séquard CE, d'Arsonval A (1887) Recherches sur l'importance surtout pour les phtisiques d'un air vicié par des exhalaisons pulmonaires. C R Acad Sci (Paris) 105: 1056–1058.

Unlike François Magendie and Claude Bernard, who had a close following of pupils, Brown-Séquard had none during his 16 years at the Collège de France. If he did, their names have not been recorded. He was reluctant to admit anyone to his laboratory. When he was away from the College, spending the summer months at Sainte-Adresse or the winter ones in Nice, he had instructed d'Arsonval to let no one enter his premises. However, several American medical historians mention that Charles Euchariste de Médecis Sajous was his pupil.

Sajous, a descendant of the Médecis, whose father was Count Charles Roustan de Médecis-Jodoigne, was born at sea in 1852. He spent his childhood in France, and was only two years old when his father died. His mother remarried and the young Charles adopted his step-father's name, Sajous. In 1878, he qualified as a doctor in medicine at the Jefferson Medical College of Philadelphia. He was interested in laryngology and was a Course Lecturer at the College from 1883 to 1891. The following year, he gave up his clinical lectureship and a flourishing practice "for the study of internal secretions with Brown-Séquard in France."[74] There is no concrete evidence that he was at the Collège de France in the early 1890s.[75] However, he remained in France until 1897. His study of internal secretions earned him the title of Father of American Endocrinology on which, in 1903, he became the first in The United States to publish a book on The Internal Secretions and the Principles of Medicine, which was dedicated to the memory of Brown-Séquard.

[74] Wagner FB (ed) (1989) Thomas Jefferson University: Tradition and Heritage. Leo and Febiger, Philadelphia, p. 370.

[75] Communication to the author from M. Yves Laporte, Professor of Neurophysiology and Administrator of the College de France.

# Chapter 18
# The Father of Hormonal Therapy: 1889–1893

Brown-Séquard devoted the last 4 years of his life to the study of the therapeutic effects of extracts of endocrine glands and other organs. As far back as 1869, while a Course Lecturer at the Paris Medical School, he had made a very interesting statement, notably that if it was possible to inject semen without danger into the veins of old men, one would obtain manifestations of regeneration with respect to intellectual work and physical powers.[1]

It was the current belief then, that the loss of semen was a cause of debility and of physical and mental ailments. In the eleventh century, Avicenna had stated that one volume of ejaculated semen was equivalent to the loss of 40 volumes of blood. This opinion still prevailed in the nineteenth century.

Brown-Séquard shared with his contemporaries the belief that physical and mental weaknesses resulted from over-indulging of coitus and masturbation. In the course of the 18th century, onanism had been held responsible for a number of morbid conditions. The term onanism is derived from the biblical personage, Onan, who broke the levirate by refusing to "go into his brother's wife" Tamar, a widow and chose rather to "spill the semen on the ground." However, it was an obscure surgeon, by the name of John Marten who, in 1712, elevated the sin of Onan—thought to be masturbation—to a devastating disease for which he sold remedies. In 1760, Simon André Tissot had published a book entitled: L'onanisme ou dissertation physique sur les maladies produites par la masturbation (Onanism or physical dissertation on diseases caused by masturbation). This book went through some three dozen editions from the time of its publication to the first decade of the twentieth century. Also, in 1836, Claude François Lallemand published his work on Des Pertes séminales involontaires (Involuntary Losses of Semen). Brown-Séquard asserted that:

[1] Brown-Séquard CE (1889) Des effets produits chez l'homme par des injections d'un liquide retiré des testicules frais de cobaye et de chien. C R Soc Biol (Paris) 41: 415–419, p. 415.

L.-C. Celestin, *Charles-Edouard Brown-Séquard*,
DOI: 10.1007/978-3-319-03020-3_18, © Springer International Publishing Switzerland 2014

> The testicles, apart from their role in reproduction, have a dynamic function of the greatest importance in man. Weakness in old men is dependent on two causes: organic changes and the lack of stimulation exercised on the nervous centres by active testicles.[2]

He compared the weakness of elderly men to the consequences that follow castration. He wrote:

> It is known that in man castration during infancy or adolescence is followed by marked alterations of the individual physically and mentally. It is particularly well known that true eunuchs are characterised by their debility and their lack of physical and intellectual activity. Moreover, it is well known that similar defects are observed in men who abuse of coitus or masturbation. These facts, besides many others, clearly show that the testicles provide to the blood, by reabsorption some substances in semen, principles which give energy to the nervous system and probably also to the muscles.[3]

Regarding these seminal principles which enter the bloodstream, he had stated in 1869, in several of his lectures at the Medical School that:

> All glands, with or without excretory ducts give to the blood, by an internal secretion, principles which are of great importance if not necessary. I showed this to be the case particularly for the kidneys, the suprarenal capsules, and the sexual glands.... I thought that if we could safely introduce the principle of internal secretion of a gland taken from a living animal into the blood of men suffering from the lack of this secretion, important therapeutic effects would thereby be obtained.[4]

To counteract losses in semen and to conserve physical strength, he had, in the past, advised his patients, especially intellectuals that:

> Each time they were going to perform some great physical or intellectual work, to get themselves into a lively state of sexual excitement, while avoiding any ejaculation of Semen. The testes acquiring temporarily a great functional activity soon followed by the desired increase in power of the nervous centres.[5]

The testicles and their secretion had interested him for a very long time. Thus, in Agassiz's laboratory at Nahant, in 1875, he had attempted to implant whole or part of guinea-pigs' testes into old dogs, and had registered some success in one case.[6] Early in 1889, he conceived the idea of injecting sub-cutaneously a liquid extract of ground up testicles of young and vigorous animals into older and weaker ones.[7] Having put the idea into practice by using rabbits as experimental animals and having noticed no harmful effects, he decided

---

[2] Brown-Séquard CE (1889) Troisième note sur les effets des injections sous-cutanées de liquide testiculaire. C R Soc Biol (Paris) 41: 430–431, p. 431.

[3] Brown-Séquard, *op. cit.*, note 1, above, p. 415.

[4] Brown-Séquard CE (1893) On a new therapeutic method consisting in the use of organic liquids extracted from glands and other organs. Br Med J 1: 1145–1147, 1212–1214, p. 1145.

[5] Brown-Séquard CE (1889) Seconde note sur les effets produit chez l'homme par des injections sous-cutanées d'un liquide retiré des testicules de cobaye et de chien. C R Soc Biol (Paris) 41: 420–422, p. 420.

[6] Brown-Séquard, *op. cit.*, note 1, above, p. 415.

[7] *Ibid.*

to perform upon myself studies which appeared to me ought to be, in every respect, more decisive than those on experimental animals.[8]

So, over a period of 15 days, in May 1889, he gave himself a course of eight sub-cutaneous injections of an aqueous extract of ground-up dogs' and guinea-pigs' testicles.[9] The extract having been treated to avoid contamination by bacteria.

The results of his self-injections of testicular extract were reported on June 1st, 1889, in a lengthy statement to the Société de biologie, of which the main interesting part is as follows:

I was 72 years old on the 8th of last April. My general strength which has been considerable, has notably and gradually diminished in the course of the last 10 or 12 years. Prior to the experiments that I am presently undertaking, I had to sit down after working half an hour standing in the laboratory. After three or four hours and even sometimes after only two hours of experimental work at the laboratory, although I remained seated, I was left exhausted. On arriving home by carriage, around six o'clock in the evening, after some hours spent in the laboratory, I have been for a number of years so tired that I had to go to bed almost immediately after taking a hasty meal. Sometimes the exhaustion was such that despite the need to sleep and a drowsiness which prevented me even reading a paper, I could not fall asleep for hours.

Today, and since the second day and above all the third day after the first injection, all that has changed and I have recovered at least all the strength that I had a number of years ago. Experimental work at the laboratory tires me very little now. I am able to the great astonishment of my assistants, to remain standing for hours without feeling the need to sit down. A few days ago, after three hours of experimental work standing, I was able, contrary to my habits of the past twenty or more years, to prepare a report for more than one and a half hour after dinner. All my friends know what this improvement means to me.[10]

Apart from a feeling of well-being, he had measured the increase in his physical strength, by recording regularly the muscular strength of his forearm by means of a dynamometer. He registered an increase in strength, on flexing his forearm over his arm. Likewise, he had noticed an increase in the distance of his propelling a jet of urine!

I have comparatively measured, before and after the first injection, the distance a jet of urine travelled to reach the toilet bowl, and I have found that… the average distance was a quarter less than it is now after the first two injections.[11]

At the conclusion of his report, he urged his colleagues, of about the same age as him, to undertake similar trials. This is what he wrote:

I hope that other physiologists of advanced age will repeat these experiments and show whether or not these effects in me depend only on my idiosyncrasy.[12]

---

8 *Ibid.*

9 *Ibid.*

10 *Ibid.*, p. 417.

11 *Ibid.*

12 *Ibid.*, pp. 418–419.

From the moment that he had reported the beneficial effects of his testicular extract on himself, the reaction in the medical world was mixed. There were those to whom his reputation as a distinguished and reliable scientist was an absolute guarantee of his good faith and there were those who were downright hostile to his report.

The most vitriolic attacks came from the German medical press. The Deutsche Medizinische Wochenschrift considered the scholar's experiments as "senile aberrations;"[13] while the Wiener Medizinische Wochenschrift's remark was most uncharitable, commenting that Brown-Séquard's report was "further proof of the necessity of retiring professors who had attained their three scores and 10 years."[14]

In France, apart from a few harmless comments in the lay press, such as that of a physician who claimed that Brown-Séquard's idea had been dug out of a 16th century pharmaceutical treatise, and who concluded his article with the commonplace Latin quotation: Nil sub sole novum[15]: several physicians followed Brown-Séquard's advice and undertook clinical trials. The first, within days of the latter's report, was Gaston Variot, a hospital consultant and a physician to the Santé Prison of Paris. He treated with appreciable results, three elderly prisoners debilitated by chronic diseases and long periods of confinement.[16] His report to the Société de biologie led other physicians to use the testicular extract, such as Auguste Charles Rémy, in charge of practical courses on histology at the Paris Medical School; Professor Mouret of Montpellier and several practitioners from various regions of France.[17]

In The United States, the medical press was at first hostile. It spoke of erotico-senile folly and discredit to the profession. In the periodical, The Open Court, a physician wrote:

> The idea is as old as stupidity, wicked as superstition, cruel as savagery; it is false in its premises, false in its logic, false in its conclusion.[18]

Some physicians used locally prepared testicular extracts for injection and for oral administration. The first report, in August 1889, amplified by the media, was very damaging for, through lack of adequate sterilization of the aqueous extracts, several cases of blood poisoning were reported. Leiden Weir, the first patient to be treated by his family doctor, had his treatment paid for by the local newspapers and ended suffering from abscesses and indurations at the sites of the injections.[19] A

---

[13] Hamilton D (1986) The Monkey Gland Affair. Chatto and Windus, London, p. 12.

[14] *Ibid.*

[15] Quoted by Olmsted JMD (1946) Charles-Edouard Brown-Séquard. A nineteenth century neurologist and endocrinologist. The John Hopkins Press, Baltimore, p. 210.

[16] Variot G (1889) Expériences sur l'action physiologique du suc testiculaire injecté sous la peau, suivant la méthode de Brown-Séquard. C R Soc Biol (Paris) 1: 451–454.

[17] Lanterne (1892) Brown-Séquard. Les Progrès de sa méthode. Paris, 8th Aug.

[18] Olmsted, *op. cit.*, note 15, above p. 210.

[19] Boston Weekly (1889) Serious results of "elixir" tests. Boston, 23rd Aug.

man, by the name of Steele, operated upon with Brown-Séquard's so-called elixir, had blood poisoning,[20] and was determined to sue his doctor for $5,000 damages. The chemist "who prepares nine-tenths of all elixir in Cincinnati, says it is dangerous if used after an hour, and rank poison after two."[21] The lack of the most basic precautions in the preparation of these extracts aroused the anger of Brown-Séquard who castigated the culprits in the following terms:

> In The United States especially, and often without knowing what I have done, nor the most elementary rules regarding subcutaneous injections of animal materials, several physicians or rather quacks and charlatans, have exploited the ardent desire of a large number of individuals and have made them run the greatest risks, if they have not done worse.[22]

As to prude Victorian England, she felt utter revulsion at the thought that semen of guinea-pigs and dogs were being injected in human beings. She was shocked that a physician could recommend sexual stimulation without ejaculation to mobilise intellectual and physical powers. For her, it was nothing short of condoning onanism. The medical press and especially its two mainstays, The British Medical Journal and The Lancet chose to remain aloof. On the other hand, Brown-Séquard's report created a stir in antivivisectionist circles, which were afraid that the use of testicular extracts would lead to mass castrations of animals. In July 1889, Edward Berdoe, a general practitioner and a member of an antivivisectionist society, circulated 6,000 copies of a printed letter among his colleagues, which said that:

> The object of these abominable proceedings is to enable broken down libertines to pursue with renewed vigour the excesses of their youth, to rekindle the dying embers of lust in the debilitated and aged, and to profane the bodies of men which are the temples of God, by an elixir drawn from the testicles of dogs and rabbits by a process involving the excruciating torture of the innocent animals, which elixir is then injected by a physician into the veins of his patient who he has caused to practice a degrading and loathing vice.... We may have also a new race of beings intermediate between man and lower animals as a remoter consequence of the boon to humanity conferred by this French physiologist.[23]

On June 22, 1889, 3 weeks after Brown-Séquard's report to the Société de biologie, the British Medical Journal reported his experiments in an article entitled "The Pentacle of Rejuvenescence."[24] The choice of such title attracted the attention of the lay press. The word 'Pentacle': a five-pointed star being the symbol, in occult terms, of the perfect man. The article compared Brown-Séquard's experiments to the "wild imaginings of medieval philosophers in search

---

[20] *Ibid.*

[21] *Ibid.*

[22] Brown-Séquard CE (1889) Du rôle physiologique d'un suc extrait des testicules d'animaux d'après nombre de faits observés chez l'homme. Arch Physiol norm pathol 1: 739–746, p. 739.

[23] Berdoe E (1889) Serious moral question. Letter for private circulation among physicians, 12th Jul. Br Med J: 1416. Also GMcCC Ms 980/67.

[24] British Medical Journal (1889) 1: 1416.

of an elixir vitae." Two weeks later, on July 6th, the same periodical, in an article entitled "Dr Brown-Séquard's Hypodermic Fluid,"[25]commented:

> The extraordinary statements made by Professor Brown-Séquard as to the efficiency of hypodermic injections of fluid expressed from the testicles of young animals in senile debility have been to a certain extent confirmed by M. Variot who made a communication to the Société de Biologie on June 29th.... M. Brown-Séquard said that M. Variot's observations disposed of the objection that the results he had observed in himself were due to suggestion.

Five weeks after, this same periodical was again content to report a 'medically unconfirmed cure' in Indianapolis in The United States, in an article entitled "The New Elixir of Youth,"[26] which said:

> Dr Brown-Séquard's rejuvenating fluid is said to have been tried in Indianapolis on a decrepit old man with marvellous effect. Four hours after the injection, the patient walked over a mile in twenty five min. He declared that he felt more vigorous than he had done for twenty five years. He read a newspaper without glasses, a thing he had not been able to do for thirty years. It should be added that no medical authority is given for the story.

As for The Lancet, it published on July 20, 1889, an article by Brown-Séquard entitled: "Note on the effects produced in man by subcutaneous injections of a liquid obtained from the testicles of animals."[27] This article was sent from Brighton, where he, his wife and daughter were spending part of the summer. But the journal wished to remain non-committal, as exemplified in the Editors' letter of July 10th to Brown-Séquard, prior to the publication of the article:

> We have not yet published any account of your experiments in the power of a liquid extracted from the spermatic glands of animals.
>
> We shall be glad to avail ourselves of your kind offer to write a short paper on the subject for publication in our columns. We think it desirable that the article should appear under your name as somewhat sensational and no doubt inaccurate paragraphh have been lately appearing in the daily press.[28]

In January 1890 the same periodical published an article from its New York correspondent, dated December 13, 1889, taking its title from a book on Brown-Séquard's therapeutic method, recently printed in America, the Elixir of Life. It commented in the following manner:

> The announcement that this distinguished physiologist had discovered a method of renewing the vigour of youth in the aged was received in this country with an incredulous smile by the profession. But there is always a class of medical men who are ready at once to test the value of any new remedy, and during the past months, the newspapers have been filled with experiments made in various parts of the country. It is surprising at the first blush to note the different results obtained as reported. In the hands of one experimenter,

[25] British Medical Journal (1889) 2: 29.

[26] British Medical Journal (1889) 2: 611.

[27] Lancet (1889) 2: 105–107.

[28] Lancet (1965) Before our time. Lancet's editors: Letter to Brown-Séquard. 1: 315.

> the paralysed immediately walk, the lame throw aside canes and crutches, the deaf hear, and the blind see. The same experiment failed altogether in the practice of another.[29]

The medical profession was not the only section of society in turmoil; the lay press had a field day at Brown-Séquard's expense. Up to then, he had made the headlines once or twice, as when he carried out blood perfusion experiments on severed arms of decapitated criminals, or when he was assaulted by an antivivisectionist activist, in the course of one of his lectures at the Collège de France. Now, he became a household name for ridicule. His experiments were the subject of crude jokes, humorous songs and satires by cabaret artistes, all over France. Newspapers' cartoons depicted him armed with a scalpel and a syringe, ready to castrate dogs, cats, rabbits and guinea-pigs surrounding him. As one French daily, L'Evénement commented: "He was without any doubt the most laughed at man of all times."[30] Such derision and abuse on the part of humorous artistes and newspapers' cartoonists did not affect him in the least, though he was acutely aware of the comments of the lay press. He wrote:

> Since the publication of the experiments that I have carried out on myself, the lay press of the Two Worlds has reported them without knowing about them and unfortunately has given rise to absurd hope, which was promptly disappointing to thousands of people debilitated by old age, by abuse of sexual power or by disease.[31]

In the autumn of 1889, Brown-Séquard published a report summarizing the results obtained by physicians with whom he was in correspondence, and who had carried out therapeutic trials in the best possible conditions in Europe and The United States. He cited the studies of Variot and Dehoux in Paris, those of Villeneuve in Marseille.[32] Those of Loomis[33] in New York, who used rams' testicles and of Hammond[34] who noticed improvements in the condition of some debilitated patients, as well as sufferers from various cardiac ailments. He quoted also the experiments of Brainerd in Cleveland—a county of the industrial region of Teeside, North-East England—and those of Grigorescu in Bucharest.

Although he did not mention the studies of his British colleagues, he was well acquainted with the results of those who had been supplied with the testicular fluid from the Laboratoire du Collège de France. Such was the case with medical practitioners like William Dakin Waterhouse; George Fenton Cameron, the author of a work On Imperfect Digestion, With Cases[35]; the ophthalmologist, Robert

---

29 Lancet (1890) Dr Brown-Séquard's "Elixir of Life" 1: 57–58.

30 Perry J (1894) Brown-Séquard. L'Evenèment, Paris, 5th Apr.

31 Brown-Séquard, *op. cit.*, note 22, above.

32 Marseille médical (1889) 30th Aug, p. 458.

33 The Medical Recorder (189) 14th Aug, p. 206.

34 Hammond WA (1889) Experiments relative to the therapeutic value of the expressed juice of the testicles when hypodermically introduced into the human system. NY Med J 50: 232–234.

35 Medical Directory for the year 1889. London.

Brudenell Carter. By mistake, d'Arsonval sent samples to Victor Alexander Haden Horsley, but it is unlikely that he used them.[36]

Both Brown-Séquard and d'Arsonval were overcome by requests for the testicular extract by elderly colleagues, scientists, writers, politicians, diplomats and influential persons. To satisfy all the demands, they hired gratuitously the services of several general practitioners, who called at the home of these celebrities to inject them with the testicular fluid . One of these ambulant practitioners was nicknamed Brown-Séquard's pricker. He was Dr Depoux, who was the husband of Françoise Jeanne Schültz, alias Felia Litvinne, a professional singer. This is what d'Arsonval has to say about him:

> One of the most enthusiastic of our dispensers was a peculiar little man, a native of Auvergne, very intelligent and sprightly, of good repute in Paris, by the name of Doctor Depoux. Being the husband of the opera singer, Felia Litvinne, he was greatly esteemed in literary and artistic circles.[37]

It was Dr Depoux who regularly injected Brown-Séquard's fluid to the great but unfortunate writer, Alphonse Daudet, protracted by excruciating pains.[38]

Daudet is the author of Lettres de mon moulin which depicts scenes of Provençal life in the 1860s and whose novels include Le Petit Chose and Tartarin de Tarascon. The Journal of the brothers Edmond and Jules de Goncourt tells the story of the treatment of Daudet, who suffered from tertiary syphilis. He complained to the Goncourts of the horrible pains brought about by the injections of Brown-Séquard's liquid which caused a contracture of his whole body, which he compared to the tightening of a hoop round a cask of wine.[39]

But the injections had "the most soothing effect on the awful sickness."[40] In 1937, d'Arsonval still had, in his possession, a telegram of Daudet, asking urgently for the "precious fluid."[41] Léon Daudet, Alphonse's son, in his book Quand vivait mon Père (When My Father Was Alive), often mentions Charcot's visits to his father's home. It appears that when the former learnt that Depoux had replaced him as Daudet's physician, there was a cooling off of relations between the eminent neurologist and the great writer.

Towards the end of his life, Brown-Séquard's pricker gave a striking proof of the power of his master's testicular fluid , by "marrying at the age of seventy-two a beautiful 18-year old shepherdess"[42] from his native Auvergne!

According to the Goncourts, the novelist Emile Zola—who drew attention to contemporary social problems in a series of novels which includes L'Assomoir,

---

[36] Delhoume L (1939) De Claude Bernard à d'Arsonval. Baillière et Fils, Paris, p. 360.

[37] Chauveau L (1937) D'Arsonval. Soixante-cinq ans à travers la Science. Editions J Oliven, Paris, p. 216.

[38] *Ibid.*

[39] Goncourt E and J (1893) Journal, vol 3. Robert Laffont, Paris, p. 731.

[40] Chauveau, *op. cit.*, note 37, above, p. 216.

[41] *Ibid.*

[42] *Ibid.*

Nana and Germinal—had recourse to Brown-Séquard's testicular fluid to "make of him a 25-year old man by the side of the young woman who had succeeded to Mrs Zola."[43] Effectively, from 1887, Zola had, as his mistress, his 20-year old servant who bore him two children.

Pasteur also subjected himself to several courses of testicular fluid . Brown-Séquard in a letter of March 25, 1893, addressed to Dr Poupinel de Valencé of Mauritius says:

> I am happy to tell you that, for the past six months, M. Pasteur has nearly fully recovered his health, thanks to the testicular fluid .[44]

Pasteur himself wrote:

> I rely more and more on Brown-Séquard's injections, and today, I think, I have the definite proof of its effectiveness. I have had eighteen prior to Roux's [Paul Emile] departure and I am in a hurry to have more.[45]

Writing to Jacques Grancher, Professor of Paediatrics at the Medical School of Paris, Pasteur strongly advised him to use the injections of testicular fluid:

> Yesterday, 6th September 1892, while listening to M Brown-Séquard's report to the Académie des sciences, I thought of you. You should try his injections. No one anymore can fail to take seriously the facts noted by him and a great number of foreign physicians.[46]

Another eminent scholar, who benefited from the testicular fluid, was the German naturalist Karl Vogt. A letter, which he wrote in 1893, ends thus:

> All that I know is that as soon as I feel an oncoming neurasthenic bout, like those that I have experienced in the past, I take hold, without hesitation of the Pravaz [syringe] and the Brown-Séquardine, without for this reason becoming a Brownnomaniac or imagining that we are in possession of a Fountain of Youth, with the difference, however, that according to the ancient saying, the whole body had to be immersed in it, whereas today, the latter serves as receptacle for a few cubic centimetres of the fluid...[47]

Brown-Séquard kept experimenting and reporting the results of his testicular extract and replying to hundreds of letters a day, sent to him by physicians from all over the world. By the end of 1889, it was reckoned that, in France, 12.000 practitioners were using the testicular fluid in the treatment of an infinite variety of ailments.

Soon, however, problems arose, Brown-Séquard accused charlatans of cashing on his discovery, by preparing so-called testicular extracts and selling them under various names. He contemplated legal action against them, only to be told that

---

[43] Goncourt, *op. cit.*, note 39, above, p. 740.

[44] Brown-Séquard CE (1893) Letter to Dr Poupinel de Valencé, 25th March. In: Lettres inédites du Brown-Séquard. Revue Historique et Littéraire de l'île Maurice, N°12, July 1894.

[45] Darmon P (1995) Pasteur. Fayard, Paris, p. 389.

[46] *Ibid.*

[47] Binet L (1954) Médecins Biologistes Chirurgiens. Segep, Paris, p. 123.

having disclosed, in medical journals, the mode of preparation and the composition of the fluid, he could not now claim the patent rights. The lay press put pressure on the government to have the fluid prepared by the Central Pharmacy of the Social Services for distribution, at cost price, to the physicians; but Brown-Séquard was informed by the Authorities that the government was not prepared to do so, and that he had to publish in extenso, the mode of preparation and sterilization of the fluid. He turned down financial propositions from pharmaceutical firms, and from 1890 to 1892, he supplied the fluid, free of charge, to any physician who asked for it, spending his own money in the process. The fluid supplied by him bore a label of the Laboratoire de Médecine du Collège de France and his name and that of d'Arsonval on the bottom part of the label.

A group of benefactors offered to fund the cost of a laboratory, exclusively for the manufacture of the testicular fluid, but Brown-Séquard was adamant. The following letter of March 1893 to Dr Charles Poupinel de Valencé of Mauritius, sums un his absolute moral integrity:

> An association of generous men put at my disposal 500,000 (half a million) francs to fund an institute after the manner of the Pasteur Institute, on condition that I supply the fluid to physicians who ask for it. I refuse on the ground that after spending 300,000 to extend my laboratory or to found a new one, there will be left only 200,000 francs, a return of only 6 or 7000 francs per year, which will suffice to prepare the fluid for 2 or 300 physicians. There are 40,000 in France and more than half will ask for it. It would be impossible for me to supply it without selling it and I cannot tarnish my name by selling anything. I have spent more than 20,000 francs of my own since May 1892 in giving away the fluid.... I am poor, but I could still continue to spend for some more months.[48]

From 1889 to 1893, reports reached Brown-Séguard from all over the world of marked improvements of various diseases treated with testicular extracts. In a communication to the Académie des sciences, on April 24 1893,[49] he and d'Arsonval listed all the affections which had been ameliorated by the fluid. They ranged from nervous complaints, such as locomotor ataxia, neuritis and neuralgia to endocrine dysfunction such as hypothyroidism to cancer and even cholera and leprosy. They pointed out that these reported improvements were not the result of a direct action of the testicular fluid on each of the mentioned morbid conditions, but that it strengthened the nervous system—a dynamogenic action, as they called it—thus enabling the body to cope with the disease.

This seemingly beneficial effect of testicular extracts on various diseases, prompted physicians, among them, members of the Paris Medical School, to ask Brown-Séguard and d'Arsonval to prepare extracts of organs other than of the testicles. In March 1891, d'Arsonval informed Brown-Séguard by letter that

[48] Brown-Séquard CE (1893) Letter to Dr Poupinel de Valencé, 2nd March. In: Lettres inédites du Brown-Séquard. Revue Historique et Littéraire de l'île Maurice, N°13, July 1894.

[49] Brown-Séquard CE, d'Arsonval A (1893) Effets physiologiques et thérapeutiques d'un liquide extrait de la glande sexuelle mâle. C R Acad Sci (Paris) 116: 856–861.

> The physicians after having cried a great deal, have in turn been struck by prurigo piquandi, they want to make use of injections of extracts of all tissues (spinal cord, liver, spleen, thymus, etc.). The testicular fluid has put them in the mood.[50]

This suggestion was, of course, not adverse to Brown-Séquard's conviction, as he wrote back to d'Arsonval a few days later:

> Like the testicles, all glands of external secretion are at the same time glands of internal secretion. The kidneys, the salivary glands, the pancreas are not exclusively organs of elimination.... They are, like the thyroid, the spleen, etc., organs giving to the blood some important principles, some directly, others by reabsorption after external secretion.[51]

His reply was but the confirmation of what he had always believed and which he had asserted in the course of his lectures at the Paris School of Medicine, nearly 20 years before:

> I have always taught that the glands with external ducts have, like the vascular glands, the function of modifying the blood by a sort of internal secretory work.[52]

Not long after this request from the medical profession, Brown-Séquard began experimenting with other organ extracts. He was interested in the treatment of diabetes mellitus and wrote to d'Arsonval:

> When the pancreas is suppressed (extirpation, ligature of the veins, etc.), diabetes follows. Would there be no diabetes if, after suppression of the functions of the gland, there were daily injections of an extract of the gland taken from a healthy animal? Moreover, would this gland's secretion taken from the pancreatic duct prevent the appearance of diabetes after the suppression of the gland, as well as an extract obtained by crushing the gland?[53]

His knowledge that extirpation of the pancreas was followed by diabetes, rested upon the experimental work carried out on a dog, the previous year, by Joseph Freiherr von Mering and Oscar Minkowski.[54] However, d'Arsonval's administration of pancreatic extracts to pancreatomized animals was not crowned with success; likewise, the experiments of researchers such as William Hale White at Guy's Hospital in London and of Emile Gley and Raphaël Lépine in Paris. It was Edouard Hédon who attributed an internal secretion to the islets of Langerhans, and it was Eugène Lindsay Opie who showed that there was a relation of cause and effect between diabetes mellitus and a lack of secretion of the islets of Langerhans. In 1909, J de Meyer gave the name insulin to the hormone secreted by the islets; but it was not until 1921 that the Canadians Frederick Grant Banting, Charles

---

[50] D'Arsonval A (1891) Letter to Brown-Séquard, 24th March. Quoted by Delhoume, *op. cit.*, note 36, above, p. 379.

[51] Brown-Séquard CE (1891) Letter to d'Arsonval, 28th March. Quoted by Delhoume, *op. cit.*, note 36, above, p. 384.

[52] Brown-Séquard, *op. cit.*, note 5, above, p. 421.

[53] Brown-Séquard (n.d) Letter to d'Arsonval. Quoted by Delhoume, *op. cit.*, note 36, above, p. 393.

[54] Arch Exp Pathol Pharmako (1890) 26: 371–378.

Herbert Best and John James Rickard Macleod isolated insulin and were awarded a Nobel Prize, for the importance of their discovery in the treatment of diabetes by the injection of insulin derived mainly from pigs' pancreases.

Brown-Séquard studied the effects of extracts of adrenal glands on the survival of adrenalectomized animals and likewise, the effect of injections of blood from healthy guinea-pigs on those deprived of their adrenal glands and registered some success.[55] He found that:

> Animals dying from the absence in the blood of the secretion of these glands (after they have been removed) can be revived, at least for a time, when they receive an injection of a liquid extracted from healthy suprarenal capsules.[56]

However, his treatment of bronzed disease (Addison's disease) with adrenal glands' extracts was far from satisfactory.[57] The reason being that the active principles of these glands do not dissolve in water. It was much later, in the late 1920s, that adrenal extracts dissolved in fat solvents, were shown to maintain life in adrenalectomized animals.

He demonstrated that injections of a renal extract improved the state of nephrectomized animals, thus foreshadowing the work of Robert Adolf Armand Tigerstedt, Professor of Physiology of the Karolinska Institute in Stockholm on the kidney hormone renin. Nowadays, it is known that renin is involved in the regulation of blood pressure. When it acts on the globulin angiotensinogen, it produces angiotensin which causes a narrowing of the small blood vessels in tissues, thereby increasing blood pressure as well as stimulating the release of the hormone aldosterone of the adrenal cortex, which also increases blood pressure. Brown-Séquard carried out a good many experiments on rabbits and guinea-pigs, to show that they survived much longer after double nephrectomy, when injections of liquid renal extracts were administered.[58] He stated that what he knew of the physiology and pathology of these organs clearly show the paramount importance of their internal secretion, the cessation of which is notably more to be dreaded than is the cessation of the external secretion.[59]

He experimented with extracts of thymus, liver, spleen, bone marrow and pituitary gland . He inferred that a pituitary gland extract would be beneficial in hypopituitarism, whenever the full symptomatology of such condition was known:

> It would be important to collect more of such facts, so as to build up the malady constituted by these special symptoms showing the absence of secretion of the pituitary gland, as there is good ground to hope that injections of a liquid extract drawn from the gland would act on these symptoms.[60]

---

[55] Brown-Séquard CE (1893) Influence heureuse de la transfusion du sang normal après extirpation des capsules surrénales chez le cobaye. C R Soc Biol (Paris) 45: 448–449.

[56] Brown-Séquard, *op. cit.*, note 4, above, p. 1231.

[57] *Ibid.*

[58] *Ibid.*, p. 1146.

[59] *Ibid.*

[60] *Ibid.*, p. 1231.

At that time, the clinical picture of what was termed hypopituitarism was a mosaic of symptoms which left both clinicians and experimentalists baffled, as none of the ten hormones secreted by the pituitary gland had been isolated, although there were reasons to believe that a type of dwarfism (caused by a deficiency of growth hormone from the anterior pituitary gland ) and acromegaly (caused by excessive secretion of the growth hormone) were due to malfunctions of the pituitary. Furthermore, recent studies by Guilio Vassale and Ercole Sacchi, had shown that the pituitary gland was essential to life and that animals deprived of their glands improved when treated by injections of extracts of the pituitary.[61]

As for bone marrow extracts, Brown-Séquard had noticed an improvement in the state of patients suffering from anaemia and other blood dyscrasias.[62]

Finally, regarding ovarian extracts, he anticipated that they would have the same effects on elderly women as testicular extracts had on old men.[63] Studies carried out by Villeneuve[64] in Marseilles and by an American woman physician by the name of Brown[65] in Paris, seemed to confirm his prediction.

By early 1892, at a time when the demand for the testicular fluid had reached an unprecedented high. Brown-Sequard was compelled to limit the supply "because of d'Arsonval, who cannot spend all his time preparing the fluid."[66] Indeed, for over 3 years, the latter had coped with an ever increasing demand for the testicular fluid . On September 5, 1892, the Laboratoire de Médecine du Collège de France issued a circular limiting the supply of the fluid to 1,200 physicians in France, to those persons who were being actively treated and to physicians who were treating them selves.

By that time, it was not just the testicular fluid which was being prescribed, but a host of other organ extracts in various diseases: extracts of spinal cord and grey matter in neurological disorders, splenic extracts in malaria, and muscle extracts in progressive muscular atrophy. The impetus given by Brown-Séquard to organotherapy, in the last 3 years, had caught the imagination of researchers all over Europe. In August 1890, Bettencourt and Serrano of Lisbon reported a marked improvement the day after grafting a sheep thyroid under the skin of a 36-year old woman, suffering from myxoedema[67] and concluded that such rapid improvement could only be explained by absorption of the thyroid juice by the patient's tissues. In November 1890, Guilio Vassale in Italy, successfully treated thyroidectomized dogs with intravenous injections of a thyroid extract, a treatment which had

[61] *Ibid.*

[62] *Ibid.*

[63] Brown-Séquard, *op. cit.*, note 5, above, p. 422.

[64] Brown-Séquard, *op. cit.*, note 4, above, p. 1145.

[65] Brown-Séquard, *op. cit.*, note 4, above, p. 1213.

[66] Brown-Séquard, *op. cit.*, note 4, above.

[67] Semaine médicale, 13th Aug 1890.

already been recommended by Charles Bouchard, a pupil of Brown-Séquard, in 1887.[68] In April 1891, Emile Gley stopped convulsions in thyroidectomized animals by injections of a thyroid extract, unaware that the convulsive fits were due to the ablation of the parathyroid glands, removed at the same time as the thyroid.[69] The parathyroid glands, four in number, are attached to the posterior surface of the thyroid gland and secrete the hormone parathormone, which regulates the level of calcium and phosphorous in the body. A deficiency of this hormone leads to a lowering of calcium blood levels with a relative increase in phosphorous levels. This is manifested clinically by the appearance of muscular spasms: tetany. It was a year later that Gley discovered the parathyroid glands, embedded in the back surface of the thyroid.

However, it was the remarkable success achieved in England, by George Redmayne Murray with a thyroid extract in a solution of glycerol, administered by subcutaneous injections, in a case of advanced myxoedema, which is acknowledged to be the first recorded success of organotherapy. Murray published his findings in October 1891, but he had been treating, since April, a 46-year old woman who went on to live until the age of 74.[70]

Following in Murray‘s footsteps were Hector Mackenzie in England who, in 1892, treated myxoedema by oral administration of fresh thyroid gland[71]; and Howitz of Copenhagen, who obtained appreciable results by feeding cooked sheep's thyroid to patients suffering from hypothyroidism.

Murray conceived the idea for his treatment after having, in April 1891, acquainted himself, in Paris, with the text of the communication of Brown-Séquard and d'Arsonval to the Société de biologie, entitled: "L'Injection des extraits liquides provenant des glandes et des tissus de l'organisme comme méthode therapeutique."[72] ("The Injection of liquid extracts of glands and tissues of the organism as a therapeutic method"). In their communication, the authors declared that active internal secretions exist in all the organs and tissues of the body and that they could be used for the treatment of disorders caused by the deficiency of a given internal secretion.

This communication is considered by many medical historians as marking the anniversary of "the foundation of Endocrinology and Hormonotherapy;"[73] for these two scholars proclaimed "that all tissues, glandular or not, provide something special to the blood, that all acts of nutrition is accompanied by an internal

---

[68] Abelous JE (1893) La physiologie des glandes à secretion interne: corps thyroïde et capsules surrénales. Revue générale des sciences pures et appliquées 4: 275–278.

[69] Gley E (1891) Note préliminaire sur les effets physiologiques du suc de diverses glandes et en particulier du suc extrait de la glande thyroïde. C R Soc Biol (Paris) 3: 250–251.

[70] Murray GR (1891) Note on the treatment of myxoedema by hypodermic injections of an extract of the thyroid gland of a sheep. Brit Med J 2: 796–797.

[71] Mackenzie HWG (1892) A case of myxoedema treated with great benefit by feeding with fresh thyroid gland . Brit Med J 2: 940–941.

[72] C R Acad Sci (Paris) 114: 1399–1405, 1892.

[73] Chauveau, *op. cit.*, note 37, above, p. 214.

secretion. We therefore believe that all tissues could and should be used, in special cases, as modes of treatment, that there is here, the prospect of creating a new therapy, whose curative agents would be the products manufactured by the various tissues of the body and that all the cells of the organism are dependent on each other by a mechanism other than the nervous system."[74]

No doubt, Murray deserves to be honoured for his successful treatment of myxoedema, but his success is due first and foremost to Brown-Séquard's studies on the therapeutic worth, false or true, of his testicular extract and on his understanding of the existence and role of internal secretions.

It was Murray's report which, in the United Kingdom, brought about a greater awareness of Brown-Séquard's researches on the therapeutic significance of organ extracts. In June 1893, the British Medical Journal published a two-part article of Brown-Séquard entitled: "On a New Therapeutic Method consisting in the Use of Organic Liquids extracted from Glands and other organs,"[75] in which, he provides an explanation of the mechanism of action of glandular and organ extracts:

> When a morbid state, such a myxoedema, or a series of symptoms such as we see in cases of deficiency to the internal secretion of any gland, exists, it is very easy to understand how the cure is obtained when glandular liquid extracts are used: we simply give to the blood the principle or principles missing in it.... The great movement in therapeutics as regard the organic liquid extracts, has its origin in the experiments which I made on myself in 1889, experiments which were at first so completely misunderstood.

He went on to say:

> Certain principles entering the blood after having been injected... give to certain tissues nutritive elements, which our food... could not furnish.... The tonic influence certainly existing when the liquid from the sexual glands, or some other liquids in a lesser degree are injected, explains how nutrition is improved, and how also morbid phenomena due to weakness can disappear. When the liquid extracted from the sexual glands are employed,... elements able to form new cells enter the organism and thereby favourable organic changes can occur. Organic extracts resemble each other on account of the presence in the blood and, necessarily, in the various tissues of elements coming from the internal secretion of all parts...

After the publication of this article, the British Medical Journal summed up Brown-Séquard's statements in a leading article entitled: "Animal Extracts as Therapeutic Agents."[76] Its comments, though guarded, were in sharp contrast to those of its derisory short reports of 1889:

> It is now some years since Brown-Séquard announced the wonderful effects which followed the subcutaneous injections of testicular extracts as exemplified in his own person, and though many jeered at him as the discoverer of the secret of perpetual youth, the notion has steadily gained ground that there is, after all, something in it. Since also, the success that has followed the injection of thyroid extract in myxoedema, we can hardly wonder that this belief has increased. Physiologists have recently been making a number

---

[74] C R Acad Sci (Paris) *op. cit.*, note 72, above.

[75] Brown-Séquard, *op. cit.*, note 4, above.

[76] British Medical Journal (1893) 1: 1279.

of observations, which show that many organs do more than what was formerly regarded as their functions. The experiments of Bradford on the kidney have shown that this organ does something else in addition to excreting urine; those of Minkowski and v. Mering on pancreatic diabetes, of Langlois and Abelous on the suprarenal capsules, and of Horsley and others on the thyroid, have led to the introduction of the expression "internal secretion."

Such volte-face on the part of the British Medical Journal shows to what extent, in the space of less than 4 years, Brown-Séquard's conception of internal secretions and replacement of their deficiencies by the administration of glandular and organ extracts had evolved. Everywhere, physicians faced with diseases that did not respond to the limited therapeutic means then available, were prepared to resort to animal gland and organ extracts.

History has proved most unkind and unfair to Brown-Séquard's researches in the field of organotherapy and hormonotherapy, through the many adverses comments made up to the present day, by medical men not fully aware of the scope of his findings. These comments have distorted the true nature and therapeutic worth of the organotherapy conceived by Brown-Séquard. No doubt that many of those, who passed judgement, were influenced by the ridicule with which his work was treated during the last 4 years of his life. As the French paper L'Evénement wrote: "Sarcasm diminished him to such an extent, that for many he is still reckoned as a common charlatan coupled with a joker of poor taste."[77]

Indeed, prior to and after his death, crude jokes on the part of ill-informed physicians, so-called medical historians and sensation-seeking journalists abounded. Thus, in 1889, at the time of his first report on the effects of the testicular fluid on his own person, he had stated: "I can also now, go running up and downstairs, as I had always done up to the age of sixty."[78] This statement was at the origin of a current joke in American medical circles, following a remark attributed to the physiologist Jacques Loeb of the Rockfeller Institute of New York: "Poor Brown-Séquard! He injected himself with testicles, ran upstairs, and died at the top."[79] Loeb, of German origin, was a pioneer of experimental parthogenesis. He obtained larvae from sea urchins' eggs by dipping them in a hyper-saline sea water solution.

Still as damaging was a Clermond-Ferrand newspaper's eulogy which, after poking fun at Brown-Séquard's experiments on the testicular extract, reminded its readers that he had once hoped to imitate Christ by bringing back from death executed criminals and whose comments ended thus:

Quite truly, he did not straighten up the hunchback, nor give back their legs to the legless; nor did he give speech back to the dumb and sight to the blind; but his speciality was far more marvellous... He has proved... that it is possible not to quite resuscitate the dead, which would be a miracle, which is not done anymore, but to give back sensitivity to the bodies of executed criminals with an injection of blood.[80]

---

77 Perry, *op. cit.*, note 30, above.

78 Brown-Séquard, *op. cit.*, note 1, above, p. 417.

79 Kruif P de (1945) The Male Hormone. Harcourt, Brace & Co., New York, p. 45.

80 Hardy J (1894) L'Actualité. La Séquardine. Le Petit Clermentois, Clermond Ferrand, 6th Apr.

An English paper wrote that Brown-Séquard was the "Madame Rachel of Medicine", an allusion to a Mademoiselle Rachael, a contemporary tragic actress of world-wide reputation.[81] Another London-based newspaper inferred that Charcot had, in his lifetime, claimed that injections of distilled water, were as effective as those of the testicular fluid .[82] Such a statement was never made by this eminent neurologist, although—as was well-known to the newspapers of the time—he had been provided with very large quantities of animal testes by several of the Paris's slaughterhouses, with which he prepared extracts to treat his many debilitated patients at La Salpêtrière. Charcot used so large quantities of testes of bulls and rams, that on learning this, Brown-Séquard wrote to d'Arsonval that Charcot might try either to prove that the fluid is worthless or that he has cured his patients by modifying the composition and strength of the extract.[83]

In America, Brown-Séquard was debased by the public, the lay press and the medical profession. There were those who objected to his "attempt at rejuvenation" on religious grounds, as pointed out by Richard Harrison Shyrock, quoting from an article which appeared in 1894:

> The tradition that old age was inevitable, that it was part of the divinely established nature of things, appeared to be confirmed. It seemed foolish at best, and perhaps somewhat occult and sacrilegious to pry into the matter.[84]

To other Americans, Brown-Séquard was classed amongst those who had made false scientific claims to feather their own nests; like Robert Koch, who advantageously marketed his tuberculine treatment of tuberculosis; of Poehl of Russia who exaggerated the rejuvenescent properties of spermine and even Charles Darwin for his "irreligious" and controversial Theory of Evolution.[85]

The most condemnatory remark was that of Harvey William Cushing who referred to physicians who treated their patients with organ extracts as "endo-criminologists." Cushing was not only the pioneer of neurosurgery, but also an endocrinologist who described the syndrome that bears his name: Cushing's syndrome, characterised by an increase in the secretion of corticosteroids most commonly due to a malignant tumour of the pituitary gland and whose symptoms include obesity, hirsutism, hypertension and osteoporosis. Moreover, Cushing christened Brown-Séquard the "Ponce de Léon" of endocrinology.[86] Juan Ponce de Léon was the Spanish explorer who discovered Florida in 1513, while searching

[81] The Star (1894) Dr Brown-Séquard, London, 3rd Apr.

[82] The Daily News (1894) Obituary of Brown-Séquard. London, 3rd April.

[83] Brown-Séquard CE (n.d.) Letter to d'Arsonval. Quoted by Delhoume, *op. cit.*, note 36, above, p. 481.

[84] Shyrock RH (1947) American Medical Research. Past and Present. The Commonwealth Press, New York, p. 180.

[85] Greenley TH (1894) The Evolution and descent of Man. American Practitioner and News 17: 291–292.

[86] Fulton JF, Wilson G (1966) Selected Readings in the History of Physiology. Charles C Thomas, Springfield, Illinois, pp. 410–411.

for an island which, he had been told, had a miraculous spring that could rejuvenate those who drank from it.

Also, another factor which contributed to the depreciation of Brown-Séquard's work in organotherapy was the proliferation of dubious elixirs—some twenty in all—prepared by private pharmaceutical firms, which abused the credulity of the general public, by marketing products, some similar to Brown-Séquard's preparation, like L'Extrait Brown-Séquardien in France. Others related to his testicular fluid by name only, such as, in England, Sequardine Serum, advertised by C. Richter & Company. Although Brown-Séquard had been dead for more than 16 years, the 1910-prospectus of this firm reads:

> If you are suffering from any nervous, organic, functional or blood disorder, a treatment with Sequardine Serum will bring you relief and restore your health in a permanent way.... The name of Dr Brown-Séquard LL.D (Cambridge), Fellow of the Royal Society and Fellow of the Royal College of Physicians (London) is sufficient guarantee of its efficiency.[87]

Other factors which contributed to diminishing Brown-Séquard's reputation were: the manner of preparation of his testicular fluid and its content, and the widely publicised failures and antics of those who, in the first three decades of the 20th century, tried to emulate him. In his lifetime, some had attributed the beneficial effects of his testicular extract to suggestion or to the influence of the imagination. Today's prevailing opinion is that it was the result of a placebo effect, and therefore that he had deluded himself, the more so, that it is unlikely that an aqueous solution of crushed testes would have contained any androgenically active principle, as androgens do not dissolve in water. This finding rejoiced his many detractors: "They danced up and down on his scientific grave. They rubbed his mistake into his modest bid for immortality."[88]

However, there are those who consider that the quantity of water used in the preparation of the testicular fluid was so minimal that a mild androgenical effect could have been due to "some active androgens complexed to protein."[89] Also, that the presence of "histamine and other biogenic amines, either present in the materials injected or endogenously released due to foreign macro-molecules injected,"[90] could have accounted for the beneficial effects reported world-wide. Others have evoked the possibility of "anaphylactic shocks causing a state of euphoria."[91]

In the years that followed Brown-Séquard's death, several pseudo-scientists and quacks used his work as a front to promote their financial interests or to give vent

87 Circular from the Medical Department of C. Richter & Co., (1910) Manufacturing Chemists, Albion House, 59–61 New Oxford Street, London.

88 Kruif, *op. cit.*, note 79, above, p. 58.

89 Emerson GM (ed) (1976) Aging. Dowden, Hutchinson & Ross Inc, Stroudsburg, Pennsylvania, p. 67.

90 *Ibid.*

91 Klein M (1973) Sur les Interférences des sciences fondamentales et de la Clinique sur l'essor de l'endocrinologie sexuelle. Clio Medica 8: 31–52, p. 32.

to their fanciful imagination. One of the first was Serge Voronoff, a physiologist of Russian origin, who was the Head of the Laboratory of Experimental Surgery at the Collège de France. He attempted to graft apes' testicles on human beings,[92] in the hope of giving them back their youth. Though his experiments failed, they were greatly and adversely talked of by the public press of the early part of the 20th century, which inaccurately linked Brown-Séquard's name to that of Voronoff.[93] Then, there was the ligature of the vas deferens, advocated by Steinach, to stimulate and store the production of the testicles' active principles. In the 1920s, the experiments of Stanley: hypodermic injections of extracts of boar, deer and rams' testicles into the inmates of the San Quentin Prison in California, and in the 1930s, Brinkley's transplantation of he-goats' testes to prop up the failing strength of elderly men.[94]

Although organotherapy was far from being a new science, having been advocated by Hippocrates and boosted in the 15th century by the Swiss physician Philippe Aureolus Paracelsus's saying: "Heart cures heart, spleen spleen, lungs lungs", Brown-Séquard is without doubt the Father of modern organotherapy having helped to promote the science of Endocrinology by a crude method of hormonal therapy. Many distinguished medical historians regard June 1st, 1889—the day Brown-Séquard made his report to the Société de biologie—as the definite birthday of the internal secretions, when he laid the cornerstone of the science of Endocrinology.

Moreover, Brown-Séquard's contribution to sexual endocrinology and to gerontology should not be ignored. It was, following his experiments with the testicular fluid, that the term sexual male hormone was coined and that important studies were undertaken in the field of sexual physiology. Together with Arnold Adolf Berthold, he anticipated the action of the male hormone, testosterone, namely its anabolic attributes in increasing the weight, the strength and the well-being of the elderly through its tissue-building properties. This was 40 years before Carl Moore and his colleagues obtained a pure sample of the male hormone in 1931 and Friedrich Johann Butenandt isolated testosterone in crystal form, which earned him the 1939 Nobel Prize.

Brown-Séquard never—unlike the medical and lay press of his time and the fallacious interpretations of many of his contemporary colleagues—claimed that his testicular fluid was a rejuvenating elixir. In 1889, in his journal Archives de physiologie normale et pathologique, he wrote:

> The question is certainly not whether the injections rejuvenate (which I believe to be impossible, as I have previously made known), the question is to know if one acquires the powers of a less advanced age, and this appears certain to me.[95]

---

92 Voronoff S (1923) Greffes testiculaires. O. Doin, Paris, 1923.

93 Hamilton, *op. cit.*, note 13, above.

94 Herman JR (1982) Rejuvenation : Brown-Séquard to Brinkely. NY State J Med 2: 1731–1739.

95 Brown-Séquard, *op. cit.*, note 22, p. 741, note 1.

Time and again, he had called the attention of the medical world to the concept of **internal secretion**. The term had been coined by Claude Bernard in 1855, to differentiate between the production of glucose within the liver and the production of bile, the liver's external secretion. Prior to 1855, the existence of internal secretions had been hinted at by Théophile de Bordeu, Julien Jean César Legallois and Albrecht von Haller, but Claude Bernard and Brown-Séquard are "clearly the founders of internal secretions."[96]

Brown-Séquard's research work on gland and organ extracts led to the discovery of "a new category of biological substances, the chemical messengers."[97] The following passage from a letter he wrote to d'Arsonval reveals that he had some sort of understanding of the role of the **hormone**—the term had not yet been coined at that time—a substance which is carried by the blood from the organ where it is produced to the organ which it affects:

> These special products enter the blood and influence… the other cells… of the organism. The result is that the various cells of the organism become jointly dependent on one another by means of a mechanism other than the nervous system.[98]

It is inconceivable to share the opinion that his organotherapeutic investigations hampered the progress of endocrinological research; that it was a disastrous incident which "proved even more disastrous for the nascent science of endocrinology"[99] and that

> For a full generation only a corporal's guard of researchers remained to carry on quietly the endocrine studies which, but for Brown-Séquard, hundreds of bright minds would have been pursuing with enthusiasm and vigor.[100]

Nor is it a regrettable episode in the history of medicine. Such an opinion originated with the comment made by Herbert McLean Evans in 1933, that: "Endocrinology suffered obstetrical deformation at birth,"[101] for:

> Growing out of his error [Brown-Séquard's], if error it was, has come a development in the field of medicine more significant than any other since the discovery of the bacterial origin of disease.[102]

---

[96] Rollestone HD (1936) The Endocrine organs in health and disease with a historical review. Humphrey Milford, Oxford University Press, London p. 21.

[97] Borell M (1976) Origins of the Hormone concept. Internal secretions and physiology research 1889–1905. Dissertation presented to the Faculty of the Graduate School of Yale University in Candidacy for the Degree of Doctor of Philosophy, 2nd December 1976, p. 2.

[98] Brown-Séquard CE, d'Arsonval A (1891) Addition à une note sur l'injection des extraits liquides de divers organs, comme méthode thérapeutique. C R Soc Biol (Paris) 43: 265–268, p. 267.

[99] Maisel AQ (1965) The Hormone Quest. Random House, New York, p. 14.

[100] *Ibid.*

[101] Quoted by Young FG. The Evolution of Ideas. Animal hormones. In: Needman J (ed) (1971) The Chemistry of Life: lectures on the History of Biochemistry. Cambridge University Press, Cambridge, p. 125.

[102] Hoskins HG (1933) The Tides of Life. The Endocrine glands in bodily adjustment. Kegan Paul, Trench, Trebner & Co., London p. 16.

Indeed, within 50 years of Brown-Séquard's death, **Endocrinology** had reached its manhood. As previously mentioned, George Oliver and Albert Sharpey-Schafer had, in 1894, described the effects of an extract of the adrenal medulla on pressure, whose active principle, **Adrenaline**, was isolated, in 1901, by the Japanese Yokichi Takamine and the American Thomas Bell Aldrich. Then came the discovery by William Haddock Bayliss and Ernest Henry Starling of **secretin,** a hormone of the mucous membrane of the duodenum and jejunum which, in response to acid from the stomach **stimulates the secretion of bile by the liver and of pancreatic juice which** helps in the digestion of proteins and fats. It was Starling who coined the term **hormone** to describe a substance produced by an organ or a group of cells which exercises a specific action, mostly remotely, on another organ or tissue. In 1909, J de Meyer gave the name **insulin** to the hormone secreted by the islets of Langerhans, a cluster of three types of pancreatic cells which also produces **glucagon** which, like insulin regulates blood-sugar levels and a third hormone, **somatostatin**, which is the antagonist of **somatotropin** or growth hormone produced by the anterior pituitary gland. In 1921, MacLeod, Banting and Best ascertained that insulin had an anti-diabetic effect. Furthermore, in 1909, William George McCallum and Carl Voegtlin differentiated between the functions of the thyroid and parathyroid glands. Three years later, Edward Calvin Kendall isolated **thyroxine**, the active principle of the thyroid gland. In the course of the second and third decades of the 20th century, Collip discovered **parathormone**, the hormone of the parathyroid and Herbert McLean Evans, collaborating with Joseph Abraham Long discovered **somatotropin,** the growth hormone of the anterior pituitary gland, essential to the normal growth and development of the body. The doors of **Endocrinology**, which Brown-Séquard had pushed ajar, were now wide open for outstanding discoveries well until the middle of the 20th century.

The following words of the eminent naturalist, Georges Cuvier, come to mind when one views the rapid development and benefits which originated with Brown-Séquard's organotherapy, and one wonders what all the jokes and laughter were about:

> When men have spent their admiration upon those who entertain them or upon those who kill them, they have none left for those who are helpful to them.

# Chapter 19
# The Last Years: 1892–1894

The 16 years that Brown-Séquard spent at the **Collège de France** were years of contentment and financial stability, brought about by his happy marriage to Emma, who cared for him and Charlotte, as if the latter were her own daughter. With these two, he lived "a peaceful and happy life as much as his incurable anxious nature allowed him to."[1] From 1883, the family divided their time between three residences. They spent the winter months in Nice at 'Villa Montplaisir', in avenue Lambert, the summer months at Saint-Adresse, a seaside resort, near Le Havre and the spring at 19, rue Francois 1$^{er}$, their Parisian apartment.

The annual departure for Nice was a great event for Brown-Séquard and his daughter, packing a great many trunks full of books, filed notes, instruments, apparatuses and confining to cages guinea-pigs and rabbits.[2] All this preparation was because he had set up a laboratory in the villa where, during the 1880s, he carried out several investigations. While experimenting in Nice, Arsène d'Arsonval lectured in his place during the winter months and part of the summer.

Ever since his days as a medical student, Brown-Séquard had many acquaintances and a settled period at the Collège de France helped him consolidate his friendship in the medical profession and elsewhere, as he was connected with wealthy, influential and titled people. His very close circle of medical men included Paul Bert, Paul Broca, Eugène Dupuy, Baron Hippolyte Larrey, Charles Robin and Alfred Vulpian, who all have been mentioned before. Other physicians and scientists he knew included Louis Pasteur, Charles Marie Benjamin Rouget, professor at the Paris Medical School; Aristide Auguste Stanislas Verneuil, who held chairs of Surgery at **La Pitié** and **l'Hôtel-Dieu** Hospitals; Pierre Carl Edouard Potain, Professor of Medicine at the Necker Hospital. The younger generation also found their way into his academic circle. These were his close friend and protégé, Charles Jacques Bouchard, Jules Déjerine, a hospital consultant who became professor of nervous diseases at **La Salpêtrière** and Georges Paul Dieulafoy.

---

[1] Le Gendre P (1924) Un Médecin philosophe. Charles Bouchard. Son Oeuvre et son temps. Mason et Cie., Paris, p. 491.

[2] Binet L (1936) Cérémonie en l'honneur de C.E Brown-Séquard. La Presse médicale N° 65:1245–1254.

L.-C. Celestin, *Charles-Edouard Brown-Séquard*,
DOI: 10.1007/978-3-319-03020-3_19, © Springer International Publishing Switzerland 2014

The rest of his acquaintances were a varied group of writers, philosophers, historians and chemists. The architect César Daly, the humanist Victor Considérant and the writer and businessman, Désiré Laverdant have also been previously mentioned. But this by no means exhausts his large group of friends which included the novelists Emila Zola and Alphonse Daudet and the latter's son, Léon, the founder of the royalist paper **l'Action Française** and the religious historian, Ernest Renan.

Brown-Séquard met Renan at the Collège de France, where the latter was the holder of the Chair of Hebraic Studies and the College's Administrator. They found that they both shared two things in common: their liberal views and the fact that both had lost their fathers at sea in more or less similar circumstances. Indeed, the mystery of his father's disappearance seems to have haunted Brown-Séquard until late in his life. In 1885, a letter written by Renan to Mountstuart Elphistone Grant Duff, the governor of Madras, seems to indicate that Brown-Séquard was searching for an explanation for his father's death. In it, Renan says:

> Our eminent colleague M. Brown-Sequard, whose fine work in physiology you certainly know about, is in need of information on a matter which I believe you can, better than anyone, throw light on. What I know of your love for the truth has prompted me to introduce this illustrious scholar to you. He will be in a better situation than I am to tell you what he wants.[3]

Although Brown-Séquard's letter to Grant Duff is not available, it is known that Captain Edward Brown loaded his cargo of rice at the port of Madras, in which case, his arrival and departure dates would have been logged by the port authorities.

Through Renan, Brown-Séquard got to know the philosopher Hippolyte Adolphe Taine and Marcelin Berthelot, whom he had met for the first time at the **Société de biologie** in 1856. The latter held a chair at the Collège de France since 1865. A brilliant chemist, he worked out the synthesis of methane, acetylene, benzene, formic acid, methyl and ethyl alcohols.

The Renans like the Brown-Séguards spent the winter months in Nice. They came to be on the most intimate terms, especially as Renan greatly admired Brown-Séquard, as evidenced by the following passage from a letter of Mme Cornelia Renan to Emma Brown-Séquard, written on December 8, 1892, thanking her for her sympathy on the death of her husband:

> He [Renan] had such a great admiration for M. Brown-Séquard! No one else understood better than he, this noble life devoted to work and to scientific discovery, in which are revealed an intuition of genius.[4]

Brown-Séquard was also well connected in the world of architectural engineering. Among his acquaintances here was Alexandre Gustave Eiffel, still a household name for his 320-m tower in Paris. His other engineering feats include

---

[3] Renan E (1885) Draft of a letter to Grant Duff. GMcCC, Ms 981/125, 19th Apr.

[4] Renan C (1892) Letter to Emma Brown-Séquard. GMcCC, Ms 981 8th December.

the Statue of Liberty frame, the viaduct of Gabarit and the Maria Pia bridge in Porto. Brown-Séquard was also friendly with Viscount Ferdinand Marie de Lesseps, the originator of the Suez and Panama Canals, whose wife, née Autard de Bragard, was a Mauritian.

Perhaps, the most colorful characters who befriended Brown-Séquard were Madame Marie Raffalovitch and Pedro II de Alcantara, Emperor of Brazil. The former was a Russian Jewess, whose husband a banker of Odessa, was established in Paris. Combining the charm and grace of a socialite with the qualities of an intellectual, Mme Raffalovitch had opened a salon, where scholars and politicians met. She had, from 1869 to 1878, been in regular correspondence with Claude Bernard for whom she gratuitously translated into French from German and Russian, current physiological and philosophical publications. Her influence was very great and her interventions on behalf of scholars at ministerial level was very often crowned with success. She was a friend of the Renans and like them and the Brown-Séguards, spent the winter months in Nice. In 1893, Brown-Séquard tried, through her intervention, to secure a chair for d'Arsonval at the Collège de France, when the Chair of Chinese became vacant and there seemed to be no candidate to fill it. He hoped that Mme Raffalovitch, who entertained Léon Victor Auguste Bourgeois, the then Minister of Public Education, could convince him to create a Chair of Biological Physics in replacement of the Chinese one, and to appoint d'Arsonval as the titular professor of this new Chair.[5] However, her intervention was to no avail, for a candidate was found for the Chair of Chinese Studies.

The story of Pedro II de Alcántara is a complicated one, which goes back to 1807 when Marshal Junot, on the orders of Napoléon conquered Portugal. John VI, who was then King of Portugal, Algarve and Brazil, fled to the latter country. After the French departed from his country, John VI returned there in 1821, leaving his son Dom Pedro in possession of Brazil, who proclaimed its independence in 1822, and was crowned Pedro I, Emperor of Brazil. However, he abdicated in 1831 in favour of his 6-year old son, who was proclaimed Emperor at the age of sixteen. Pedro II was the second and last Emperor of Brazil. During his 49-year reign, Brazil experienced a period of stability, prosperity and growth. He abolished slavery—it is said on the advice of Brown-Séquard—and instituted free and compulsory education by building schools and colleges. He established government institutions based on the British representative system. A highly cultured man, he spoke six European languages and was versed in the Natural Sciences. He admired the philosophy of Auguste Comte. Particularly interested in science and literature, he made several journeys to Europe, where he enjoyed the company of intellectuals, befriending Claude Bernard, Louis Pasteur, Jean-Martin Charcot, Charles Jacques Bouchard and Victor Hugo. In 1887, he attended a session of the Société de biologie as a guest of Brown-Séquard. His rule of Brazil was

[5] Godart J (1950) Bernard C. Lettres Beaujolaises. Editions du Cuvier. Villefranche-en-Beaujolias, pp. 249–252.

overthrown two years later by a republican revolt, so he took refuge in France, where he lived until his death in 1891.[6]

It is to Pedro II that is owed one of the three existing photographs—all studio portraits—of Brown-Séquard. The reason why there are so few photographs of him was his dislike of being photographed, especially in France. There is one taken when he was about 40. However, the photograph most commonly reproduced was especially taken in 1882, to be sent as a gift to Pedro II, in exchange of his own. The third one is rather rare and depicts a patriarchal figure at the age of 75. In 1890, when Brown-Séquard was approached by Hercule Bianchou for a photograph, which he wanted to include in his book **Nos Grands Médecins d'aujourd'hui (Our Eminent Physicians of Today)**, the former wrote to explain that he did not have a spare one. In place of a portrait, Bianchou published a photography of the reply to his request.

> You will be surprised to learn that I cannot satisfy your request, for the simple reason that I do not have a single photograph of myself to give you. Wanting to avoid being "sold and bought", I have never been photographed in France, and when my photograph was taken abroad, I only gave my patronymic - which is not renowned - so that no one has been tempted "to exhibit and sell me."[7]

Apart from the photographs, there is one oil painting of him in existence. It is the work of the Mauritian-born, Paris-based artist, Louis Serendat de Belzim, painted in the late 1880s.

Brown-Séquard dressed in the same manner for all his studio portraits: a black tail coat, a white shirt and a black bow tie. It seems that he wore these white shirts with starched front and cuffs quite often, as they gave rise to an amusing story. He used to jot down notes on any piece of paper he could get his hands on[8] and when he could not find any paper, he would scribble on his left cuff. One day, during a cab journey, he scribbled down some notes on his cuff, and promptly forgot about having written them. When he remembered, he looked for his shirt, but it had already been collected by the laundress. He immediately took a cab to the washhouse in Puteaux, on the outskirt of Paris, but the laundress had left to deliver laundry to her customers. He paid the washer-women 100 francs to look for his shirt and bring it back to him unwashed as soon as possible. The next morning, a shirt was duly delivered, unwashed, with this message on the cuff: "At four o'clock, go and give a mouthful to Eugénie, ask for my togs, and give her a clout in the face!"[9]

---

[6] Pedro II. Letters to Brown-Séquard from February 1876 to October 1885. GMcCC, Mss 981/121–131. For information on the life and career of Pedro II, consult Freitas DG de (1978) Le Voyage de l'empereur Pierre Second (D. Pedro II) en France. His Sci Med (Paris) 12:91–99. Also: Rogers JA (1972) Don Pedro II "The Magnanimous" Brazilian Emancipator (1825–1892) In: Clarke JH (ED) World's Great Men of Color. Collier Macmillan Publisher, London, vol 2, pp. 203–210.

[7] Published by Société d'Editions Scientifique, Paris, 1891.

[8] Dauriac J (1894) Nécrologie: Brown-Séquard. Le Progrès medical 190:270–271.

[9] Unidentified newspaper cutting entitled: Courier de Paris, no date, GMcCC, Ms 1000/86.

Another anecdote, from this period of his life, arose from the visit of an Anglo-Mauritian. Paris was host to a sizeable Mauritian colony—over 1,500—and Brown-Séquard was often visited by Mauritian newcomers to the capital. The visit of Frédéric Condé-Williams, a Judge of the Supreme Court of Mauritius, in October 1891, was recorded in some detail. He went to the Collège de France to make the acquaintance of the man whom he had read so much in the Mauritian newspapers. He asked the concierge, at the College, for 'Mr. Brown', only to be told that there was nobody of that name there. After lengthy insistence by Condé-Williams, the concierge realized that the visitor may have been asking for 'Monsieur Broune', as he had misunderstood Condé-Williams's correct English pronunciation of the name. The latter eventually received a warm welcome from Brown-Séquard and left a sympathetic description of the man at the age of 74:

> I found him a gentle, modest white-haired old man, rather below the middle height, of manners quiet and unassuming and of a smile full of kindness.[10]

Despite having been away from Mauritius for most of his life, Brown-Séquard never lost contact with the island and through his correspondence with his Mauritian friends and colleagues, he was never short of local news. On April 29, 1892, Mauritius made international headlines, having been hit by its worst cyclone in living memory. In a matter of hours, the island was devastated by a typhoon which caused extensive damage and claimed over a thousand lives in the Port Louis area. Newspapers in Great Britain and France launched an appeal for public donations to help the victims. In order to raise money for his compatriots, Brown-Séquard delivered a lecture at the Hôtel Continental in Paris, on June 15. It was very well attended by government officials and by diplomats of many nations, eager not only to hear him speak, but to see him in the flesh, as evidenced by the following note, he received from Prince Loubetsky, equerry of Czar Alexander III of Russia:

> The Prince sends his offering to M. le Professeur for his unfortunate compatriots of Mauritius, and takes the liberty of asking to have an admission ticket sent to him for the Lecture of tomorrow, Wednesday 15th June 1892.[11]

To this lecture, the Mauritian community of Paris, representing the various branches of arts and science, came in force.[12] The sculptor Prosper d'Epinay was there, as was the painter Serendat de Belzim , the poet Albert Mallac, the journalist Charles Giraudeau, the actor and director of the Opéra Comique, Léon Carvaille, alias Carvalho, the gallery owner Elias Daruty, who was reckoned to own more than 15 million francs worth of old masters. The Mauritian Paris-based medical profession was represented by Eugène Dupuy, d'Hotman de Villiers, Le Juge de Segrais, d'Abaddie de Barreau and Raffray. Also present were the members of 'Le Tout Paris Mauricien': Mme Ferdinand de Lesseps, daughter of the Judge Autard

---

[10] Rouget FA (1930) Brown-Séquard et son oeuvre. Esquisse biographique. General Printing & Stationary C., Port Louis, Mauritius. pp. 153–155.

[11] Prince Dvoutsky Loubetsky (1892) Letter to Brown-Séquard. GMcCC, Ms 999/6, 14th June.

[12] Tomel G (1892) Au jour le jour. La Colonie mauricienne. Le Figaro, 17th June.

**Fig. 19.1** Brown-Séquard's bust in the jardin de la compagnie, Port Louis, Mauritius © Celestin

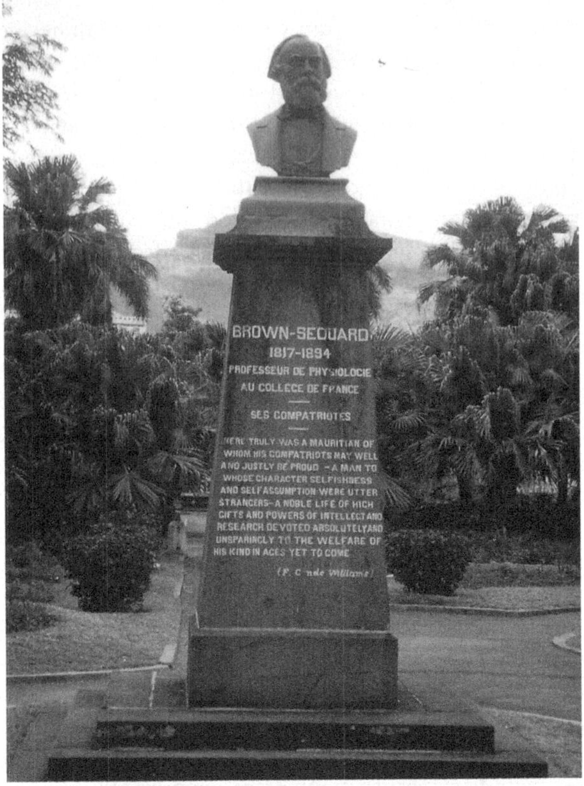
BROWN-SEQUARD
1817-1894
PROFESSEUR DE PHYSIOLOGIE
AU COLLEGE DE FRANCE
SES COMPATRIOTES
TRULY WAS A MAURITIAN OF
WHOM HIS COMPATRIOTS MAY WELL
AND JUSTLY BE PROUD – A MAN TO
WHOSE CHARACTER SELFISHNESS
AND SELF ASSUMPTION WERE UTTER
STRANGERS – A NOBLE LIFE OF HIGH
GIFTS AND POWERS OF INTELLECT AND
RESEARCH DEVOTED ABSOLUTELY AND
UNSPARINGLY TO THE WELFARE OF
HIS KIND IN AGES YET TO COME

**BROWN-SEQUARD'S BUST IN THE JARDIN DE LA COMPAGNIE,PORT LOUIS, MAURITIUS.**

de Bragard; the Count and Countess de Rochecouste; Mme Schneider, the wife of the industrialist Henri Schneider; Mme Vermeulen, renowned for her beauty, the great-grand-daughter of the Bailli de Suffren and the wife of a Belgian diplomat. Even though the event took place in high summer, when most of the wealthy people were away from Paris, the lecture still managed to generate a great deal of money. In a letter to Dr Charles Poupinel de Valencé of Mauritius, Brown-Séquard wrote:

> I have been deeply grieved by the news of your cyclone. I have done everything I could to come to the help of those who have been ruined. Unfortunately, I have found a long time since, the means of staying poor, and I could only give a very small sum, but I have given without stint my time and my labour. My lecture has brought in a fairly large sum. It would have been much larger at any other time of the year: Paris was nearly empty.[13]

[13] Brown-Séquard CE (1892) Letter to Dr Poupinel de Valencé, 11th July. In: Lettres inédites de Brown-Séquard. Revue Historique et Littéraires de l'île Maurice N°12, 1894.

At the age of 72, Brown-Séquard's health began to fail. In the autumn of 1889, he started suffering from pain and swelling of the joints of the hands and wrists, probably caused by rheumatoid arthritis, as well as from osteoarthritis of the hip and benign prostatic hypertrophy. During the winter, when he was in Nice, he suffered from a persistent, paroxysmal and enervating cough, which was diagnosed as whooping cough.[14] At that time, he was treating himself regularly with injections of his testicular fluid. There is a note that he wrote on his health, in 1892, where he refers to himself as a patient of 75 years of age. He analyses the beneficial effects of the injections of the fluid and notes that his 'patient' has previously suffered from whooping cough and has had laryngeal spasms and had barely recovered from an attack of gastroenteritis which has considerably weakened him.[15]

The state of Emma's health also became a cause for concern during the summer of 1893, when they were at Sainte-Adresse. When they moved to Nice that December, her health took a turn for the worse and from then on, she was in the final stages of a terminal illness. To make matters worse, Brown-Séquard was confined to bed or a sofa, suffering from phlebitis of the right leg, for most of December of that year and January 1894. On January 18th, Emma passed away at the age of 56.[16] Her husband's grief was uncontrollable and for 2 months he ate little, slept badly and closeted himself in the Villa Montplaisir, still suffering from phlebitis.

Against the advice of d'Arsonval, and not yet recovered from his leg ailment, he returned to Paris at the beginning of March. He was a pitiful sight: a frail old man, shattered by grief, mumbling over and over again: "I can't work anymore. It's all over."[17] Unable to face the familiarity of the rue Francois 1er apartment, he bedded down for a couple of days in a tiny room adjacent to his laboratory in the Collège de France. He had made the journey because he had to travel to London, in order to settle Emma's estate. She had made a will in August 1888, while on a visit to London, leaving her estate to her husband and, in the eventuality of his death, to Charlotte and her future children.[18] However, on March 23rd, he wrote to d'Arsonval, explaining that he could not leave for England, because of the state of his leg.[19]

The next day, which was a Saturday, his health grew much worse. He was taken suddenly with vertigo and his eyesight was affected. This was followed, next morning, by a period of confusion, semi-consciousness and amnesia, which lasted for a couple of hours. Eugène Dupuy was summoned but he was unable to

---

[14] Lancet (1890) 1:96.

[15] Brown-Séquard CE (n.d.) Note in his handwriting. GMcCC, Ms 987/12.

[16] Unidentified handwritten note. GMcCC, Ms 987/12.

[17] Dupuy E (1894) Notice sur M. Le professeur Brown-Séquard, ancient Président de la Société de biologie. Revue Scientifique (Paris) 2:737–743.

[18] New York Herald Tribune (May 1894) Mrs Brown-Séquard. Probate of her will.

[19] Delhoume L (1939) De Claude Bernard à d'Arsonval, Baillière et Fils, Paris. Quoting a letter of Brown-Séquard to d'Arsonval, 23rd March 1894.

persuade Brown-Sequard to rest in bed. Instead, he spent the next two days writing letters, one of which was a remarkable one to Dr William Dakin Waterhouse of West Hampstead, London, who was Emma's relative. It is a unique letter, not because of the writer's lucidity, even though, he was a few days from death, but it contains a remarkable analysis of all the symptoms he was experiencing:

> My leg being much worse, I have had to give up the hope of going to England. But the bad state of my leg (swelling and pain) is nothing in comparison with the very grave cerebral symptoms that have come since. In the first place, my sight has become almost suddenly very poor - this is persistent: and another slight trouble, almost constant, but not absolutely so, exists; it is a complete loss of sight in a small part of the vision field constituting hemiopia, limited to a small part of the left of the two retinae. This is, of course, of cerebral origin, but it does not seem to be of organic origin, because it is not absolutely constant. Most likely, there is either inhibition or a vascular spasm, which destroys at time the power of sight in two small parts of the retinae. This began on Sunday. The next morning something worse occurred. My life, and all that occurred for many months lately, became suddenly a blank ... I found, I was in my small library; but, although recognizing the room and the various objects in it, I did not know where to locate that room, at Nice, in Paris, or in some other place. This lack of memory of everything lasted at least two or three hours. I knew I was mentally suffering in some way, but nobody found that there was something wrong about me, except a faithful servant who had been with us since 1876, to whom I said I was not well and might be suddenly struck with loss of consciousness (apoplexy), paralysis, or convulsions, and I advised her what to do if anything very bad occurred.... Yesterday, I had a good many visitors (when they came the attack was over), and I talked rationally with them, saying but little of what had occurred. To-day, I have perhaps less of the hemiopia, but the dullness of sight is at times as great as yesterday. No other symptoms, no paralysis, no rigidity, no numbness, no alteration of the power of speech, no titubation.... There may have been a very small focus of softening or haemorrhage, but the principal direct cause of the symptoms must have been a vascular trouble or some purely inhibitory effect due to the constant irritation of the brain...[20]

The Lancet added that "on March 29th, he wrote again to Dr Waterhouse, recapitulating the above letter; and on Friday, the 30th yet again, mentioning his intention of coming immediately to London."

He was visited and examined by Professor Pierre Carl Edouard Potain and Dr Joseph Jules Djérine who were called by Eugène Dupuy, but they could not convince Brown-Séquard to eat and rest. On Friday 30th, he took small quantities of milk, bread and meat and seemed to be in a cheerful mood, but that evening, his vertigo and eye affection worsened gravely. Even in this distressing state, he crawled around the rooms of his apartment commenting on his symptoms and analyzing the prognosis of his case as if he were dealing with one of his patients. During the night, he was seized by vomiting and by the morning of Saturday, March 31st, he was unable to speak and his left arm and the right side of his face were paralyzed. At two o'clock in the morning, on Sunday 1st April, he was unconscious and a coma set in. The end came peacefully that night, near midnight. His death was due to a slowly progressing cerebral haemorrhage over a period of one week.

---

[20] Lancet (1894) Obituary: Professeur Brown-Séquard. 1:975–977, p. 977.

The news of his death was received with grief and shock by the general public and by his many colleagues. The Eleventh International Medical Congress was meeting in Rome and Professor Jacques Bouchard, his friend, pupil and protégé broke the news at a Physiology session, with tears streaming down his cheeks. The President of the Congress, Professor Guido Bacelli, immediately sent a telegram of sympathy to the Académie des sciences, where on Monday April 2, the Members had adjourned, after meeting for five minutes, to pay homage to Brown-Séquard's memory.[21] His death was particularly honoured and grieved in his native Mauritius. When the telegram arrived with the sad news, all the newspapers of the island were issued with black frames. The Mayor of Port Louis, Eliacin François, flew the flag at half mast over the Town Hall, and orders were issued to Mr. Adam, the agent of the Port Louis Municipal Council, in Paris, to lay a wreath on Brown-Séquard's coffin. Eulogies were read at the Town Hall by Dr Eugène Laurent, at the Medical Society by Dr Alfred Lesur, and at the Royal Society of Arts and Sciences by Dr Charles Poupinel de Valencé.[22]

Brown-Séquard had made specifications for the nature of his funeral, which took place on the Wednesday following his death. He wrote that it

> Be as simple as possible (like a fourth class one). No letters of announcement, no military honors, despite my decoration of the Legion d'honneur, no flowers on the hearse or on the coffin, no speech at the grave (except should Pasteur Fontanès be present and wishes to), no religious ceremony should I die in Paris (or not far from Paris). My coffin to be laid in the vault where lies already the mortal remains of my poor mother and of a daughter whom I lost in 1860, and where also will be, as soon as I can have them brought here, the mortal remains of my poor wife, which are at present in Nice.[23]

For a pauper's funeral, it was well attended. The government representatives were Hector Depasse, principal private secretary to the Minister of Public Education and Louis Lépine, chief commissioner of the Paris Police. The learned societies were well represented. The Académie des sciences sent its President, Maurice Loewy and its Secretary, Louis Bertrand. The Société de biologie its General Secretary, Amédée Dumont-Pallier, while the Collège de France was represented by its Administrator, Gaston Boissier. The official representative for Mauritius was the sculptor Prosper d'Epinay, but the Mauritian community of Paris were out in force. The great majority of the mourners,however, were from the medical world. Mme Bouchard and Mme Renan accompanied the under-age Charlotte, Brown-Séquard's daughter.

It was difficult for the mourners to observe all of the conditions set out in Brown-Séquard's will. There was also the problem of religious observance in the ceremony. Brown-Séquard was a lapsed Roman Catholic and an atheist, but it seems that he had his daughter's feelings in mind when he made the concession, in his second will, allowing Pasteur Fontanès to say some words at the funeral. The

---

21 Journal des dèbats (1894) Académie des sciences. Séance du 2 avril, 3rd Apr.

22 Rouget, *op. cit.*, note 10, p 154.

23 McCausland C (n.d.) Notebook in her handwriting. GMcCC, Ms 999/7, p 55.

pastor had been a regular visitor to the Paris apartment, as Emma was a practicing Anglican. The French radical press however, accused the deceased of reneging on his atheistic principles, unlike his two intimate friends, who had recently died: Victor Considérant and César Daly. It concluded that, may be, the family had turned what was meant to be a strictly secular funeral into a religious one. This is what one of the newspapers had to say:

> Materialist he was, and he did not hide it... He ought to have been taken to his last resting place without the escort of a representative of some cult, as was the case with his two old and excellent friends: Victor Considérant and César Daly. Prayers were mumbled by a protestant pastor. Treason or concession without weight, no doubt, on the part of the family.[24]

Pasteur Fontanès chose to pronounce an oration, the day before the funeral, at the family's apartment. Avoiding any reference of a religious nature, he paid tribute to the deceased's character, mentioning a selflessness "rare in our time when the needs of life leads us to compromise, to small deeds of cowardice and to great injustice", going on to say that:

> Lives like that of Brown-Séquard are rich in teaching and provide new motives to ennoble us and make us devote ourselves with more ardour to the happiness of humanity.[25]

The only flowers at the funeral were gifts from Mauritius. These were two wreaths, decorated with ribbons of silk. The one, which was laid on the coffin by the Port Louis Municipality agent, Mr. Adam, was inscribed simply: "Mauritius to Brown-Séquard." The other wreath bore the inscription : Société Royale des Arts et des Sciences de Maurice. Besides the tomb at Montparnasse Cemetery, Pasteur Fontanès read quietly from a psalter.

Brown-Séquard's will left his estate to his daughter Charlotte, after deduction of a sum of six thousand francs. This sum to be given to the "daughter of my son (the only child that he has up to now) Ellen Grace Brown-Séquard."[26] He nominated Jacques Bouchard and his wife to be Charlotte's guardians, should she be unmarried or under-age at the time of his death. They had to consult Charlotte as to whether she would live in France or in Great Britain, where it is understood that her guardian would be the physician, William Dakin Waterhouse. Charlotte also inherited her adoptive mother's estate. Emma's will stated that she wished her family to treat "my dear daughter with the same regard as if she were my own child."[27]

Over the years, Charlotte kept in touch with Mme Bouchard, who was widowed in 1915. She married an Anglo-Irish physician, Richard Bolton McCausland of Dublin. They had a son named Charles Edward, who received his military call-up to the Western Front in 1918. When Mme Bouchard learned the news that this young man was to be in France, she wrote to Charlotte:

---

[24] Maubourg (1894) Hommes et Choses. Brown-Séquard. Le Radical, 6th Apr.

[25] Unidentified newspaper cutting, 6th Apr, 1894. GMcCC 987/13.

[26] McCausland, *op. cit.*, note 23, above.

[27] Brown-Séquard CE (n.d.) Note in his handwriting. GMcCC, Ms 997/78a.

> Should he come to France, I hope to make the acquaintance of the grandson of a man whom my husband loved and venerated, and whom I equally loved with all my heart.[28]

The First World War over, Charles Edward McCausland left the Army to become a physician, following in his father's and grandfather's footsteps. His parents left Dublin for England for the following reasons, as explained by Charlotte in a letter to Dr Rouget of Mauritius, in 1930:

> We have left Ireland since 1923, life was no more possible for the Loyalists. Our lives were threatened, especially because our only son, who had trained at Sandhurst Military School, joined the Irish Guards and had taken part in the last battles against the Germans, his heart being all for France.[29]

Charles Edward McCausland practiced in the Sheffield area, then in Folkestone, where he died in 1971, and is survived by a son and daughter.

Today, there remains few memorials to the life of Brown-Séquard. His resting place at Montparnasse cemetery was well looked after by his daughter during her lifetime, and the original grey-granite pyramid was still there in the early 1970s, though its seven-line gold-lettered inscription was somewhat worn out.[30] It read:

BROWN-SÉQUARD
DOCTEUR EN MEDECINE
PROFESSEUR AU
COLLEGE DE FRANCE
MEMBRE DE L'INSTITUT
1$^{ER}$ AVRIL 1894
77 ANS

Nowadays, on a horizontal slab which has replaced the original seven-line inscription, is to be found only a large-lettered inscription:

BROWN SÉQUARD

Taking into consideration a fixed number of years' concession in French cemeteries, it is likely that this will sooner or later disappear. Then the only memorials that will be left are a plaque and two busts. On November 18, 1938, a plaque was set into a wall in Nice, at the Centre Universitaire Méditerranéen at the same time that a street was renamed after Brown-Séquard, to commemorate his stay in that city.[31] One bust—of which both are in Mauritius—has its own story. In 1898, a bust in imitation marble was unveiled in Port Louis by the then Mayor,

---

[28] Bouchard Mrs (1918) Letter to Charlotte McCausland, 13th Jan. GMcCC, Ms 982/24.

[29] McCausland C (1930) Letter to Dr FA Rouget. In: Rouget, *op. cit.*, note 10, above, pp. 146–147.

[30] Blanchard R (1905–1915) Epigraphie médicale. Corpus inscriptorum and medicinam biologiamique spectantum. Asselin et Monzeau, Paris.

[31] Le Temps (1950) A la mémoire de Brown-Séquard, 20th Aug. Also Binet, *op. cit.*, note 2, above.

**Fig. 19.2** Brown-Séquard's bust fronting Brown-Séquard Hospital, Quatre Bornes, Mauritius © Celestin

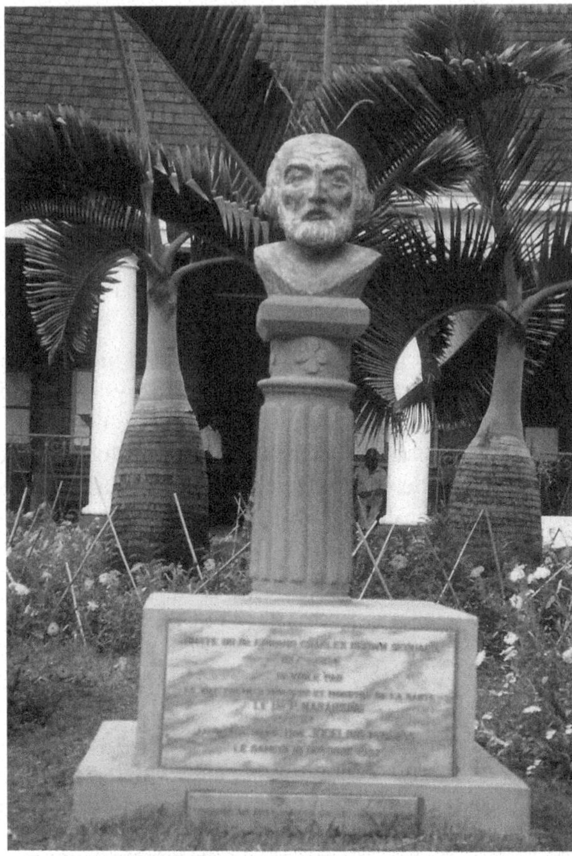

BROWN-SEQUARD'S BUST FRONTING BROWN-SEQUARD HOSPITAL,QUATRE BORNES, MAURITIUS.

Thomy Pitot de la Beaugardière, only to be shattered by the cyclone of 1924. The island's inhabitants decided to make up for the accident as well as for the cancellation of celebrations to mark the Centenary of Brown-Séquard's birth, due to the First World War, by erecting a bronze bust by the sculptor Georges Clément De Swiecinski, which was unveiled in Port Louis on August 13, 1928, in the Jardin de la Compagnie.[32] It stands on a massive grey-granite pedestal with an inscription in French and below it a passage in English from a eulogy of Judge Condé-Williams of the Supreme Court of Mauritius (Fig. 19.1). It reads:

[32] Read J (1938) Letter to Charlotte McCausland, 26th Dec. GMcCC, Ms 999/6. Also Vinson (1928) A la mémoire de Brown-Séquard, Discours prononcé lors de l'inauguration du bronze de Brown-Séquard. Le Radical, Port Louis, Mauritius, 13th Aug.

BROWN-SEQUARD
1817–1894
PROFESSEUR DE PHYSIOLOGIE
AU COLLEGE DE FRANCE

---

SES COMPATRIOTES

---

HERE TRULY WAS A MAURITIAN OF
WHOM HIS COMPATRIOTS MAY WELL
AND JUSTLY BE PROUD—A MAN TO
WHOSE CHARACTER SELFISHNESS
AND SELF ASSERTION WERE UTTER
STRANGERS—A NOBLE LIFE OF HIGH
GIFTS AND POWER OF INTELLECT
AND RESEARCH DEVOTED ABSOLUTELY
AND UNSPARINGLY TO THE WELFARE
OF HIS KIND IN AGES TO COME

The second bust is in the town of Quatre Bornes and fronts the entrance to the BROWN-SEQUARD HOSPITAL, devoted to the care and relief of nervous and mental diseases (Fig. 19.2).

Brown-Séquard's life and achievements have been the subject of very few studies, none of a comprehensive nature. In May 1994, a whole session of the First International Congress of the History of the Neuro-sciences, held in London, was devoted to some aspects of his work and discoveries, to commemorate the Centenary of his death. In Mauritius, his memory lives on unabated. He is not, by far, the only distinguished Mauritian medical man, but he is, no doubt, the greatest of them all.

# References

## Archives & Records

**Mauritius: Civil Status, Church & Census Records**

The Registrar General's Office, Civil Status. Extracts from the Register of the Acts of the Civil Status:

(1813) Copy of the marriage certificate of Charles Edward Brown and Henriette Perrine Charlotte Séquard.

(1817) Copy of the birth certificate of Charles Edward Brown.

Diocese of Port Louis, Mauritius. Register of Births, Baptisms, Marriages and Deaths:

(1787) Copy of the marriage certificate of Pierre Paul Séquard and Marie Jeanne Elizabeth Geneviève Nativel.

(1790) Copy of the joint baptismal certificate of Henriette Perrine Charlotte and Marie Louise Gillone Séquard.

(1817) Copy of the baptismal certificate of Edouard Charles Brown.

Census Returns:

(1796) Record the arrival of Pierre Paul Séquard in the Isle de France.

(1821) List the occupants of Charlotte Brown's house, that is herself, her son, her slaves, their spouses and their children.

**Virginia Medical College, Richmond, USA**

(1854-55) The four months that Brown-Séquard spent there, as professor, is the subject of an article by HB Hagg, (listed hereafter), who consulted the Medical College records.

**The National Hospital for Neurology & Neuro-Surgery, Queen's Square, London**

(1860-63) This period of Brown-Séquard's life has been fully documented by Dr William Gooddy, who studied the Hospital records. His articles are listed below.

**Harvard Medical School: Archives & Records**

(1864-1867) The foremost source for Brown-Séquard's professorship at Harvard is an article by HR Tyler and KL Tyler. These authors have consulted the Harvard Archives, the Harvard Medical Library Archives, the Countway Library Collection of the Harvard Medical Library and the Minutes and Records of the Medical Faculty of Medicine of Harvard. Their article is listed hereafter.


DOI: 10.1007/978-3-319-03020-3, 

**Collège de France: Archives & Records of the Minutes of the Professors' Assemblies:**

(1878-1894) Brown-Séquard's file in the Archives of the College is a modest one comprising only three items:

(1858) Letter to the College Administrator, 17th Dec. Ms-G-IV-C, 32B.

(1878) Catalogue of his work compiled in that year: Indication des principaux travaux originaux du Dr E. Brown-Séquard. Ms-G-IV-C, 32C.

(1878) A copy of the 1878 Presidential decree: Appointment of Brown-Séquard as Professor of Medicine.

Minutes of Professors' Assemblies

(1855) Appointment of Claude Bernard as Professor of Medicine. 9th Dec.

(1878) Appointment of Brown-Séquard as Professor of Medicine. 26th May.

**Archives of the Library of the Royal College of Physicians of London – The Gooddy McCausland Collection** (hereafter abbreviated GMcCC)

This collection is made up of the private and personal papers of Brown-Séquard. It was the property of Brown-Séquard's daughter, Charlotte McCausland and was passed on to her son Dr Charles Edward McCausland. Consisting of over 1,550 items, it was consulted item by item over a period of 18 months.

**Personal papers**: they comprise two groups:

Documents collected in the lifetime of Brown-Séquard:

Offprints and copies of and extracts from a large number of his articles and lectures.

Stenographic transcripts of two of his unpublished lectures.

Notes in Brown-Séquard's handwriting relating to his lectures and articles on the physiology and pathology of the nervous system, on vivisection, hygiene, testicular extract, etc.

Documents collected by his daughter from 1894 to 1940:

Newspaper cuttings relating to Brown-Séquard's life and those of his colleagues and contemporaries.

A considerable number of obituary notices from newspapers all over France.

Biographical notices of Brown-Séquard published from 1894 to 1937 by Maurice Arthus, Marcelin Berthelot, Léon Binet, Frédéric Damrau, Eugène Dupuy, Emile Gley, Eugène Laurent, François Auguste Rouget, Beverley Rudolph Tucker and Henry Crosnier de Varigny.

**Private papers**: Made up of two groups:

Letters and documents dating from the time of Brown-Séquard.

Brown-Séquard's letters and correspondence:

(1852-1864) 43 letters to his first wife, Ellen Fletcher.

(1872-1873) 22 letters to his second wife, Maria Rebecca Carlisle.

(1876-1880) 162 letters to and from his third wife, Emma Elizabeth Doherty, née Dakin.

(1838-1839) 10 letters to his friends in Mauritius.

(1884-1893) 29 letters to and from Arsène d'Arsonval.

(1865-1874) 6 letters from Désiré Laverdant.

Other documents include:

Letters of Charlotte Brown to her Mauritian friends.

Letters of Ellen Fletcher to her family.

Correspondence relating to members of Brown-Séquard's family, to births, marriages, deaths, nationality and change of name.

Two copies of Brown-Séquard's birth certificate.

Brown-Séquard's appointments, honorary appointments and awards.

Testimonials and letters of introduction for Brown-Séquard's application for a physicianship at the National Hospital.

A large number of letters – over 100 – from some 40 eminent colleagues and distinguished contemporaries, among them: Arsène d'Arsonval, Louis Rodolphe Agassiz, Paul Bert, Jacques Alexandre Bixio, Paul Broca, Jean-Martin Charcot, Charles Darwin, Eugène Dupuy, Gustave Eiffel, Marshall Hall, Oliver Wendell Holmes, Thomas Henry Huxley, John Hughlings Jackson, Ferdinand de Lesseps, Napoléon III, James Paget, Louis Pasteur, Charles Sumner, Joseph-Désiré Tholozan and Alfred Vulpian.

Letters & correspondence of Charlotte McCausland:

Letters of Brown-Séquard's biographers or would-be biographers, such as Binet and Olmsted.

Letters concerning Brown-Séquard's tombstone in Montparnasse Cemetery.

Photos of Brown-Séquard as a young man; of his certificate of candidature for election to the Royal Society and of his signature to the Obligation of the Fellows of the Royal Society.

**Department of Western Manuscripts, Wellcome Institute for the History of Medicine**

Brown-Séquard's file contains 21 letters, 20 in his handwriting, among which, is one to Neil Arnott and two to James Paget.

One letter is from Auguste Désiré Waller. Emile Gley's file contains one letter of Brown-Séquard, dated 1892.

**BROWN-SÉQUARD'S ORIGINAL WORK**

The abbreviation, **MGcCC**, followed by the manuscript number, used throughout the listings of the lectures and articles published by Brown-Séquard, stands for the **McCausland Collection** of the private and personal papers of Brown-Séquard, placed in the Archives of the Library of the Royal College of Physicians of London. There is no collection of Brown-Séquard's writings. All his original work was published by him in books, booklets and in articles in numerous medical and scientific journals. Very little of his work has remained unpublished.

**Doctoral Thesis**

(1846) Recherches et Expériences sur la Physiologie de la Moelle Épinière. Thèse pour le Doctorat en Médicine. Rigoux, Imprimerie de la Faculté de Mèdecine, Paris.

**Books**

(1853) Experimental researches applied to Physiology and Pathology. H. Baillière, New York.

(1857) Researches on Epilepsy. Its Artificial Production in animals and its Etiology. Its Nature and Treatment in Man. Clapp, Boston.

(1860) Course of lectures on the Physiology and Pathology of the Central Nervous System. Delivered at the Royal College of Surgeons of England in May 1858. Lippincott, Philadelphia.

(1861) Lectures on the Diagnosis and Treatment of the Principal Forms of Paralysis of the Lower Extremities. William & Norgate, London.

(1864) Leçons sur le Diagnosis et le Traitement des Principales Formes de Paralysie des Membres Inférieurs. Traduit de l'anglais par Richard Gordon. Mason, Paris.

(1868) Lectures on the Diagnostic and Treatment of Functional Nervous Affections. William & Norgate, London.

(1872) Leçons sur les nerfs vaso-moteurs, sur l'épilepsie et sur les actions réflexes, normales et morbides. Traduit de l'anglais par le Dr Béni-Barde. G. Mason, Paris.

(1882) Recherches expérimentales et clinques sur l'inhibition et la dynamogénie. Applications des connaissances fournies par ces recherches aux phénomènes principaux de l'hypnotisme et du transfert. G. Mason, Paris.

**Lectures**

The majority of Brown-Séquard's lectures have been published in enlarged versions in articles or gathered in bookform. A few have appeared in booklets and a couple have remained unpublished.

(1862) Lectures on diseases of the brain. Lectures I-V, Lecture VI missing. Delivered in Philadelphia. GMcCC Ms 999/10.

(1864) Lecture on hospital practice. Stenographic transcript of lecture delivered at the Smithsonian Institution, 14th June. GMcCC Ms 991.

(1864) Lecture on the relations between muscular irritability, cadaveric rigidity, and putrefaction. Gulstonian Lecture. Proceedings of the Royal Society, 16th May. Available also in GMcCC Ms 1011/40.

(1865) Lecture on the importance of the application of physiology to the practice of medicine and surgery. Delivered at the College of Physicians of Ireland on 3rd of Feb. 1865. John Falconer, Dublin. Also available in GMcCC Ms 999/57.

(1866) Advice to students. An address delivered at the opening of the medical lectures of Harvard University, 7th Nov. John Wilson & Sons, Cambridge, Massachusetts. Available also in GMcCC Ms 999/58.

(1874) Lectures on the nerves. Delivered at the Lowell Institute, Boston. February-March. Extracts from the New York Daily Tribune: Lecture and Letters Extras, No15, 9th Apr. Available also in GMcCC Ms 999/43.

(1875) Lecture on the localisation of functions of the brain. Delivered in the rooms of the Boston Society of Natural History. 1st June. Boston Medical and Surgical Journal 43: 119-124. Available also in GMcCC Ms 999/30.

(1878) Lecture on the dual character of the brain. Smithsonian Miscellaneous Collection 15: 1-21.

(1878) Leçon inaugurale. Collège de France. Doctrines relatives aux principales actions du centre nerveux. Leçon d'ouverture du cours de médicine au Collège de France. Fait le 2 décembre 1878. Mason, Paris. Available also in GMcCC Ms 999/31 & 999/63.

(n.d.) Leçon d'hygiène. Unpublished. Stenographic transcript. GMcCC Ms 992.

**Articles**

Brown-Séquard published over 600 original articles from 1846 to 1893. Many of these underwent consecutive revisions. Each revision clarifying his original thinking or introducing new ideas, new findings and new concepts. Moreover, many of these papers were translations from and into English and French. These articles appeared in over two dozen American, English and French periodicals. The largest number is to be found in the following journals: Archives de Physiologie Normale et Pathologique, Paris (1868-1893); Archives of Scientific and Practical medicine, New York (1873); Boston Medical and Surgical Journal (1852-1875); British Medical Journal (1880-1893); Comptes-rendus de l'Académie des sciences, Paris (1846-1893); Comptes-rendus de la Société de biologie (1849-1893). Dublin Journal of Medical Science (1877-1880); Gazette de Médecine et de Chirurgie, Paris (1855-1889); Journal de Physiologie de l'Homme et des Animaux, Paris (1859-1865); Lancet, London (1856-1893).

Hereafter is a comprehensive and representative selection of his articles, listed according to their subjects. They highlight his life achievements. Several lists of these articles are a available, compiled by Brown-Séquard himself. These lists are enumerated here, prior to his articles.

**Lists of articles compiled by Brown-Séquard**

(1855) Notes sur les travaux de M. E. Brown-Séquard. Imprimerie Masticot, Paris. Available also in GMcCC Ms 999/55.

(1864) Notes sur les travaux originaux (spécialement ceux de physiologie) du Docteur Brown-Séquard. Mason, Paris.

(1867) Liste des auteurs des mémoires originaux ou des mémoires traduits ou analysés dans les six volumes du Journal de physiologie de l'homme et des animaux. Publiés de janvier 1861 à décembre 1865, sous la direction du Dr Brown-Séquard. Mason, Paris. Available also in GMcCC Ms 999/59.

(1878) Notice sur les travaux scientifiques de M C. E. Brown-Séquard. Mason, Paris. Available also in GMcCC Ms 999/62.

(1883) Notice sur les travaux scientifiques de M C. E. Brown-Séquard. Mason, Paris.

(n.d) List compiled by someone other than Brown-Séquard: Bibliography of work by Brown-Séquard. Typescript. GMcCC Ms 983/6.

**Brown-Séquard's Articles**

**Adrenal Glands**

(1851) Influence d'une partie de la Moelle épinière sur les capsules surrénales. C R Soc Biol (Paris) 3: 146-148.

(1856) Recherches expérimentales sur la physiologie et la pathologie des capsules surrénales. C R Acad Sci (Paris) 44: 422-425, 542-546. Pages 422-425 availible in GMcCC Ms 999/29.

(1857) Nouvelles recherches sur l'importance des fonctions des capsules surrénales. C R Acad Sci (Paris) 45: 1036-1039.

(1893) Influences heureuse de la transfusion de sang normal après l'extirpation des capsules surrénales chez le cobaye. C R Soc Biol (Paris) 45: 448-449.

**Analgesia, Laryngeal**

(1882) Production d'anesthésie générale sous l'influence de l'irritation de la muquese laryngée par de l'acide carbonique ou du chloroforme. C R Soc Biol (Paris) 34: 799-819.

(1882) Production d'anesthésie surtout dans une des moitiés du corps par une irritation du larynx, après la section d'un des nerfs laryngés supérieurs. C R Soc Biol (Paris) 34: 816-819.

(1883) Analgesia by the proposed method. Letter to the editor of the Lancet. Lancet 2: 598.

(1891) Recherches sur l'inhibition de la sensibilité aux causes de la douleur sous l'influence d'une irritation de la muquese laryngée par de l'acide carbonique. Arch Physiol norm pathol 3:646-660.

**Animal Heat & Hibernation**

(1853) On the causes of the torpidity of the Tenrec (*Erinaceus ecaudatis*). In: Experimental Researches applied to physiology and pathology. H. Baillière, New York pp 25-26.

(1853) On the normal degree of temperature of man. In: Experimental Researches applied to physiology and pathology. H. Baillière, New York pp 30-31.

(1858) Note sur la basse température de quelques palmipèdes longipennes. J Physiol (Paris) 1 : 42-43.

(1858) In collaboration with J-D Tholozan: Recherches expérimentales sur quelques uns des effets du froid sur l'homme. J Physiol (Paris) 1: 497-499.

**Aphasia**

(1877) Aphasia as an effect of brain disease. Dublin J Med Sci 63: 209-255. Available also in GMcCC Ms 999/60.

(1884) Persistance de la parole, dans le chant, dans les rêves et dans le délire chez des aphasiques. C R Soc Biol (Paris) 36: 256-257.

**Arterial and Venous Blood**

(1857) Recherches expérimentales sur les propriétés physiologiques et les usages du sang rouge et du sang noir et de leurs principaux éléments gazeux, l'oxygène et l'acide carbonique. C R Acad Sci (Paris) 45: 552-566, 925-928.

(n.d.) Production de globules sanguins semblables à ceux des mammifères dans diverses parties du corp d'animaux de cette classe, lorsqu'on y injecte du sang d'oiseau, même longtemps après la mort. GMcCC Ms 999/36.

**Auditory Nerve**

(1858) Course of lectures on the physiology and pathology of the central nervous system. Lecture XII. Lancet 2: 625-626.

(1861) Note sur la production de symptômes cérébraux à la suite de certaines lesions du nerf auditif. Gaz Hebd Med 8: 56-58.

(1869) La section des canaux semi-circulaires ne cause le tournoiement que parce qu'elle s'accompagne d'une irritation du nerf auditif. C R Soc Biol (Paris) 21: 157-159.

**Autonomous Nervous System & Vaso-Motor Nerves**

(1853) Researches on the influence of the nervous system upon the function of organic life. In: Experimental Researches applied to physiology and pathology. H. Baillière, New York pp 6-16.

(1854) Sur les resultats de la section et de la galvanisation du nerf grand sympathique au cou. C R Acad Sci (Paris) 38: 72-80.

(1858) Course of lectures on the physiology and pathology of the central nervous system. Lecture IX. Lancet 2: 441-443.

**Cerebral Localization of Functions**

(1875) On localisation of functions in the brain. Boston Med Surg J 93: 119-124. Available also in GMcCC Ms 999/30.

(1875) Sur les localisations des fonctions cérébrales. C R Soc Biol (Paris) 24: 400-401.

(1876) The localisations of the functions of the brain applied to the use of the trephine. Lancet 2: 107-108.

(1888) Cerebral localisation of functions. Forum pp 166-177. Available also in GMcCC Ms 999/56.

(1892) Localisation prétendue de fonctions diverses dans les centres nerveux et surtout dans certaines parties des organes auditifs. Arch Physiol norm pathol 4: 366-368.

**Chloral Hydrate & Chloroform**

(n.d.) Sur le rôle des nerfs cutanés et de la moelle épinière dans la production de l'anesthésie, de la stupeur, et d'autres phénomènes, après des applications de chloroforme sur la peau. GMcCC Ms 999/64.

(1880) Nouvelles preuves que c'est à une irritation des nerfs cutanés que sont dus les effets inhibitoires et autres que produit le chloroforme appliqué sur la peau. C R Soc Biol (Paris) 32: 376-377. Available also in GMcCC Ms 999/64a.

(1880) Nouveaux faits relatifs à l'action du chloroform appliqué à la périphérie du système nerveux (peau et conduit auditif externe.) GMcCC Ms 999/64b.

(1880-1881) Cutaneous application of chloroform. Lancet 2: 900-902, 1880; 1: 1036-1037, 1881.

(1881) Des phénomènes unilatéraux inhibitoires et dynamogéniques dus à une irritation des nerfs cutanés par le chloroforme. GMcCC 999/56.

(1880) Effets produits par le chloral liquid pur (anhydre) appliqué sur la peau. C R Soc Biol (Paris) 33: 2-4.

(1882) D'un effet syncopal particulier causé par l'application du chloral anhydre sur la peau. C R Soc Biol (Paris) 35: 18.

**Digestion & Dyspepsia**

(1858) In collaboration with FG Smith: Expériences sur la transformation de l'amidon en glucose dans l'estomac. J Physiol (Paris) 1: 158-161.

(1873) On a new mode of treatment of functional dyspepsia, anaemia and chlorosis. Arch Sci Pract ed (NY) 1: 30-38.

**Duality of the Brain**

(1871) Différences entre les deux moitiés du cerveau, montrant que le côté droit devient surtout un centre de nutrition et le gauche un centre de vie intellectuelle. C R Soc Biol (Paris) 22: 27-29, 97-98; 23: 96-98.

(1871) Symptômes variables suivant le côté de l'encéphale qui est le siège des lesions. C R Soc Biol (Paris) 23: 98-100.

(1874) The brain power of man. Has he two brains or has he only one? Cincinnati Lancet & Observer 17: 330-333.

(1887) Dualité du cerveau et de la moelle épinière, d'après des faits montrant que l'anesthésie, l'hyperesthésie, la paralysie et des état varies d'hypothermie et d'hyperthermie, dus à des lésions organiques du centre cérébro-spinal, peuvent être transférés d'un côté à l'autre du corps. C R Acad Sci (Paris) 105: 642-652.

(1887) Recherches sur les deux principaux fondements des doctrines reçues à l'égard de la dualité cérébrale dans les mouvements volontaires. C R Acad Sci (Paris) 105: 840-845.

(1887) Sur l'existence dans chacun des hémisphères cérébraux de deux séries de fibres capable d'agir sur les deux moitiés du corps, soit pour y produire des mouvements, soit pour déterminer des phénomènes inhibitoires. C R Acad Sci (Paris) 39: 261-264.

(1890) Have we two brains or one ? Forum 9: 627-643. Available also in GMcCC Ms 999/66.

**Epilepsy, Artificially Induced**

(1850) D'une affection convulsive consécutive à la section transversale de la moelle épinière. C R Acad Sci (Paris) 2: 169-170.

(1850) D'une affection convulsive qui survient chez des animaux ayant la moitié latérale de la moelle épinière coupée. C R Acad Sci (Paris) 2: 195-196.

(1856) Recherches expérimentales sur la production d'une affection convulsive, épileptiforme à la suite de lésions de la moelle épinière. C R Acad Sci (Paris) 42: 86-89, 542-546.

(1858) Course of lectures on the physiology and pathology of the central nervous system. Lecture XI. Lancet 2: 571-673.

(1858) Note sur des faits nouveaux concernant l'épilepsie consécutive aux lésions de la moelle épinière. J Physiol (Paris) 1: 472-478.

(1869) Nouvelles recherché sur l'épilepsie due à certaines lesions de la moella épinière et des nerfs rachidiens. Arch Physiol norm pathol 2: 211-220, 422-441, 496-503.

(1870) Remarques sur l'épilepsie causé par la section du nerf sciatique chez les cobayes. Arch Physiol norm pathol 3: 153-160.

(1870) Faits nouveaux concernant la physiologie de l'épilepsie. Arch Physiol norm pathol 3: 516-522.

(1885) Production d'épilepsie spinale par une lésion du cervelet. C R Soc Biol (Paris). Available also in GMcCC Ms 999/32.

**Heredity of Acquired Characters**

(1859) De la transmission par hérédite chez les mammifères, et particulièrement chez les cochons d'Inde, d'une affection épileptiforme produite chez les parents par des lesions traumatiques de la moelle épinière. C R Soc Biol (Paris) 11: 194-196.

(1859-1860) Hereditary transmission of an epileptiform affection accidentally produced. Proc R Soc Lond 10: 297-298.

(1870) Modifications des mères par leur embryons, d'après des faits observés chez le cobaye C R Soc Biol (Paris) 22: 5-6.

(1875) On the hereditary transmission of effects of certain injuries to the nervous system. Lancet 1: 7-8.

(1880) Transmission par hérédite de certaines altérations des yeux chez les cobayes. C R Soc Biol (Paris) 32: 358-359.

(1882) Faits nouveaux établissant l'extrême fréquence de la transmission par hérédité d'états organiques morbides, produits accidentellement chez des ascendants. C R Acad Sci (Paris) 94: 697-700.

**Hypnotism**

(1882) Recherches expérimentales et cliniques sur l'inhibition et la dynamogénie. Application des connaissances fournies par ces recherches aux phénomènes principaux de l'hypnotisme, de l'extase et du transfert. Gaz Hebd Med 19: 35-37, 53-55, 75-76. 105-107, 136-138.

(1889) Le sommeil normal, comme le sommeil hypnotique, est le résultat d'une inhibition de l'activité intellectuelle. Arch Physiol norm pathol 1: 333-335.

**Iris, Effect of Light upon the**

(1847) Note complémentaire d'un mémoire sur l'action de la lumière et d'un changement de température sur l'iris. C R Acad Sci (Paris) 25: 508-510.

(1850) Lettre au Secrétaire de la Société de biologie concernant la stimulation par la lumière des tissus de l'iris chez l'anguille. 23rd Aug. GMcCC Ms 995/2

(1856-57) Researches on the action of certain parts of the solar spectrum upon the iris. Proc R Soc Lond 8: 233-234.

(18590 Recherches expérimentales sur l'influence excitatrice de la lumière, du froid et de la chaleur sur l'iris dans les cinq classes d'animaux vertébrés. J Physiol (Paris) 2: 281-294, 451, 460.

**Nervous System: Influence on Nutrition & Blood Composition**

(1859) Remarques sur le mode d'influence du système nerveux sur la nutrition. J Physiol (Paris) 2: 112-114.

(1862) Première note sur l'existence du sang rouge dans les veines et sur l'influence du système nerveux sur la couleur du sang veineux. J Physiol (Paris) 5: 566-574.

(1869) De l'influence du centre nerveux cérébro-rachidien sur les échanges entre le sang et les tissus. C R Soc Biol (Paris) 21: 98-99.

(1880-82) Researches on some of the physiological and pathological influence of the nervous system on nutrition. Br Med J 2: 915-916, 1880; 1: 313, 1882.

**Nervous System: Inhibition & Dynamogenesis**

(1873) On the mechanism of production of symptoms of disease of the brain. Arch Sci Pract Med (NY) 1: 117-122, 251-266.

(1882) Faits montrant que certaines parties du système nerveux peuvent agir de façon à augmenter plus ou moins soudainement les propriétés d'autres parties de ce système. C R Soc Biol (Paris) 34: 16-17.

**Nervous System: Physiology & Pathology**

(1858) Course of lectures on the physiology and pathology of the central nervous system. Lancet 2: 1-4, 27-31, 53-56, 108-112, 137-140, 165-168, 219-220, 245-247, 271-274, 295-297, 345-347, 367-369, 391-393, 415-416, 441-443, 467-468, 493-494, 519-520, 545-547, 571-573, 599-601, 625-626, 651-653.

(1860) Lectures on the diagnosis and treatments of the principal forms of paralysis of the lower extremities. Lancet 1: 389-390, 415-417, 437-438, 511-512, 563-564, 613-614; 2: 27-28, 77-78, 155-156, 229-230, 377-378, 451-452.

(1861) Lectures on the diagnosis and treatment of the various forms of paralytic, convulsive and mental affections considered as effects of morbid alterations of the blood, or the brain or other organs. Being a continuation of the Gulstonian Lectures delivered at the Royal College of Physicians in February 1861, and of the Clinical Lectures at the National Hospital for the Paralysed and Epileptics. Lancet 2: 1-2, 29-30, 55-56, 79-80, 153-154, 199-200, 391-392, 415-416, 611-613.

(1866) Recent advances of our knowledge on the diagnosis and treatment of functional nervous affections. Lancet 2: 85-87, 139-141, 247-250.

(1877) Anasthesia and amaurosis as effects of brain disease. Reprinted from Dublin Journal of Medical Science, February 1877. GMcCC 999/61.

(1877) Lectures on the pathology of the brain. Lancet 2: 39-40, 77-79, 117-119, 155-157, 265-267, 339-340, 485-486, 599-601, 709-712, 827-829.

(n.d.) Introduction à une série de mémoires sur la physologie et la pathologie des diverses parties de l'encéphale. VI. Extract from Archives de physiologie normale et pathologique. Deuxième série, pp 655-694. GMcCC Ms 999/71.

(n.d.) Introduction à une série de mémoires sur la physologie et la pathologie des diverses parties de l'encéphale. IX. Extract from Archives de physiologie normale et pathologique. Deuxième série, pp 409-423. GMcCC Ms 999/72.

(n.d.) Recherches sur l'excitabilité des lobes cérébraux, Extract from Archives de physiologie normale et pathologique. Deuxième série, pp 854-865. GMcCC Ms 999/73.

**Nervous Tissues: Regeneration**

(1849) Cas de régeneration complète du nerf sciatique. C R Soc Biol (Paris) 1: 137-138.

(1850) Régeneration des tissues de la moelle épinière. C R Soc Biol (Paris) 2: 3-5.

(1851) Sur plusieurs cas de cicatrisation de plaies faites à la moelle épinière avec retour des fonctions perdues. C R Soc Biol (Paris) 3:77-79.

(1859) Possibility of repair and of return to function after a partial or complete division of the spinal cord in man and animals. Letter to the Editor of the Lancet. Lancet 1: 96-97.

(1882) Régeneration du nerf sciatique dans une longuer de douze centimètres dans l'espace de deux semaines, chez un petit singe. C R Soc Biol (Paris) 34: 30-32.

(1892) De la régeneration de la moelle épinière d'après l'expérimentation et des faits cliniques. Arch Physiol norm pathol 4: 410-413.

**Organotherepy: Extracts other than testicular**

(1890) Remarques sur les effets produits sur la femme par des injections sous-cutanées d'un liquide retiré d'ovaires d'animaux. Arch Physiol norm pathol 2: 456-457.

(1892) Quelques notes sur l'histoire du traitement du myxoèdeme par des injection d'un liquide extrait de la thyroïde. Arch Physiol norm pathol 4: 752-753.

(1892) Influence de l'extrait aqueux de capsules surrénales sur des cobayes presque mourants à la suite de l'ablation de ces organes. C R Soc Biol (Paris) 44: 410-411.

In collaboration with Arsène d'Arsonval:

(1891) Recherches sur les extraits liquides retirés des glands et d'autres parties de l'organisme et sur leur emploi, en injections sous-cutanées, comme méthode thérapeutique. Arch Physiol norm pathol 3: 491-506.

(1891) De l'injection des extraits liquides provenant des glandes et des tissus de l'organisme comme méthode thérapeutique. . C R Soc Biol (Paris) 43: 248-250, 265-268.

(1891) Innocuité de l'injection dans le sang d'extraits liquides de pancréas, du foie, du cerveau et de quelques autres organs. C R Soc Biol (Paris) 43: 722-725.

(1892) Des injections sous-cutanées ou intraveineuses d'extraits liquides de nombre d'organes, comme méthode thérapeutique. C R Acad Sci (Paris) 114: 1399-1405.

(1893) Remarques sur le traitement du diabète par les liquids pancréatiques et testiculaires. C R Soc Biol (Paris) 45: 371-373.

(1893) Traitement de l'acromégalie par certains liquids organiques. C R Soc Biol (Paris) 45: 527.

**Organotherapy: Testicular Extract**

(1889) Des effets produits chez l'homme par des injections d'un liquide retiré des testicules frais de cobaye et de chien. . C R Soc Biol (Paris) 41: 415-419.

(1889) Seconde note sur les effets produit chez l'homme par des injections sous-cutanée d'un liquide retiré des testicules de cobaye et de chien. C R Soc Biol (Paris) 41: 420-422.

(1889) Troisième note sur les effets des injections sous-cutanée de liquide testiculaire. . C R Soc Biol (Paris) 41: 430-431.

(1889) Remarques à l'occasion du travail de M. Variot, sur les injections du liquide testiculaire chez l'homme. . C R Soc Biol (Paris) 41: 454-455.

(1889) Du rôle physiologique et thérapeutique d'un suc extrait de testicules d'animaux d'après nombre de faits observé chez l'homme. Arch Physiol norm pathol 3: 739-746.

(1891) Exposé de faits nouveaux montrant la puissance du liquide testiculaire contre l'affaiblissement dû à certaines maladies et en particulier la tuberculose pulmonaire. Arch Physiol norm pathol 3: 224-229.

(1891) Faits montrant combien est grande et variée l'influence curative du liquide testicularie dans un grand nombre d'affections locales ou générales, organiques ou fonctionnelles. Arch Physiol norm pathol 3: 747-761.

(1892) Effets produits sur de nombreux états morbides par des injections sous-cutanée d'un extrait liquide retiré des testicules. C R Acad Sci (Paris) 114: 1318-1321.

(1892) Note sur le traitement du cancer et du choléra par le liquid testiculaire. C R Acad Sci (Paris) 115: 375-377.

(1893) Notes sur les conclusions physiologiques et cliniques qui ressortent de certaines expériences dans lesquelles l'ataxie locomotrice ou la paralysie dues à des lésions de la moelle épinière ont été guéries ou ameliorées par des injections de liquid testiculaire. C R Soc Biol (Paris) 45: 365-367.

In collaboration with Arsène d'Arsonval:

(1892) Remarques sur l'emploi du suc testiculaire par plus de douze cents médecins et en particulier sur l'influence favorable exercée par ce liquide dans vingt et un cas de cancer et dans quelques autres affections. C R Soc Biol (Paris) 44: 815-818.

(1893) Effets physiologiques et thérapeutiques d'un liquide extrait de la glande sexuelle mâle. C R Acad Sci (Paris) 116: 856-861.

**Perfusion of dead tissues & Relations between muscular irritability, cadaveric rigidity & putrefaction**

(1851) Sur la persistence de la vie dans les members atteints de rigidité qu'on appelle cadavérique. C R Acad Sci (Paris) 32: 855-857.

(1851) Recherches sur le rétablissement de l'irritabilité musculaire chez un supplicié. C R Acad Sci (Paris) 32:897-902.

(1851) Recherches sur le rétablissement de l'irritabilité musculaire chez un second supplicié, plus de quatorze heures après la mort. C R Soc Biol (Paris) 3: 103-107.

(1862) On the relation between muscular irritability, cadaveric rigidity and putrefacation. Proc R Soc Lond 204-214. Available also in GMcCC Ms 1011/40.

(1885) Recherches sur l'augmentation de la tonicité musculaire et sur l'inhibition de la propriété essentielle des tissus contractiles. GMcCC Ms 999/35.

**Sensory Pathways in the Spinal Cord & the Brown-Séquard Syndrome**

(1849) De la transmission des impressions sensitives dans la moelle épinière. C R Soc Biol (Paris) 1: 192-194.

(1850) Mémoire sur la transmission des impressions sensitives dans la moelle épinière. C R Acad Sci (Paris) 31: 700-702.

(1850) De la transmission croisée des impressions sensitives dans la moelle épinière. C R Soc Biol (Paris) 2: 33-34.

(1855) Recherches expérimentales sur la voie de transmission des impressions sensitives dans la moelle épinière. C R Acad Sci (Paris) 41: 118-122.
(1855) Recherches sur la voie de transmission des impressions sensitives dans la moelle épinière. C R Soc Biol (Paris) 7: 51-65.
(1855) Recherches expérimentales sur la distribution des fibres postérieures dans la moelle épinière et sur la voie de transmission des impressions sensitives dans cet organe. C R Soc Biol (Paris) 7: 77-89.
(1856) The discoveries of Sir Charles Bell and M. Brown-Séquard in the nervous system. Letter to the editor of the Lancet. Lancet 1: 465-466.
(1858) Course of lectures on the physiology and pathology of the nervous system. Lecture I & II. Lancet 2: 1-4, 27-31.
(1863) Recherches sur la transmission des impressions sensitives dans la moelle épinière. Extract from Mémoires originaux pp 581-646. GMcCC Ms 999/42.

**Spine, Fracture of**
(1863) Trephining in cases of fracture of the spine. Lancet 1:477.

**Suckling Reflex**
(1849) L'action de têter est indépendante du cerveau. C R Soc Biol (Paris) 1: 119-120.

**Strychnine**
(1848) Recherches sur l'action de la strychnine. C R Soc Biol (Paris) 1: 119-121.

**Tuberculosis & Vitiated Air**
In collaboration with Arsène d'Arsonval:
(1887) Confined air and development of phtisis. Lancet 2: 1195.
(1887) Recherches sur l'importance surtout pour les phtisiques d'un air non vicié par des exhalaisons pulmonaires. C R Acad Sci (Paris) 105: 1056-1060.
(1887) Démonstrations de la puissance toxique des exhalaisons provenant de l'homme et du chien. C R Soc Biol (Paris) 39: 814-818.
(1888) Recherches démontrant que l'air expiré par l'homme et les mammifères, à l'état de santé, contient un agent toxique très puissant. C R Acad Sci (Paris) 106: 106-112.
(1888) Nouvelles recherches démontrant que les poumons secrètent un poison extrêmement violent qui en sort avec l'air expiré. C R Soc Biol (Paris) 40: 35-37.
(1888) Resemblance entre l'action toxique de certaines ptomaïnes et celle du posion pulmonaire. C R Soc Biol (Paris) 40: 108-110.
(1888) Sur quelques points importants relatifs à la durée de survie des lapins après injection du liquide contenant le poison de l'air expiré. C R Soc Biol (Paris) 40: 151-152.
(1889) Nouvelles recherches démontrant que la toxicité de l'air expiré ne dépend pas de l'acide carbonique. C R Acad Sci (Paris) 108: 267-272.
(1893) Nouvelles recherches démontrant que la toxicité de l'air expiré dépend d'un poison provenant des poumons et non de l'acide carbonique. Arch Pysiol norm pathol 6: 113-124.

**Vagus Nerve**
(1850) De l'influence des nerfs vagues sur les battements du coeur. C R Soc Biol (Paris) 2: 45-46.
(1853) Des effets de la section des nerfs vagues sur la force du coeur. C R Soc Biol (Paris) 5: 152-153.
(1853) Nouveau fait relatif à l'arrêt du coeur par la galvanisation du nerf vague. C R Soc Biol (Paris) 5:155.
(1854) Sur les resultants de la section et de la galvanisation du nerf grand sympathique au cou. C R Acad Sci (Paris) 3: 72-73.
(1862) Remarques sur l'action du nerf vague sur le coeur. J Physiol (Paris) 5: 295-296.

**Works Containing References to Brown-Séquard's Life and Work**


Ackerknecht EH (1974) The history of the discovery of the vegetative (autonomous) nervous system. Med Hist 18: 1-18.

Agassiz EC (1885) Louis Agassiz. His life and correspondence. Houghton, Miffin & Co. Vol 2, p 782. French edition: Agassiz CE (1887) Louis Agassiv. Sa vie et sa correspondence (trans. A Meyer) Librairie Fishbacher, Paris, p 590.

Albanese A (1989) Extrapyramidal system and extrapyramidal disorder. In: Rose EC (ed) Neuroscience across the centuries. Smith Gorgon, London pp 97-109.

Aminoff MJ (1993) Brown-Séquard. A visionary of science. Raven Press, New York.

Aminoff MJ (1996) Introduction to Brown-Séquard centenial. J Hist Neurosc 5: 5-6.

Aminoff MJ (1996) Brown-Séquard and his syndrome. J Hist Neurosc 5: 14-20.

Andres E (1939) Contribution of Brown-Séquard on spinal and trauma pathology. Brain Res Bull 22: 3-5.

Arthus M (1894) Brown-Séquard. Rev encyclo (Paris) 4: 509-513.

Arthus M (1898) Brown-Séquard et son oeuvre. In: Le Blanc (ed) Brown-Séquard. Imprimerie Roussel et Cie, Port Louis, Mauritius.

Atkinson WB (1878) Brown-Séquard. In: Physicians and surgeons of the United States. Charles Robin, Philadelphia, pp 700-701.

Atwarer EC (1967) The Lifelong Sickness of Francis Parkman (1832-1893). Bull Hist Med 41: 413-439.

Bendiner E (1988) Brown-Séquard's triumph and fiascos. Hosp Pract 28: 127-131, 134, 139-140.

Bernard C (1960) Cahiers de notes, 1850-1860. Edition intégrale du "Cahier Rouge" présentée et commentée par Mirko Drazen Grmek. Gallimard, Paris, pp 225-226, 234-235.

Bernard C (1950) Lettres Beaujolaises. Publiées et annotées par Jules Godard. Editions du Cuvier, Ville-Franche-en-Beaujolais, pp 249-252.

Bernard T (1894) Contes à renversement. Arrivée de Brown-Séquard au paradis. Le Journal, 3rd Apr.

Bert P (1885) Prix Lallemand. C R Biol (Paris) 100: 535-537.

Berthelot MPE (1898) Notice sur la vie et les traveux de M Brown-Séquard. Typographie Firmin-Didot et Cie, Paris. English edition: Berthelot MPE (1900) The life and work of Brown-Séquard. Government Printing Office, Washington, pp 677-697.

Bianchou H (1891) Nos grands médecins d'aujord'hui. Société d'Editions Scientifiques, Paris, pp 45-49.

Binet L (1930) Cérémonie en l'honneur de Brown-Séquard (La vie et l'oeuvre) Presse médicale N° 65: 1243-1245.

Binet L (1943) Brown-Séquard, médecin et physiologiste. Bio méd (Paris) 33 (4,5,6).

Binet L (1947) Brown-Séquard. In: Dusmenil R, Bonnet-Rof (eds) Les médecins célèbres. Editions d'art Lucien-Mazenod, Paris pp 182-183

Binet L (1954) Brown-Séquard ou le rêve de Faust. In: Binet L (ed) Médecins Biologistes Chirurgiens. Segep, Paris, pp 115-125.

Blanchard R (1905-15) Epigraphe médicale. Corpus Inscriptorum and Medicinam Biologianque Spectantum. Asselin et Houzeau, Paris p 263.

Blanton WB (1933) Medicine in Virginia in the nineteenth century. Garett & Massie Incorporated, Richmond, p 51.

Bliss (1982) The discovery of insulin. Macmillan Press, London, p 27.

Blumenthal (1975) American and French culture 1800-1900. Interchange in Art, Science, Literature and Society. Louisiana States University Press, Baton Rouge, p 241.

Blunstein BE (1993) Book Review: Michael Aminoff: Brown-Séquard. A visionary of science. New York, Raven Press, 211 pages. Bull Hist Med 68: 165-166.

Borell ME (1975) Origins of the hormone concept: Internal secretions and physiological research 1889-1905. Dissertation presented to the Faculty of the Graduate School of Yale University in candidacy for the degree of Doctor of Philosophy. pp 1-57.

Borell ME (1976) Brown-Séquard's organotherapy and its appearance in America at the end of the nineteenth century. Bull His Med 50: 309-320.
Borell ME (1976) Organotherapy, British physiology and discovery of the internal secretions. J Hist Biol 9: 235-268.
Borell ME (1978) Setting the standards for a new science. Edward Schafer and Endocrinology. Med Hist 22: 252-290.
Borell ME (19850 Organotherapy and the emergence of reproductive endocrinology. J Hist Biol 18: 1-30.
Boston Medical & Surgical Journal:
(1856) Brown-Séquard's discoveries. 55: 252-254.
(1857) Honor to science. 56: 52.
(1869) Medical Miscellany 68: 444.
(1894) Brown-Séquard's teaching. 134: 370-371.
Boston Weekly (1889) Serious results of "Elixir" test. Boston, Massachussets, 23rd Aug.
Bowditch HP (1902) Memoir of Charles-Edouard Brown-Séquard 1817-1894. Biographical memoirs of the National Academy of Sciences 4: 93-97.
Bower JZ, Purcell BF (1976) Advances in American Medicine: Essays at the Bicentennial. Jossica Marcy, New York, pp554-558.
Brasse A (1895) La Méthode de Brown-Séquard, traité et histothérapie, la thérapeutique des tissus, compendium des médications par les extraits d'organes d'animaux. Rothschild, Paris.
British Medical Journal:
(1869) Brown-Séquard. 1: 52.
(1880) The honorary degree. 2: 304-305.
(1881) Festivities of the Congress. 2: 303-304.
(1882) Brown-Séquard. Paper to the Académie des sciences. Arrêt des échanges entre le sang et les tissus. 1: 313.
(1883) Brown-Séquard. 2: 536.
(1889) Pentacle of rejuvenescence. 1: 1416.
(1889) Brown-Séquard's hypodermic fluid, 2: 29.
(1889) Recent experiments of Dr. Brown-Séquard. 2:229.
(1889) Brown-Séquard's experiments. A member of the medical public writes. 2: 347.
(1893) Animals extracts as therapeutic agents. 1: 1279.
(1894) Death of Brown-Séquard. 1: 776.
Broca PP (1855) Rapport sur les expériences de M. Brown-Séquard relatives aux propriétiés et aux fonctions de la moelle épinière. Mém Soc Biol (Paris) 7: 23-50.
Broca PP (1886) Correspondence 1841-1857, Vol 2. Typographie Paul Schmidt, Paris pp 337-338.
Brody LA, Wilkins H (1968) Brown-Séquard's syndrome. Arch Neurol 19: 347-348.
Brooks C, Cranefield P (1959) The historical development of physiological thought, The Haffner Publishing Co., New York, pp 184, 190-191.
Brown GH (1955) Brown-Séquard, Charles-Edouard. In: Lives of the Fellows of the Royal College of Physicians of London, 1826-1925. Published by the College, London, pp 124-126.
Carmichael E (1972) Charles Edward Brown-Séquard, physician, endocrinologist, neurologist, physiologist. Ala J Med Sci 9:224-237.
Chauvois L (1937) D'Arsonval. Soixante-cinq ans à travers la science. Editions J. Oliven, Paris, pp 114-117, 212-217.
Cier JF (1982) Brown-Séquard.L'homme et le physiologiste. In: Conférence de la médecine de l'université Claude Bernard. Lyon, Cycle 1981-82. Fondation Mérieux, Lyon, pp 175-195.
Cier JF (1982) Brown-Séquard. L'homme et le physiologiste. Lyon Pharmaceutique 33: 443-450.
Cileuls J de (1978) André Role: La vie étrange d'un grand savant, le professeur Brown-Séquard. Hist Sci Med (Paris) 12: 115-117.

Clarke E, Dewhurst K (1996) An Illustrated history of brain function. Imaging the brain from antiquity to the present, 2nd edn. Norman Publishing, San Francisco, p 149.
Corner GW (1965) Two centuries of medicine. A history of the School of Medicine, University of Pennsylvania. JB Lippincott, Philadelphia, p 121.
Critchley M (1960) The beginning of the National Hospital, Queen's Square 1859-1860. Brit Med J 1: 1829-1837.
Daily News (1894) Obituary. Dr. Brown-Séquard. London, 3rd Apr.
Daintich J, Mitchell S, Tootal E (eds) (1981) Brown-Séquard. In: Chambers Biographical Encyclopaedia of scientists. W & R Chambers, Edinburgh, Scotland, pp 72-73.
Damrau F (1937) Brown-Séquard. In: Pioneers of neurology. Dois Chemical Co., St Louis, Missouri, pp 9-17.
Darmon P (1995) Pasteur. Fayard, Paris, pp 388-389.
Darwin C (1868) The variation of animals and plants under domestication, vol 2. John Murray, London, p 101.
Daudet L (1927) Un maître méconnu. Brown-Séquard. L'Action Française, Paris, 7th Oct.
Daudet L (1930) La mort du savant. L'Action Française, Paris, 1st Aug.
Dauriac J (1894) Nécrologie: Brown-Séquard. Le Progrès médical 19: 270-271.
De Jong RN (1982) A history of American neurology. Raven Press, New York, pp 8-12, 51-52 & 54.
Delhoume L (1939) De Claude Bernard à d'Arsonval. Baillière et Fils, Paris.
Denny-Brown D, Rose AS, Sabs A (eds) (1975) Centenial anniversary volume of the American Neurological Association, 1875-1975. Springer Publishing Co., New York, pp 91-93, 388-389.
Dingwall EJ (1968) Abnormal hypnotic phenomena. A survey of nineteenth century cases, vol 2. J & A Churchill Ltd, London, p 129.
Dunbar N (ed) (1889) The "Elixir of Life". Dr. Brown-Séquard's own account of his famous alleged remedy for debility and old age, Dr. Variot's experiments and contemporaneous comments of the profession and the press. JG Cupple Co,. Boston.
Dupuy E (1894) Notice sur M. le professeur Brown-Séquard, ancient Président de la Société de biologie. Mém Soc Biol (Paris) 46: 759-777.
Dutray M (1894) Brown-Séquard. Sa méthode à Marseille. Le Petit Provençal de Marseille, 4th Apr.
Eclaireur de l'Est (1894) Brown-Séquard. Rennes, France, 3rd Apr.
Egli N (1970) Der "Montyon de physiologie expérimentale" in 19 Jahrhundert. Juris + Druck Verlag, Zurich, pp 23-24.
Enclyclopedia Britannica (1910) Brown-Séquard, vol 4, p 674.
Emerson GM (1978) Aging. The Brown-Séquard's reports and reactions. Replacement therapy in nineteenth century geriatrics. Dowden, Hutchinson & Ross Inc., Stroudsburgh, Pennsylvania, pp66-105.
Fearing F (1930) Reflex action. A study in the history of physiological psychology. The Wilkins Co., Baltimore, p 64.
Finger S (1994) Origins of the neurosciences. A history of exploration into the brain function. Oxford University Press, Oxford, pp 52-53, 153-154 & 397.
Francis SW (1866) Biographical sketches of distinguished living New York physicians. C.E. Brown-Séquard, M.D., F.R.S., etc. Med Sur Rep (Philadelphia) 15: 169-172.
Fulton JF, Wilson LG (1966) Selected readings in the history of physiology. Charles C Thomas, Springfield, Illinois, pp 297-298, 392-393, 410-411.
Fye WB (1983) Weir Mitchell, Philadelphia "Lost Physiologist". Bull Hist Med 57: 188-202.
Gasser J (1988) Charcot et la découverte des localisations motrices chez l'homme. Gesnarus 45: 501-520.
Gasser J (1995) Aux origines du cerveau moderne. Fayard, Paris, pp 82-89.
Gavault P (1894) Le secret de Jouvence. Voltaire, Paris, 5th Apr.

Gazette hebdomadaire de médecine (1894) Bulletin, Paris 6 août: Brown-Séquard N°14: 157-159.
Genty M, Nicole-Genty G, Chapuis M (1972). Index biographique des members, des associés et des correspondants de l'Académie de médecine de 1820 a 1970, 2nd edn. Dion, Paris, pp 27-28.
Gley R (1900) La Vie et l'oeuvre de C.E. Brown-Séquard (1817-1894). Arch Physiol norm pathol 26: 501-516.
Gley E (1899) Cinquantenaire de la Société de biologie. C R Soc Biol (Paris) 51: 1011-1080.
Goetz CG, Bonduelle M, Gelford T (1995) Charcot constructing neurology. Oxford University Press, pp 157-158, 303: note 23.
Goizet LH (1910) The transfusion of life. A continuation of the method established by Dr Brown-Séquard. Richter & Co., London.
Goncourt E & J (1898) Journal, vol 3. Robert Laffont, Paris, pp 731 & 740.
Gooddy W (1970) Brown-Séquard in space and time. Proc Aus Asso Neurol 7: 1-5.
Gooddy W (1982) Charles-Edouard Brown-Séquard. In: Rose EC, Bynum NS (eds) Historical aspects of neurosciences. A Feschrift for McDonald Critchley. Raven Press, New York, pp 371-378.
Gooddy W (1994) Much more due to Brown-Séquard. Lancet 1: 809-810.
Gooddy W (1996) Dr C.E. Brown-Séquard, M.D., F.R.C.P., F.R.S London, The Casting of the die. J Hist Neurosc 5: 7-13.
Gooddy W (1964) Some aspects of the life of Dr C.E. Brown-Séquard. Proc Soc Med 57: 189-192.
Greenley TB (1894) Evolution and descent of Man. American Practitioner and News 17: 291-292.
Gremk MD (1970) Charles Edouard Brown-Séquard. In: Gilepsie CC (ed) Dictionary of scientific biography. Charles Scribner & Sons, New York.
Guévin CA (1896) Brown-Séquard. In: Le Blanc (ed) Brown-Séquard. Imprimerie Roussel & Cie, Port Louis, Mauritius, back cover.
Haag HB (1959) Charles Edouard Brown-Séquard: His Richmond sojourn. Virginia Med Monthly 86: 311-313.
Haller JS (1931) American medicine in transition 1840-1910. University of Illinois Press, Chicago, p 357.
Hamilton D (1986) The monkey gland affair. Chatto & Windus, London, pp 12-13.
Hardy J (1894) L'Actualité. La Séquardine. Le Petit Clermontois, Clermond Ferrand, France, 6th Apr.
Harrington A (1987) Medicine, mind and the double brain. A study in nineteenth century thought. Princeton University Press, Princeton, New Jersey, pp 2,86,105,114-116,263.
Harrington TF (1905) The Harvard Medical School. A history, narrative and documentary, vol 2. Lewis Publishing Co., New York.
Hawkings C (1856) Address to the Royal Medical and Chirurgical Society. Lancet 1: 348-349.
Herman H (1952) A propos d'un centenaire. Comment se fit la découverte des nerfs vasomoteurs. Biologie médicale, Paris 41: 201-230.
Herman JR, Schulte H (1978) Charles Edouard Brown-Séquard (1817-1894). Invest Urol 15: 432.
Herman JR (1982) Rejuvenation: Brown-Séquard to Brinkely. NY State J Med 82: 1731-1739.
Hoff HE (1940) The history of vagal inhibition. Bull Hist Med 8: 461-496.
Holmes C (n.d.) The National Hospital, Queen Square 1860-1948. Livingstone, Edinburgh.
Hoskins HG (1933) The tides of life: the endocrine glands in bodily adjustments. Kegan Paul, Trench, Trebner & Co., p 16.
Howard AV (1951) Brown-Séquard. In: Dictionary of scientists. W & H Chambers, London p78.
Huguet F (1991) Les professeurs de la faculté de medicine de Paris. Dictionnaire biographique, 1794-1939. Editions du CRNS, Paris, pp 534-535.
Jacobson M (1993) Foundations of neurosciences. Plenum Press, New York, p 319.

Janin J (1851) Feuilleton du Journal des débats. Journal des débats, 7th July.
Jefferson M (1952) Brown-Séquard. A biographical essay. Lancet 1: 760-761.
Joly C (1894) Statues à élever. Le Moniteur du Puy du Dôme, Clermond Ferrand, France, 6th Apr.
Journal of the Amercian Medical Association (1960) Double-hyphenated neurologist. The Editorial, 178: 756-757.
Keele KD (1994) Brown-Séquard, Charles Edouard. In: William T (ed) A biographical dictionary of scientists. Harper Collins, Glasgow, p 80.
Kelly HA (1912) Brown-Séquard. In: A Cyclopedia of American biography. Comprising the lives of eminent deceased physicians and surgeons from 1610 to 1910, vol 1. W.Saunders, Philadelphia, pp 119-122.
Kelly HA, Burrage WL (1920) Brown-Séquard. In: The American Medical Biogrpahy. The Norman Remington Co., Baltimore, pp 155-157.
Klein M (1973) Sur les interférences des sciences fondamentales et de la clinique sur l'essor de l'endocrinologie sexuelle. Clio Medica 8: 31-52.
Koehler PJ, Endtz LJ (1986) The Brown-Séquard syndrome: true or false. Arch Neurol 43: 921-924.
Koehler PJ, Kruiters RRF (1986) Brown-Séquard syndrome caused by a spinal subarachnoid hematoma due to anticoagulant therapy. Sur Neurol 25: 191-193.
Koehler PJ (1989) Het localisatie concept in de neurologie von Brown-Séquard. Uitgiver, Rodopi, Amsterdam.
Koehler PJ (1989) Brown-Séquard's localisation concept: the relationship with Sherrington "integrative action" of the neurosystem. In: Rose PC (ed) Neurosciences across the centuries. Smith-Gordon, London, pp 135-138.
Koehler PJ (1991) Brown-Séquard spinal epilepsy. Part of a paper presented at the 3rd European Meeting of The History of Neurology. Veyrier-du-Lac, Annecy, France, May 23rd-24th .
Koehler PJ (1994) Brown-Séquard spinal epilepsy. Med His 38: 189-203.
Koehler PJ (1996) Brown-Séquard and cerebral localisation as illustrated by his ideas of aphasia. J Hist Neurosc 5: 26-33.
Koukle A (1977) Standard history of the medical profession of Philadelphia, 2nd edn. AM Press, p 243.
Kruif P de (1945) The male hormone. Harcourt, Brace & Co., New York, pp 55-60.
La Démocracie du Cher (1894) Obsèques de M. Brown-Séquard. Bourges, France, 4th Apr.
Lancet 1:
(1856) Doctrine of Charles Bell. 1: 377-378.
(1858) Brown-Séquard's lecture. 2: 25.
(1859) Lecture on the physiology and pathology of the central nervous system. 1: 271-272.
(1859) Medical news: Brown-Séquard. 1: 549.
(1860) Journal de physiologie de l'homme et des animaux. Publié sous la direction du Dr Brown-Séquard, vol 3, Baillière, London. 1: 374.
(1860) Clinical lectures on paralysis and epilepsy. 1:475.
(1861) Lecture on the diagnosis and treatment of the principal forms of paralysis. By C.E. Brown-Séquard. 1: 486-487.
(1863) Brown-Séquard's clinical lectures on paralysis and epilepsy. 1: 105.
(1864) Notice sur les traveux originaux (spécialement de physiologie) du Dr. Brown-Séquard. 2: 719.
(1869) Lectures on the diagnosis and treatment of the principal forms of paralysis of the lower extremities. 1: 400.
(1870) British Association for the Advancement of Science. Meeting of Liverpool, September 14th to 21st. 2: 436-439.
(1879) Brown-Séquard. Cerebral localization. 1: 924.
(1880) Accidents are often important factors in scientific discovery. 2: 900-902.
(1881) Brown-Séquard. Effect of application of chloroform to the skin. 1: 183.

(1881) Brown-Séquard's researches. 1: 715.
(1881) Brown-Séquard's experiments. 1: 1036-1037.
(1881) The International Medical Congress. The opening meeting 2: 244-246.
(1881) The International Medical Congress. Section II. Physiology. 2: 326-328.
(1881) Prize awarded to Dr. Brown-Séquard. 2:168.
(1887) Brown-Séquard. Puncture of the fourth ventricle. 1: 937-938.
(1887) Confined air and the development of phthisis. 2: 1195.
(1887) Microbes and expired air. 2: 1245.
(1890) Brown-Séquard's "Elixir of Life" (New York, from our correspondent) 1: 57-58.
(1894) Death of Professor Brown-Séquard. 1:906-907.
(1894) Obituary: Professor Brown-Séquard. 1: 975-977.
(1908) National Hospital for the paralysed and epileptic. Queen Square. 1: 120.
(1919) Great Mauritians. 2: 491.
(1965) Before our time. Letter of the Lancet's editors to Brown-Séquard. 1: 315.

Lanterne (1892) Brown-Séquard. Les Progrès de sa méthode. Paris, 6th Aug.

La Patrie (1894) Brown-Séquard. Mort de l'illustre savant. Détails biographiquues. Ses obsèques. Paris, 4th Apr.

Laporte Y (1996) Brown-Séquard and the discovery of the casoconstricter nerves. J Hist Neurosc 5: 21-25.

La Réforme Belge (1894) Brown-Séquard. L'homme et le savant. Découvertes sensationnelles. Bruxelles, 4th Apr.

La République:
(1894) Chronique. Paris, 6th Apr.
(1894) Désinteressement d'in grand savant. Paris, 19th Aug.

La République Française:
(1894) Mort de Brown-Séquard. Paris, 4th Apr.
(1894) Anecdotes. Paris, 11th Apr.

Laurent E (1898) Biographie de Brown-Séquard. In: Le Blanc M (ed) Brown-Séquard. Imprimerie Roussel et Cie, Port Louis, Mauritius, pp 6-7.

L'Avenir de Rennes (1894) Mort de Brown-Séquard. Rennes, France, 3rd April.

Laverdant GD (1878) Lettre au Cernéen. Le Cernéen, Port Louis, Mauritius, 1st June.

Leake CD (1956) Some founders of physiology. Contributors to the growth of functional biology. 20th International Congress, Washington DC, p 54.

Le Blanc M (1898) Brown-Séquard. Imprimerie Roussel et Cie, Port Louis, Mauritius.

L'Eclair (1894) La nationalité de Brown-Séquard. Comment il se fit naturaliser. L'étudiant pauvre. Les expériences d'un jeune docteur. Les cochons d'Inde de M. Daly. Le jugement de M. Pasteur. Paris, 4th Apr.

Le Figaro:
(1894) Début de Brown-Séquard. Paris, 5th Apr.
(1894) Lettre inédite de Brown-Séquard. Paris, 5th Apr.

Le Gaulois (1894) Brown-Séquard. Paris, 9th Apr.

Le Gendre P (19240 Un Médecin philosophe. Charles Bouchard. Son oeuvre et son temps 1837-1915. Mason & Cie, Paris, p 490-493.

Légue G (1894) Mort d'un grand savant. Le Journal, Paris, 3rd Apr.

L'Homme L (1894) La mort de Brown-Séquard. Le Journal de Maurice, Port Louis, Mauritius, 5th Apr.

L'Independance Belge (1894) Courrier de l'étranger. France. Notes du jour, Paris 2 Avril. Bruxelles, 4th Apr.

Le Journal de Chartres (1894) Lettres de Paris. Paris 3 Avril. Chartres, France, 5th Apr.

Le Journal de Maurice (1894) Mort de Brown-Séquard. Port Louis, Mauritius, 5th Apr.

Le Journal de Rouen (1894) Lettres de Paris, Paris 3 avril. Rouen, France, 5th Apr.

Le Journal des débats (1894) Académie des sciences. Séance du 2 avril. Brown-Séquard 3rd Apr.

Le Matin:
(1885) Le Fait du jour. M. Brown-Séquard. Paris, 30th June.
(1894) Brown-Séquard. Mort du célèbre professeur de physiologie. L'homme et le savant. Modestes débuts. Amour pour la France. Découvertes sensationnelles. La dernière oeuvre. Paris, 3rd Apr.
(1894) Débuts de Brown-Séquard. Paris, 5th Apr.
(1894) Nécrologie: Brown-Séquard. Paris, 5th Apr.
(1894) Brown-Séquard, Paris, 6th Apr.
Le Mauricen (1854) Leçon physiologique de M. Le docteur Brown-Séquard. Port Louis, Mauritius, 10th Oct.
Le Monde (1894) Nécrologie: Brown-Séquard. Paris, 4th Apr.
Le Petit Caporal (1894) Obsèques de M. Brown-Séquard. Paris, 5th Apr.
Le Petit Parisien (1894) Mort de Brown-Séquard. Paris, 3rd Apr.
Le Rappel (1894) Brown-Séquard. Paris, 4th Apr.
Le Siècle (1894) Nécrologie: M. Brown-Séquard. Paris, 4th Apr.
Leskind MC (1958) The Evolution of medical research in the United States. In: Martin-Ibanez (ed) History of American Medicine. A symposium. MS Publications. New York, pp 119-132.
Le Soir (1894) Mort de Brown-Séquard. Paris, 3rd Apr.
Le Temps:
(1894) Mort de Brown-Séquard. Paris, 3rd Apr.
(1938) A la mémoire de Brown-Séquard. Paris 20th Aug.
Le Tourneur ST (1957). Brown-Séquard. In: Prévost M, d'Amat R (eds) Dictionanaire de biographie française, vol 7. Librairie Letouzey et Ané, Paris, pp 459-460.
Lewis (1918) New life for old London. Sunday Dispatch, 15th May.
Lupovici C, Chapuis M, Chapuis J (1979) Paul Bert, 1883-1886. Centenaire de "La Pression barométrique". Académie de medicine, Paris, p 13.
Maisel AQ (1965) The Hormone Quest. Random House, New York, pp 13-16.
Major EH (1943) Charles-Edward Brown-Séquard. In: Essays in honour of Herbert Evans. University of California Press, Berkeley & Los Angeles, pp 369-377.
Marcou (1896) Life, letters and works of Louis Agassiz. Macmillian & Co., New York, pp 158, 165, 213-215.
Maubourg J (1894) Hommes et choses. Brown-Séquard. Le Radical, Paris 5th Apr.
Mauritius Sentential (1854) Leçon physiologique. Port Louis, Mauritius, 9th Oct.
McMenemy W (1967) International Congress of medicine 1867 and some of the personalities involved. Brit Med J 3: 487-489.
M.D.C. Editor of the Daily Chronicle (1894) Dr. Brown-Séquard. Daily Chronicle, London, 6th Apr.
Medical Recorder (NY) (1894) Charles Edward Brown-Séquard, M.D. 45:429.
Medvei VC (1993) The history of clinical endocrinology. A comprehensive account of Endocrinology from the earliest times to the present day. The Parthenon Publishing Groups. New York, pp 127, 159-162, 164-166 & 412-414.
Morgan TH (1907) Experimental zoology. Macmillan, New York, p 54.
Moulton CW (1906) A biographical cyclopaedia of medical history. The Salfield Publishing Co. New York, p48.
Mulmig G (1980) Charles-Edouard Brown-Séquard ou l'obstiné voyageur. Revue Med (Tours) 13: 1253-1255.
Nature (1894) Charles Edward Brown-Séquard. London, 49: 557-559.
New York Daily Tribune (1894) Brown-Séquard. The story of his life. New York, 22 Apr.
New York Herald Tribune:
(1892) What the doctors say. Dr Brown- Séquard's experiments with injections of liquid extracts of organs. Goitre and Addison's disease. Successful treatment of myxoedema and diseased surrenal capsules by this method. Paris, 10th July.

(1894) Brown-Séquard dead. The great physician succumbs to congestion of the brain. His life and work, New York, 3rd Apr.
(1894) Mrs Brown-Séquard. Probate to her will. New York, 1st May.
Ogle JN (1894) Further remarks on Dr. Brown-Séquard's last illness: Lancet 1: 1391.
O'Leary J, Golding S (1976) Science and epilepsy. Neuroscience gain in epilepsy research. Raven Press, New York, pp 87-90.
Olmsted JMD (1939) Claude Bernard physiologist. Cassell, London, pp 210-212.
Olmsted JMD (1943) The Aftermath of Charles Bell famous "ideas". Bull Hist Med 14: 341-351.
Olmsted JMD (1946) Charles Edouard Brown-Séquard. A nineteenth century neurologist and endocrinologist. The John Hopkins Press, Baltimore.
Olmsted JMD (1970) Charles Edouard Brown-Séquard. In: Haymaker WE, Schiller F (eds) The Founder of Neurology, 2nd edn. Charles C. Thomas, Springfield, Illinois, pp 181-186.
Ott I (1896) Brown-Séquard. Med Bull (Philadelphia) 28: 361-366.
Paris (1894) Mort de Brown-Séquard. L'Elixir de longue vie. La régénération par le jus de lapin. Un grand savant. Les résultats de sa découverte. Le XIXe siècle. Paris, 4th Apr.
Perry J (1894) Brown-Séquard. L'Evénement, Paris 5th Apr.
Pierce EL (1895) Memoirs and letters of Charles Sumner, 1877-1893, vol 3. pp 564-565.
Pilatte E (1894) Causerie scientifique. Quelques mots sur Brown-Séquard. L'Eclair de Nice, Nice France, 9th Apr.
Power d'Arcy (1917) Brown-Séquard, Charles Edouard. In: Dictionary of National Biography, vol 22. Oxford University Press, London, pp 319-321.
Putnam TJ (1894-95) Charles Edouard Brown-Séquard. Proc Amer Acad Arts 30: 589-592.
Queen Square and the National Hospital, 1860-1960 (1960). Edwards Arnold, London, pp 63-65.
Revue historique et Littéraire de l'île Maurice (1894) Attribution à Brown-Séquard de la Croix de St Michel et de St George, p 13.
Richet C (1897) Brown-Séquard. In: Dictionanaire de physiologie, vol 2. Félix Alcan, Paris, pp 256-261.
Richter C (1914) Circular from the Medical Department of C. Richter & Co., Manufacturing Chemist, Albion House, 59-61, New Oxford Street, London.
Riese W (1929) The early history of aphasia. Bull Hist Med 21: 322-324,
Robinson V (1929) Pathfinders in medicine. Medical Life Press, New York, pp 368, 582-593.
Roche P (1894) Mort de Brown-Séquard. Le Gaulois, Paris, 3rd Apr.
Role (A) La Vie étrange d'un grand savant. Le professeur Brown-Séquard. Plon, Paris.
Rollestone HD (1936) The endocrine organ in health and disease with a historical review. Humphrey Milford, Oxford University Press, London, pp 21-28.
Romanes GJ (1892) Darwin and after Darwin. An exposition of the Darwinian Theory and a discussion of past- Darwin questions, vol 2. Longmans, Green and Co., London, p 104.
Rondot P (1969) Syndrome of central motor disorder. In: Vinkin PJ, Bruyn W (eds) Handbook of neurology: Disturbances of nervous function, vol 1. North Holland Publishers Co., Amsterdam, pp 200-201.
Rouget FA (1930) Brown-Séquard et son oeuvre. Esquisse biographique. The General Printing & Stationary Cy, Port Louis, Mauritius.
Rouget FA (1931) Brown-Séquard et son oeuvre. Renseignements supplémentaires. The General Printing & Stationary Cy, Port Louis, Mauritius.
Ruch TC (1946) Charles Edouard Brown-Séquard (1817-1894). Yale J Biol Med 18: 227-228.
Sakula A (1881) Baroness Burdett-Coutt's garden party. The Internation Medical Congress, London, 1881. Med Hist 26: 183-190.
Sawin TC (1988) Defining thyroid hormones. Its nature and control. In: McCann (ed) Endocrinology. People and ideas. American Physiology Society, Bethseda, Maryland, pp 155-156.
Schiller F (1979) Paul Broca, founder of French anthropology. Explorer of the brain. University of California Press, Berkeley & Los Angeles, pp 112-116.

Schiller J (1966) Claude Bernard and Brown-Séquard. Chair of general physiology and the experimental method. J Hist Med 21: 260-270.
Schoenberg DG, Schoenberg ES (1976) Eponym: Brown-Séquard syndrome. Southern Medical Journal 69: 8
Sherrington CS (1893) Sur une action de l'écorce cérébrale. Rev Neur 1: 318-319.
Shoemaker JV (1890) Brown-Séquard. Med Bull (Philadelphia) 12: 6-10.
Shyrock RH (1947) American Research. Past and present. The Commonwealth Fund, New York, p 167.
Singh D (19940 Charles Brown-Séquard- one of Mauritius medical pioneer. Mauritius International, July-Sept. p 15.
Talbot JH (1970) Biographical history of medicine. Excerpts and essays on the men and their work. Grune & Stratton, New York, pp 820-823.
Taylor WH (1913) Old days at the old college. Old Dominion Journal of Medicine and Surgery, 17: 57-100.
The Advertiser (1894) The Elixir of life. Boston Massachusetts, 10th Apr.
The Echo (1894) Brown-Séquard. London, 3rd Apr.
The Harvard Medical School 1782-1906 (1906). Boston, p 89.
The Practitioner (1901) Heroes of medicine. Charles Eduoard Brown-Séquard, 66: 550-554.
The Standard (1894) Death of Brown-Séquard. London, 3rd Apr.
The Star (1894) Brown-Séquard, London 3rd Apr.
The St. James Gazette (1894) Late Professor Brown-Séquard. The anecdotes of a great physician. London, 4th Apr.
The Times (1894) Brown-Séquard. 3rd Apr.
Théodorides J (1965) Histoire de la biologie. Presses Universitaires de France, p 105.
Tholozan J-D (1855) Propriétés des faisceauz postérieurs de la moella. Expérience de M. Brown-Séquard. Gaz med Fr, pp 641-642, 13th Oct.
Thuilier J (1995) Monsieur Charcot de la Salpêtrière. Robert Laffont, Paris, pp 239-240.
Tizard E (1959) Theories on brain localization from Flourens to Lashley. Med Hist 31: 133-145.
Tomel G (1892) Au jour le jour. La colonie mauricienne. Le Figaro, 17th June.
Tourgis E (1938) Brown-Séquard avait raison. Les coqs le prouvent quand les physiologists leur coupent la voix. Le Petit Parisen, 8th June.
Tucker KE (1937) Charles Edouard Brown-Séquard (Read as the Chairman address of the historical section of the Richmond Academy of medicine.) April 13, 1939 at Richmond, Virginia. Enlarged from an article in the Bulletin of the Richmond Academy of Medicine.
Tucker WM (1973) The history of neurology in the State of Virginia (1854-1973) Virg Med Monthly 100; 927-929.
Tyler HR, Tyler KL (1984) Charles Edouard Brown-Séquard, Professor of physiology and pathology of the nervous system at Harvard Medical School. Neurology 34: 1231-1236.
Valence C Popinel de (1894) Lettres inédites du Dr. Brown-Séquard. Revue Historique et Littéraire de l'île Maurice. Port Louis, Mauritius. N° 12 & 13.
Varigny H Crosnier de (1894) Le mouvement scientifique. Mort de Brown-Séquard. Revue des Revues, 1st May.
Vinson L (1928) A la mémoire de Brown-Séquard. Discours prononcé à l'inauguration du bronze de Brown-Séquard. Le Radical, Port Louis, Mauritius, 18th Aug.
Vulpian EEA (1866) Leçon sur la physiologie générale et comparé du système nerveux faites au Muséum d'histoire naturelle. Baillière, Paris, p 459.
Vulpian EFA (1882) Prix Lacaze. C R Acad Sci (Paris) 94: 321-323.
Wagner FD (ed) Thomas Jefferson University: Tradition and heritage. Lea & Febiger, Philadelphia, 369-370.
Walton J, Beeson PB, Scott RB (1981) Brown-Séquard. In: The Oxford Companion to medicine, vol 1. Oxford University Press, London, p 158.
Waterhouse WD (1892) Brown-Séquard's injections. Br Med J 1: 8.

Westacott E (1949) A Century of vivisection and anti-vivisection. A study of their effects upon science, medicine and human life during the past hundred years. The C.W. Daniel Co., Ashington, Rochford, Essex, England, p 44.
William R (1949) Brown-Séquard. In: The Healing Touch. Jonathan Cape, London, pp 221-271.
York GK (1996) Brown-Séquard's theory of recovery. J Hist Neurosc 5: 34-42.
Young FG (1978) The evolution of ideas about animal hormones. In: Needman J (ed) The chemistry of life: Lectures on the history of biochemistry. Cambridge University Press, p 125.

**Works Consulted for Background Information to the Life, Time and Work of Brown-Séquard**

Abelous JE (1893) La physiologie des glandes à secretion interne. Corps thyroide et capsules surrénales. Revue générale des sciences pures et appliquées 4: 275-278.
Abraham HJ (1966) Extinct medical schools of nineteenth century Philadelphia. University of Pennsylvania Press, Philadelphia.
Achard CH (1924) Eloge de Paul Broca. Prononcé à l'Académie de médecine dans la séance annuelle du 9 décembre 1924. Mason et Cie, Paris.
Ackerneth EH (1957) Medical education in 19th century France. J Med Educ 32: 128-153.
Ackerneth EH (1982) A short history of medicine. The John Hopkins University Press, Baltimore.
Addison T (1849) Anemia: disease of the suprarenal capsules. London Medical Gazette 49: 577-578.
Addison T (1855) On the constitutional and local effects of disease of the suprarenal capsules. S. Highley, London.
Aldrich TBA (1901) A preliminary report on the active principle of the suprarenal gland. Amer J Physiol 5: 457-461.
Allen RB (1989) Economic marginality and the rise of the free population of colour in Mauritius, 1767-1836. Slavery & Abolition 10: 126-150.
Anderson DE (1918) The epidemics of Mauritius: with a descriptive and historical account of the island. HK Lewis, London.
Armand F (1948) Les Fouriéristes et les lutes révolutionnaires de 1848 à 1851. Presses Universitaires de France, Paris.
Astuc P (1946) 1848 et la médcine. Progrès médical. N°12: 268-281 & N°13: 297-302.
Barnwell PJ, Toussaint A (1949) A short history of Mauritius. Longmans Green and Co., London.
Bartholomew R (1974) Experimental investigations into the functions of the human mind. Am J Med Sci 67: 305-313.
Bazire PV (1865) On a case of partial disease of the left half of the spinal cord, causing anaesthesia on one side, and paralysis of movement on the other: with remarks on the transmission of sensitive impressions in the spinal cord. Lancet 2: 116-118.
Bedingfell E (1856) Report of the committee appointed by the government to investigate the history and particular of the cholera epidemeic of 1854. Special Commitee, Port Louis, Mauritius.
Beecher HK, Altsynde MD (1977) Mecidine at Harvard. The first 300 years. The University Press of New England, Hanover, New Hampshire.
Berdoe E (1889) Serious moral question. Letter for private circulation among physicians.. 12th July. GMcCC Ms 980/67.
Bernard C (1852) Influence du grand sympathetique sur la sensibilité et la calorification. C R Soc Biol (Paris) 3: 163-164.
Bernard C (1852) Expérience sur les fonctions de la partie céphalique du grand sympathique. C R Soc Biol (Paris) 4: 155-156.
Bernard C (1853) Recherches expérimentales sur le grand sympathique et spécialement sur l'influence que la section de ce nerf exerce sur la chaleur animale. Mem Soc Biol (Paris) 5: 77-107.
Bernard C (1856) Mémoire sur le pancréas et sur le rôle du suc pancréatique dans les phénomènes digestifs, particulièrement dans la digestion des matières grasses neutres, Paris.

Bernard C (1856) Recherches sur une nouvelle fonction du foie considerée comme organe producteur de matières sucrées chez l'homme et les animaux. Thèse de la faculté des sciences, Paris.
Bernard C (1872) De la physiologie générale. Librairie Hachette, Paris.
Bert P (1878) La Pression barométrique: Recherches de physiologie expérimentale. Mason, Paris. English edition: Bert P (1943) Barometric pressure. Researches in experimental physiology (trans: MB & FA Hitcock), Columbus, Ohio.
Bibby (1972) Scientist extraordinary. The life and scientific work of Thomas Huxley, 1825-1895. Pergamon Press, Oxford.
Bonnefin F (1851) Recherches expérimentales sur l'action des principaux poisons. Thèse pour le doctorat en médecine, Paris.
Bouillaud J-B (1825) Recherches cliniques propes à démontrer que la perte de la parole correspond à la lésions des lobules antérieurs du cerveau, et à confirmer l'opinion de M. Gall sur le siège de l'organe du langage articulé. Archives generals de medecine 8: 25-45.
Bowman L (1991) Mauritius. Democracy and development in the Indian Ocean. Darthmouth Publishing Co Ltd, London.
Boylan JW (1971) Founders of experimental physiology. Biographies and translations. J P Lehmans, Munich.
Bravais LF (1827) Recherches sur les symptôms et le traitement de l'épilepsie hemiplégique. Thèse de la Faculté de méecine. N°118, Paris.
Bramwell JM (1921) Hynotism. Its history, practice and theory. William Rider & Son, London.
Brazier MAP (1984) A history of neurophysiology in the 19th century. Raven Press, New York.
British Medical Journal:
(1867) Obituary: P.V. Bazire. 2: 144.
(1891) The New elixir of youth. 2: 796-797.
(1897) The late Sir Joseph Tholozan. 2: 728.
(1897) The late Sir Joseph Tholozan. 2: 1760.
Broca PP (1861) Perte de la parole, ramollisement chronique et destruction parteille du lobe antérieur gauche. Bull Soc d'Anthr (Paris) 2: 235-238.
Broca PP (1861) Remarques sur le siège du langage articulé, suivies d'une observation d'aphémie (perte de la parole). Bull Soc d'Anthr (Paris) 330-357.
Browne EG (1962) Arabian medicine. Cambridge University Press, Cambridge.
Carson JA (1869) History of the medical department of the University of Pennsylvania. Lindsay & Blakiston, Philedelphia.
Cavaribert R (1931) La Vie et l'oeuvre de Rayer (1793-1867). Thèse pour le doctorat en médecine. Librairie médicale et scientifique, Paris.
Caventou (1890) Profil biographique: le Dr Désiré Tholozan, médecin de S.M. le shah de Perse. A Lahore, Paris.
Cawadia AP (1952) The mid-nineteenth century clinical school of Paris. Proc R Soc Lond 45: 305-310.
Charcot J-M (1893) Oeuvres complètes, vol 4. Progrès médical et alcan, Paris.
Child T (1889) The Institue of France. Harper's New Monthly Magazine 78:501-520.
Clerihew G (1856) Report of the medical committee appointed for the purpose of drawing up short practical recommendations for general observation during the cholera epidemic. Special committee, Port Louis, Mauritius.
Corlieu A (1895) Centenaire de la faculté de médecine de Paris, 1794-1894. Imprimerie nationale, Paris.
Corvisart FRL (1852) De la contraction des extrémités ou tétanie. Thèse de la faculté de médecine, N° 223, Paris.
Coste JB (1851) Recherches expérimentales et observations cliniques sur le rôle de l'encéphale et particuliérement de la protubérance annulaire dans la respiration. Thèse pour le doctorat en médecine, Paris.
Courcy C (1967) l'Ecole de l'Hôtel Dieu de Paris au XIXe siècle. Clio Medica 2: 307-326.

Cowper (1984) Blessed Jacques Laval: Apostle of Mauritius. The Incorporated Catholic Trust Society, London.
Crosby AW (1965) American trade with Mauritius in the age of the French Revolution and Napoleon. Neptune 25: 5-17.
Dupuy E (1873) Examen de quelques points de la physiologie du cerveau. Thèse pour le doctorat en médecine, Paris.
Eccles JC, Gibson WC (1979) Sherrington. His life and thought. Springer International, New York.
Elgood CE (n.d.) Medicine in Persia. Clio Medica, London.
Ferrier D (1876) The functions of the mind. Smith, Elder & Co, London.
Fitzsimons JT (1976) Physiology during the nineteenth century. The Journal of Physiology 263: 16P-25P.
Freitas DG de (1978) Le Voyage de l'empereur Pierre Second (D. Pedro II) en France. Hist Sci Med (Paris) 12: 91-99.
French RD (1975) Antivivisection and medical science in Victorian Society. Princeton University Press, Princeton.
Fritsch G, Hitzig E (1870) Uber die elektrische Erngbarkeit des Grosshirns. Arch f Anat Physiol und wiss Med 37: 300-332.
Fye WB (1982) Why a physiologist? Henry P Bowditch. Bull Hist Med 56: 19-29.
Gazzaniga MS, Bogen JE, Sperry RW (1965) Observations on visual perception after disconnexion of the cerebral hemisphere in Man. Brain: 88: 221-226.
Gazzaniga MS (1970) The Bisected Brain. New York.
Gley E (1891) Note préliminaire sur les effets physiologiques du suc de diverses glandes et en particulier du suc extrait de la glande thyroïde. C R Soc Biol (Paris) 43: 250-251.
Gley E (1899) Cinquantenaire de la Société de biologie. C R Soc Biol (Paris) 51: 1011-1080.
Golgi C (1883) Continuation of the study of the minute anatomy of the central organs of the nervous system. Alienist & Neurologist 6: 383-416.
Gomez M (1932) Trousseau (1801-1867). Librairie médicale et scientifique, Marcel Vigné, Paris.
Goodfield GJ (1960) The growth of scientific physiology. Hutchinson, London.
Grandille M & MS (1979) Le père Jacques Laval, médecin et prêtre normand, missionaire à l'île Maurice. Hist Sci Med (Paris) 13: 219-225.
Gratiolet P (1856) Note sur les effets qui suivent l'ablation des capsules surrénales. C R Acad Sci (Paris) 43: 904-906.
Guillian G (1955) J-M Charcot (1825-1892). Sa Vie, son oeuvre. Mason & Cie, Paris.
Harley G (1857) Supra-renal capsules. Lancet 2: 550.
Hassenforder (1954) Les Médecins militaries français fondateurs et organisateurs de l'enseignement médical et de la santé publique en Iran. His Med (Paris) 4: 57-63.
Horsley V (1856) Epileptic guinea-pigs. Lancet 2; 975.
Hutchinson J (1911) The late Dr Hughlings Jackson. Recollection of a lifetime friendship. Br Med J 2: 1551-1554.
Huxley L (1901) Life and letters of Thomas Henry Huxley. Appleton & Co., New York.
Huxley TH (1888) Science and culture. Macmillan, London.
Imbault-Huart (1887-88) Concepts and realities of clinical teaching in France in the late 18th and early 19th centuries. Clio Medica 21: 59-70.
Jackson HJ (1881) Epileptiform convulsions from cerebral disease. Trans Int Med Cong 2: 6-15.
Jackson HJ (1915) On the nature of the duality of the brain. Reprinted from Medical Press & Circular. Brain 38: 80-86.
Kahn PS (1990) The Curse of Icarus. The health factor in air travel. Routledge, London.
Konke BA (1997) Standard history of the medical profession of Philadelphia, 2nd edn. AMS Press, Philadelphia.
Laffort L (1949) Médecins devant la Révolution de 1848. Librairie Le François, Paris.
Lancet:

(1854) Cholera in Mauritius. 2: 96.
(1867) Obituary: P.V. Bazire. 2: 213-214.
(1897) Sir Joseph Désiré Tholozan. 2: 554.
(1897) The late Sir J. Tholozan. 2: 690.
Launder-Lindsay (1871) Insanity in the lower animals. Brit For Med Chir Rev 48: 172-213.
Leake CD (1956) Some founders of physiology. Contribution to the growth of functional biology. International Union of Physiological Sciences and the American Physiological Society, Washington DC.
Léchelle A (1827) Cours d'exercises anglais, avec des notes grammaticales et une table des verbes irréguliers. Imprimerie Vallet et Cie., Port Louis, Mauritius.
Levy J, Treverthan C, Sperry RW (1965) Perception of bilateral chimeric figures following hemisphere disconnection. Brain 95: 61-78.
Lurie E (n.d.) Louis Agassiz. A life in science. The University of Chicago Press, Chicago.
Macdonald W (1929) William Birney. In: Dictionary of American biographies, vol 2. Oxford University Press, London, p 94.
Mackenzie HWG (1892) A case of myxoedema treated with great benefit by feeding with fresh thyroid gland. Brit Med J 2: 940-941.
Magendie F (1822) Expériences sur les fonctions des racines des nerfs rachidiens. J Physiol Exp Pathol (Paris) 2: 274-279.
Magendie F (1822) Expériences sur les fonctions des racines des nerfs qui naissent de la moelle épinière. J Physiol Exp Pathol (Paris) 2: 366-371.
Marie P (1906) Révision de la question de l'aphasie: que faut-il penser des aphasies souscorticales (aphasies pures) ? Semaine médicale pp 493-510.
Marie P (1906) Révision de la question de l'aphasie de 1861 à 1866: essai critique historique sur la génèse de la doctrine de Broca. Semaine médicale, pp 565-571.
Marin G (1948) La Révolution de 1848, Paris. Presses Universitaries de France, Paris.
Martial A (1939) Conférence de M. Arthur Martial. L'Essor N° 220 pp 93-99, Port Louis, Mauritius.
Mesulam MM (1985) Pattern in behavioural neuroanatomy: association areas, the limbic system and hemispheric specialisation. In: Mesulam MM (ed) Principles of Behavioural Neurology. F.A. Davis, Philadelphia.
Meyer A (1978) Les religieuses Augustines de l'Hôtel Dieu et leur passage à l'hôpital Broussais (1897-1975). Hist Sci Med (Paris) 12: 277-281.
Monakow C von (1911) Lokalisation der Hirufunktionen. Jornal fur Psychologie und Neurologie 17: 188-200.
Murray GR (1891) Note on the treatment of Myxoedema by hypodermic injections of an extract of thyroid gland of a sheep. Bri Med J 2: 796-797.
O'Connor WJ (1991) British physiologists 1855-1914. A biographical dictionary. Manchester University Press, Manchester.
Oliver G, Schafer EA (1895) The physiological effects of extracts of suprarenal capsules. Journal of Physiology 18: 230-276.
Olmsted JMD (1943) French medical education as a legacy from the Revolution. In: Essays in biology in honour of Herbert Evans. University of California Press, Berkeley & Los Angeles, pp 451-470.
Owen ARC (1971) Hysteria, hypnosis and healing. Dennis Dobson, London.
Philipaux JM (1856) Sur l'extirpation des capsules surrénales chez les rats albinos (*Mus retus*). C R Acad Sci (Paris) 43: 1155-1156.
Philipaux JM (1857) Ablation successive des capsules surrénales, de la rate et du corps thyroïde sur des animaux qui survivent à l'opération. C R Acad Sci (Paris) 44: 396-398.
Prince M (1919) Cerebral localization from the point of view of functions and symptoms. Journal of Nervous & Mental Diseases 37: 337-354.
Riedman SR (1973) Masters of the Scalpel. The story of surgery. Bailey & Swifen Ltd., Folkestone, England.

Rivière L (1982) Historical dictionary of Mauritius. Scarecrow Press, Metuchen, New York.
Rogers JA (1972) Dom Pedro II "The Magnanimous". Brazilian Emancipator (1825-1891). In: Clarke JH (ed) World's Great Men of Color, vol 2. Collier Macmillan Publishers, London, pp 203-210.
Rogoff JM, Stewart GN (1928) Studies on adrenal insufficiency in dogs. Amer J Physiol '4: 660-662.
Rogoff JM, Stewart GN (1928) Suprarenal cortical extracts in suprarenal insufficiency. JAMA 92: 1569-1571.
Roll-Hansen (1978) Drosophila genetics. A reductionist research program. J Hist Biol 11: 159-210.
Rostan LL (1848) Les bienfaits de la République et les devoirs qu'elle impose. Gaz des Hop, 15th Apr.
Rothschuh KE (1973) History of physiology. Robert E Kraeger Publishing Co, New York.
Ryder RD (1975) Victims of Science. The use of animals in research. Davis-Poynter, London.
Scherer AL (1990) La Réunion, 3rd edn. Presses Universitaires de France, Paris.
Schmitter C (1992) La Société de biologie. Les rapports de Claude Bernard avec cette société: histoire d'une conversion physiologique. His Sci Med (Paris) 26: 225-232.
Schneider (1911) La Médecine persane. Les Médecins francais en Perse. Leur influence. Société anonyme des imprimeries. Welhoff & Rrhore, Paris.
Simonoff LN (1866) Die Hemmungsmechanismen der Saugethiere experimentell bewiesen. Arch Anat Physiol (Leipzig) 33: 545-564.
Sinding C (1989) The history of resistant rickets. A model of understanding the growth of biological knowledge. J Hist Biol 22: 461-495.
Snow J (1849) On the mode of communication of cholera. John Churchhill, London.
Sperry RW, Gazzaniga MS (1967) Language following surgical disconnection of the hemisphere. In: Millikan CA, Darloey FL (eds) Brain mechanism underlying speech and language. Grune-Straton, London.
Thèodorides J (1991) Pierre Rayer, fondateur de la physiologie comparée, son activité à la Société de biologie (1849-1863). Hist Sci Med (Paris) 25: 293-296.
The Times (1897) Obituary: Sir Joseph Tholozan, 10th Aug.
Tholozan JD (1870) Origine nouvelle du choléra asiatique ou Début et développement en Europe d'une grande épidémie cholérique. V Masson et Cie, Paris.
Tholozan JD (1861) Traité d'auscultation, de percussion et de palpation. (Edité en langue persane) Téhéran, Iran.
Tinker H (1977) Between Africa, Asia and Europe: Mauritius. Cultural marginalism and political control. African Affairs 76: 304-323.
Toussaint A (1954) Early American trade with Mauritius. Esclapon. Port Louis, Mauritius.
Toussaint A (1966) A History of the Indian Ocean. Routledge Kegan Paul, London.
Toussaint A (1972) Histoire des Mascareignes. Berger-Levrault, Paris.
Toussaint A (1977) History of Mauritius. Macmillan Education, Basingstoke, England.
Traverthan C (1990) Brain circuits and functions of the mind. Essays in honor of Roger W. Sperry. Cambridge University Press, Cambridge.
Variot G (1889) Trois expériences sur l'action physiologique du suc testiculaire injecté sous la peau, suivant la méthode de M. Brown-Séquard. C R Biol (Paris) 41: 451-454.
Virtanen R (1960) Claude Bernard and his place in the history of ideas. University of Nebraska Press, Lincoln, USA.
Voronoff S (1923) Greffes testiculaires. O.Doin, Paris.
Vulpian A (1856) Note sur quelques réactions propres à la substance des capsules surrénales. C R Acad Sci (Paris) 43: 663-665.
Vulpian (1869) Epilepsie observée chez un cochon d'Inde qui avait subi la section d'un des nerfs sciatiques. Arch Physiol norm pathol 2: 297-299.
Wigan AL (1849) A new view of insanity: the duality of the mind proven by the structure, functions and diseases of the brain, and by the phenomena of mental derangement, and shown to be essential to moral responsibility. Reprint in 1965 by Joseph Simon, USA.

# Onomastic Index




DOI: 10.1007/978-3-319-03020-3, © Springer International Publishing Switzerland 2014

# Subject Index



L.-C. Celestin, *Charles-Edouard Brown-Séquard*,
DOI: 10.1007/978-3-319-03020-3, © Springer International Publishing Switzerland 2014

The manufacturer's authorised representative in the EU is Springer Nature Customer Service Centre GmbH, Europaplatz 3, 69115 Heidelberg, Germany. If you have any concerns regarding our products, please contact ProductSafety@springernature.com

Printed and bound by CPI Group (UK) Ltd, Croydon, CR0 4YY
25/09/2026
02222859-0016